BRITISH MEDICAL BULLETIN
VOLUME 56   NUMBER 4   2000

GW00507909

Allergy and allergic diseases:
with a view to the future

Scientific Editor

A B Kay

Series Editors
L K Borysiewicz PhD FRCP
M J Walport PhD FRCP

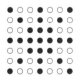

PUBLISHED FOR THE BRITISH COUNCIL BY
THE ROYAL SOCIETY OF MEDICINE PRESS LIMITED

ROYAL SOCIETY OF MEDICINE PRESS LIMITED
1 Wimpole Street, London W1G 0AE, UK
207 E. Westminster Road, Lake Forest, IL 60045, USA

British Library Cataloguing in Publication Data
A catalogue record for this book is available from the British Library
ISBN 1–85315–459–8
ISSN 0007–1420

Subscription information *British Medical Bulletin* is published quarterly on behalf of the British Council and is distributed by surface mail within Europe, by air freight and second class post within the USA*, and by various methods of air-speeded delivery to all other countries. Subscription orders and enquiries for 2001 should be sent to: Oxford University Press, Great Clarendon Street, Oxford OX2 6DP, UK (Tel +44 (0)1865 267907; Fax +44(0)1865 267485; E-mail: jnl.orders@oup.co.uk)

*Periodicals postage paid at Rahway, NJ. US Postmaster: Send address changes to *British Medical Bulletin*, c/o Mercury Airfreight International Ltd, 365 Blair Road, Avenel, NJ 07001, USA.

Back numbers of titles published 1996–2000 (see inside back cover) are available from The Royal Society of Medicine Press Limited, 1 Wimpole St, London W1G 0AE, UK. (Tel. +44 (0)20 7290 2921; Fax +44 (0)20 7290 2929); www.rsm.ac.uk/pub/bmb/htm).

Pre-1996 back numbers: Contact Jill Kettley, Subscriptions Manager, Harcourt Brace, Foots Cray, Sidcup, Kent DA14 5HP (Tel +44 (0)20 8308 5700; Fax +44 (0)20 8309 0807).

This journal is indexed, abstracted and/or published online in the following media: Adonis, Biosis, BRS Colleague (full text), Chemical Abstracts, Colleague (Online), Current Contents/ Clinical Medicine, Current Contents/Life Sciences, Elsevier BIOBASE/Current Awareness in Biological Sciences, EMBASE/Excerpta Medica, Index Medicus/Medline, Medical Documentation Service, Reference Update, Research Alert, Science Citation Index, Scisearch, SIIC-Database Argentina, UMI (Microfilms)

Editorial services and typesetting by BA & GM Haddock, Ford, Midlothian, Scotland
Printed in Great Britain by Bell & Bain Ltd, Glasgow, Scotland.

BRITISH MEDICAL BULLETIN — Volume 56 Number 4 2000

Allergy and allergic diseases:
with a view to the future

Scientific Editor: A B Kay

Acknowledgements

The planning committee for this issue of the *British Medical Bulletin* was chaired by Professor Barry Kay and also included Professor Fan Chung, Professor Hannah Gould, Professor Tak Lee and Professor Andrew Wardlaw.

The British Council and the Royal Society of Medicine Press are most grateful to them for their help and advice and particularly for the valuable work of the Scientific Editor in completing this issue.

Overview of 'Allergy and allergic diseases: with a view to the future'

A B Kay

Imperial College School of Medicine, National Heart & Lung Institute, London, UK

Allergic rhinitis, asthma and atopic eczema are among the commonest causes of chronic ill-health. These allergic diseases are increasing in prevalence and they add considerably to the burden of health-care costs. For example, in Sweden the number of children with allergic rhinitis, asthma or eczema roughly doubled over a 12 year period[1], and in the US the annual cost of treating asthma is about $6 billion[2].

The term 'allergy' was introduced in 1906 by Von Pirquet[3], who recognized that in both protective immunity and hypersensitivity reactions the antigen had induced 'changed reactivity'. With the passage of time, the word allergy has become corrupted and is now frequently used synonymously with IgE-mediated allergic disease. This restricted meaning was not as von Pirquet originally intended. He proposed that the term should apply to the 'uncommitted' biological response which in the individual may lead either to immunity (which is beneficial) or allergic disease (which is harmful).

As discussed by Dr Ewan (p 1087), allergists deal with the common allergic diseases that produce sneezing, wheezing, itching and digestive disorders. Most of their work involves the diagnosis and treatment of seasonal allergic conjunctivorhinitis ('summer hay fever'), perennial allergic rhinitis, allergic asthma (including occupational asthma), allergy to stinging insects (notably wasps and bees), food anaphylaxis and intolerance, allergy to drugs and allergy-related skin disorders like urticaria, angioedema and atopic eczema.

The term atopy from the Greek *atopos*, meaning 'out of place' is often used when describing IgE-mediated diseases. Thus, atopic individuals have an hereditary predisposition to produce IgE antibodies against common environmental allergens and have clinical manifestations of one, or more, atopic diseases (*i.e.* allergic rhinitis, asthma and atopic eczema). Some allergic diseases (*e.g.* contact dermatitis and hypersensitivity pneumonitis) operate through IgE-independent mechanisms and in this sense can be considered as non-atopic, allergic conditions. This issue reviews the cellular and molecular basis of atopic allergy, the diseases with which it is associated, and certain approaches to treatment.

Correspondence to:
Prof. A.B. Kay,
Head, Allergy and Clinical
Immunology, Imperial
College School of
Medicine, National Heart
& Lung Institute,
Dovehouse Street,
London SW3 6LY, UK

Atopy and Th2 cells

All of us inhale aero-allergens such as those derived from pollen, house dust mite and cat. In general, non-atopic adults and children mount a low grade immunological response; they produce allergen-specific IgG_1 and IgG_4 antibodies[4] and *in vitro* their T cells respond to the allergen with a modest degree of proliferation and production of interferon-gamma (IFN-γ) which is typical of Th1 cells[5-7]. Atopic individuals, by contrast, mount an exaggerated allergen-specific IgE response; they have elevated serum levels of IgE antibodies and positive skin tests to extracts of common aero-allergens. Several studies have shown that T cells from the peripheral blood respond to allergen *in vitro* by producing cytokines of the Th2-type, *i.e.* interleukin-4 (IL-4), IL-5 and IL-13[5,7], rather than cytokines of the Th1-type (IFN-γ and IL-2). There are many exceptions to this rule. For example, T cells from atopic subjects have been found to produce a mixed (Th0) cytokine pattern when challenged *in vitro* by an allergen from house dust mite[8,9]. Nevertheless, the immunopathological hallmark of allergic disease is the infiltration of affected tissue by cells with a Th2-type cytokine profile[10-12].

The early life events associated with allergic sensitisation are described by Warner and Warner (p 883) in this issue. T cells from virtually all new-

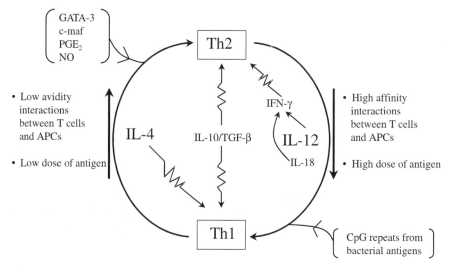

Fig. 1 Immunological and cellular factors regulating expression of the Th1/Th2 phenotype. Polarisation to Th1 or Th2 is dependent on IL-4 and IL-12, respectively. Other factors include the avidity of interactions between T-cells and APCs as well as the dose of antigen[15,16]. In addition, CpG repeats derived from bacteria favours Th1 whereas transcription factors such as GATA-3 are involved in Th2 commitments[104] as are c-maf and PGE_2. Nitric oxide (NO) favours Th2 by being less inhibitory to Th2 than Th1 cells. In human systems, IL-10 and TGF-β generally dampen Th1 and Th2 responses. IFN-γ inhibits Th2 responses; IL-12 and IL-18 release IFN-γ from T-cells. IL-4 inhibits Th1 cells and drives Th2 responses. Inhibitory effects of the cytokines are shown by the interrupted lines.

born infants are primed *in utero* to common environmental allergens and produce an immune response that is dominated by Th2 cells[13]. It has been proposed that during subsequent development the normal (*i.e.* non-atopic) subject's immune system there is a shift in favour of a Th1 response to inhalant allergen (a process termed 'immune deviation')[14]. On the other hand, in potential atopics, there is further boosting of fetally primed Th2-polarized immunity. It has been suggested that the major stimulus for developing protective Th1-like immunity is microbial exposure. Engulfment by macrophages of a wide range of microbes, including *Mycobacteria* and *Lactobacilli*, leads to the secretion of IL-12. IL-12 (by inducing Th1 cells and natural killer cells to produce IFN-γ) drives the immune system to an 'allergy-protective' Th1 response.

Other factors may also influence whether Th1 or Th2 cells dominate the response, including the dose of allergen and length of exposure as well as the avidity of allergen-specific interactions between T cells and antigen-presenting cells (Fig. 1)[15,16]. Anjana Rao and Orly Avni (p 969) describe the molecular aspects of T cell differentiation in terms of signalling pathways and transcription factors underlying the Th1 and Th2 response. There is evidence that cytokine gene expression is, in part, 'epigenetic', *i.e.* at the level of chromatin accessibility through modification of nucleosomal histones.

Rising trends in allergic disease

The marked increase in the prevalence of atopic disease in Western Europe, the US and Australasia during recent years indicates the importance of environmental influences. The role of various outdoor and indoor factors is discussed by Strachan (p 865). An interesting example of environmental as opposed to genetic changes is the incidence of seasonal allergic rhinitis and asthma after the unification of Germany. These disorders were less common in East Germany than West Germany before unification[17], whereas after unification the prevalence of atopy and hay fever, but not asthma, has increased in children who spent their early childhood in East Germany[18]. This phenomenon raises the possibility that a 'Westernised life-style' accounts for the increases in prevalence. It has been suggested that in Western countries the developing immune system is deprived of the microbial antigens that stimulate Th1 cells, because the environment is relatively clean and because of the widespread use of antibiotics for minor illnesses in early life[19].

Several epidemiological studies support this theory. For example, evidence for bacteria colonising the gastrointestinal tract preventing atopic sensitization was provided by studies by 1-year-old infants living in countries with a low (Estonia) and high (Sweden) prevalence of atopy.

Lactobacilli and *Eubacteria* predominated in Estonian infants whereas *Clostridia* were more frequent in Swedish infants[20]. At 2 years of age, allergic children were colonised less often by *Lactobacilli*, and harboured higher counts of aerobic bacteria (coliforms, *Staphylococcus aureus*) than non-allergic children[21]. Moreover, atopy and allergic asthma were less frequent in people exposed to agents in soil, air and water such as *H. pylori, T. gondii*, hepatitis A virus. Therefore, these microbes, by producing an IL-12-rich environment could drive a Th1 response. Such findings may explain, for instance, why in Europe and Africa a farming life-style, where there is increased exposure to bacteria in stables where livestock is kept, is protective against the development of atopic disease[22].

Other related factors which may encourage the Th2 phenotype include a date of birth around the pollen season, and alterations in infant diet[23]. Furthermore, atopic allergic diseases are less common in younger siblings, having three or more older siblings, and in those who have had measles and hepatitis A indicating that repeated 'immune stimulation' (*e.g.* by viruses) may be protective[24]. This is supported by the study of Ball *et al*[25] who provided evidence that exposure of young children to older children at home, or to other children at day-care centres, protected against the development of asthma and frequent wheezing in childhood.

Set against the hygiene hypothesis is the finding of increased prevalence, among poor blacks in the US, of atopic asthma in association with sensitization to cockroaches and the house dust mite[26,27]. However, more data are required on infection by foodborne and orofaecal microbes on inhabitants of inner American cities before these apparent inconsistencies can be explained. Thus, poor inner city dwellers may have the compounding effect of gut flora that do not protect against atopy and heavy exposure to allergens which may explain this paradox.

The development of specific allergic diseases may be related to alterations in the target organ. For example, the co-factors required for the development of an asthmatic attack may include respiratory virus infections and exposure to increased allergens, tobacco smoke, and air pollutants[28]. These factors alone, or in combination, may alter immuno-regulatory mechanisms at mucosal surfaces in ways that promote a Th2 cell-mediated allergic inflammatory response (Fig. 2).

Nature of allergens

Many allergens are soluble proteins which often have enzymatic function, such as proteolytic activity, in their natural state. Allergenic properties may be related to the latter (*e.g.* the augmentation of mucosal permeability) and to aerodynamic properties which in turn depend on

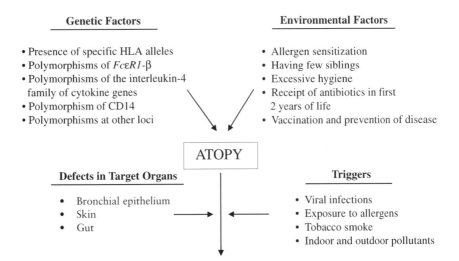

Genetic Factors

- Presence of specific HLA alleles
- Polymorphisms of *FcεR1*-β
- Polymorphisms of the interleukin-4 family of cytokine genes
- Polymorphism of CD14
- Polymorphisms at other loci

Environmental Factors

- Allergen sensitization
- Having few siblings
- Excessive hygiene
- Receipt of antibiotics in first 2 years of life
- Vaccination and prevention of disease

ATOPY

Defects in Target Organs

- Bronchial epithelium
- Skin
- Gut

Triggers

- Viral infections
- Exposure to allergens
- Tobacco smoke
- Indoor and outdoor pollutants

ATOPIC ALLERGIC DISEASE
(Th2 cell-mediated allergic inflammation)

Fig. 2 Factors influencing the development of atopy and atopic allergic disease. The inception of atopy is dependent on interactions between genes and the environment. The induction of atopic allergic disease may require further interaction between target organ defects and/or various environmental triggers.

particle size. The major allergens of Western industrialised countries are Der p 1 and Der p 2 from house dust mite (*Dermatophagoides pteronyssinus*), Fel d 1 from cat (*Felis domesticus*), several tree allergens including Bet v 1 from birch tree (*Betula verrucosa*) and many grasses such as Phl p 1 and Phl p 5 from timothy grass (*Phleum pratense*). The ragweed allergens; Amb a 1, a 2, a 3, a 5 and a 6 from short ragweed (*Ambrosia artemisiifolia*) and Amb t 5 from giant ragweed (*Ambrosia trifida*) are important seasonal allergens in North America. Allergies to Hev b 1-7 from latex, the milky sap harvested from the rubber tree (*Hevea brasiliensis*), and Ara h 1-3, which are highly allergenic peanut proteins, are increasingly important problems[29].

Genetics

As discussed by Feijen, Gerritsen and Postma (p 894), atopic allergic diseases are familial and have a genetic basis. The difficulties of conducting genetic studies in allergy are due, in part, to the multiple markers for atopy and allergic diseases. For instance. atopy manifested by positive skin prick tests and elevated serum IgE and asthma (manifested by airway hyper-responsiveness) are not always inherited together. Techniques used to identify genes that are relevant to allergy and asthma include the candidate gene approach, which depends on polymorphism in a known gene, and positional cloning, which links the inheritance of a specific chromosomal region with the inheritance of a disease[23]. Candidate gene studies have linked several loci to atopy, but the clinical relevance of these findings is unclear. Examples are the associations between an allele of the HLA-DR locus and reactivity to the ragweed allergen Ra 5[30], and the linkage of atopy to a polymorphism of the β-chain of the high affinity receptor for IgE (FcεRI-β)[31] and also to the IL-4 family of cytokine genes on chromosome 5[32]. By contrast, certain alleles of tumour necrosis factor (TNF) gene complex, while linked to asthma, were independent of serum IgE levels and other measures of atopy[33].

Polymorphisms of the FcεRI-β gene appear equally associated with severe atopy, asthma and eczema. Also, positional cloning indicates that chromosomes 2q, 5q, 6q, 12q and 13q contain loci linked to both asthma and atopy[23]. The link between the gene encoding the high affinity receptor for bacterial lipopolysaccharide (CD14) and total serum IgE may help to explain the association between childhood infections and the development of atopy[34].

Several of the genes and genetic regions that have been linked to atopy and asthma, have also been implicated in rheumatoid arthritis (chromosome 2) and inflammatory bowel diseases (chromosome 2 and 12)[23]. There has been recent interest in loci with pharmacological relevance.. As discussed by Drazen, Silverman and Lee (p 1054), polymorphisms within the promoter region of the 5-lipoxygenase gene[35] and in the β-adrenergic receptor may regulate the response to 5-lipoxygenase inhibitors and β-adrenergic agonists[23]. These findings raise the possibility that genotyping will become useful in planning therapy for asthma and other allergic diseases.

Immunoglobulin E and its receptors

The interactions between IgE and its receptors are discussed by Sutton, Beavil and Beavil (p 1004). Acute allergic reactions result from the release of preformed granule-associated mediators, membrane-derived lipids, cytokines and chemokines when an allergen interacts with IgE that is bound to mast cells and basophils by the α-chain of the high affinity IgE receptor (FcεRI)[36]. This receptor also occurs on antigen-presenting cells, where it can facilitate IgE-dependent trapping and presentation of allergen to T cells[37]. Eosinophils also possess FcεRI-α, but in these cells it is almost entirely intracellular; following release by degranulation of the eosinophil it may participate in regulating local concentrations of IgE[38].

The most important inducers of IgE production are IL-4 and IL-13. These cytokines initiate transcription of the gene for the epsilon class of immunoglobulin heavy chain constant regions. Production of IgE also requires two transcription factors, nuclear factor κB (NF-κB) and STAT-6; the former pathway involves the co-stimulatory molecules CD40 and CD154 and the latter is activated when IL-4 binds to the high-affinity α-chain of the IL-4 receptor[39]. Gould, Beavil and Vercelli (p 908) address the biochemically complex processes involved in immunoglobulin class switching in the context of IgE isotype determination. Essentially this involves germline gene transcription, DNA recombination and B cell differentiation.

Allergens, including products of some infectious micro-organisms (*e.g. Aspergillus fumigatus*), and helminthic parasites evoke Th2-mediated responses characterized by high serum IgE levels, whereas other bacterial antigens (*e.g. Listeria monocytogenes* and *Mycobacteria tuberculosis*) elicit a Th1-mediated response that is dominated by cellular immunity (cytotoxic T cells and delayed hypersensitivity). In these latter kind of organisms, the DNA contains repeating sequences of cytidine and guanosine nucleosides termed CpG repeats. These CpG repeats can bind to receptors on antigen-presenting cells and trigger the release of IL-12. This cytokine, which is produced almost exclusively by antigen presenting cells, drives and maintains the Th1 response. Furthermore the IFN-γ produced by activated Th1 cells[40] and IL-18 (IFN-γ-inducing factor, from macrophages[40]) join forces to suppress the production of IgE antibodies[41]. Therefore, at least theoretically, IFN-γ, IL-12 and IL-18, either alone or in combination, have therapeutic potential for inhibiting IgE synthesis. Furthermore (as discussed below), CpG repeats may redirect allergens to produce Th1, rather than a Th2, immune response.

The physiological relevance of the low affinity IgE receptors (FcεRII, CD23) remains speculative. It may be involved in antigen trapping and presentation, so effectively augmenting IL-4/IL-13 production[42]. On the other hand, CD23 can provide an inhibitory signal which eventually over-rides the positive effects of antigen presentation by combining with excess IgE and antigen in situations where high levels of IL-4 produce up-regulation of CD23[43].

Allergic inflammation

When the skin, nose or airways of atopic subjects are provoked with a single dose of allergen this produces, respectively, and within minutes, either an immediate cutaneous weal and flare reaction, sneezing and runny nose, or wheezing. Depending on the dose of allergen, these immediate-type hypersensitivity responses are followed by a late-phase reaction (LPR) which is slow to peak (6–9 h) and slow to resolve. In the skin, LPRs are characterized by an oedematous, red and slightly indurated swelling, in the nose by sustained blockage and, in the lung by further wheezing.

Thus, immediate-type hypersensitivity is the basis of acute allergic reactions. It is caused by molecules released by mast cells or basophils when an allergen interacts with membrane-bound IgE. There is a detailed account of mast cells and basophils in acquired immunity by Wedemeyer and Galli (p 936). The allergen/IgE/FcεRI complex on the mast cell surface triggers a non-cytotoxic, energy-dependent release of preformed granule-associated histamine, tryptase, and the membrane-derived lipid mediators, leukotrienes, prostaglandins and platelet activating factor. These mast cell mediators play a critical role in anaphylaxis, rhinoconjunctivitis and urticaria. The role of histamine in chronic asthma and eczema is probably minimal, however, as shown by the ineffectiveness of histamine antagonists in these conditions. The three cysteinyl (cys-) leukotrienes ($LTC_4/LTD_4/LTE_4$) cause smooth muscle contraction, vasodilatation, increased vascular permeability and mucous hypersecretion when they bind to specific cys-LT receptors[44]. In addition to mast cells, eosinophils, macrophages and monocytes are also major sources of cysteinyl leukotrienes. Mast cells also contain tryptase, a four chain neutral protease-tryptase which can activate the protease-activated receptors (PAR-2) on endothelial and epithelial cells. Activation through the PAR-2 receptors releases a cascade of events including up-regulation of adhesion molecules which selectively attract eosinophils and basophils[28].

The human cutaneous LPR is associated with an accumulation of eosinophils and neutrophils followed by a later infiltration of CD4+ T-cells and basophils[45]. Late-phase asthmatic[46] and nasal reactions[47] are also associated with a similar pattern of cellular infiltration, although basophils are less prominent in the airways[48].

Depending on the target organ, late-phase reactions can be provoked by activating mast cells or T cells. In the skin of both atopic and non-atopic subjects cross linking of mast cell bound IgE with an anti-IgE antibody provokes both early and late-phase reactions[49]. Late-phase reactions can be induced in atopic asthma without a preceding immediate-type, mast cell component. Haselden et al induced these reactions in patients with asthma who were allergic to cats by an intradermal injection of peptides derived from a cat allergen[50]. The fact that these late reactions were IgE-independent and MHC class II-restricted indicates that T cell activation alone is sufficient to initiate airway narrowing in allergic asthma.

Antigen presenting cells play a critical role in both initiating and controlling allergic inflammation. Dendritic cells (DC) and cutaneous

Table 1 Cytokines from Th2 cells in chronic allergic inflammation

Event	Type 2 cytokines	Other factors
Production of IgE	IL-4, IL-9, IL-13	[IFN-γ, IL-12, IL-18]
Eosinophil and basophil accumulation and development	IL-4, IL-5, IL-9, IL-13	IL-13, GM-CSF, Eotaxin 1-3, RANTES, MCP-3, MCP-4, VCAM-1
Development of mast cells	IL-4, IL-9, IL-13	IL-3, SCF
Airway hyperresponsiveness	IL-9, IL-13	IL-11 and growth factors involved in remodelling
Overproduction of mucus	IL-4, IL-9, IL-13	Histamine, LTC_4/D_4, SP, CGRP

Th2 cytokines and allergic inflammation. IL-4, IL-5, IL-9 and IL-13 (together with other cytokines, chemokines, growth factors, neuropeptides and pharmacological mediators) lead to IgE production, eosinophil/basophil development, mast cell development, airway hyperresponsiveness and mucus overproduction

Langerhans cells are particularly important in asthma and atopic eczema, respectively. They present antigen to CD4+ Th2 cells in an MHC class II-restricted fashion. Overexpression of the granuloctye/macrophage colony-stimulating factor (GM-CSF), which occurs in the asthmatic airway mucosa, leads to enhanced antigen presentation and increases in the local population density of these cells[14]. Alveolar macrophages from asthmatic patients obtained by broncho-alveolar lavage, present allergen to CD4 T cells and stimulate the production of Th2-cytokines[51]. Alveolar macrophages from the control subjects lacked this property.

As described by Robinson (p 956), Th2-type cytokines influence a wide range of events associated with chronic allergic inflammation. In addition to stimulating IgE production (IL-4, IL-13) these effects include maturation of eosinophils (IL-5, IL-9), up-regulation of the eosinophil/basophil selective adhesion molecule VCAM-1 (IL-4, IL-13), mast cell development (IL-3, IL-9, stem cell factor), airway hyper-responsiveness (IL-9, IL-13 (52)) and mucus overproduction (IL-4, IL-9, IL-13) (Table 1). Eosinophils can injure mucosal surfaces by releasing toxic basic proteins, cysteinyl leukotrienes and platelet activating factor, they can also damage inhibitory M_2 muscarinic receptors which in asthma may allow unchecked cholinergic responses[53]. On the other hand, eosinophils may also function as repair cells since they produce fibrogenic growth factors and matrix metalloproteinase involved in airway tissue remodelling in asthma[54].

IL-5 releases mature (and immature) eosinophils from the bone marrow[55], regulates the expression of the transmembrane isoform of its own receptor (IL-5-Rα)[56] and is essential for terminal differentiation of the committed eosinophil precursor[57]. Preferential accumulation of eosinophils occurs through a combination of selective adhesion molecules ($\alpha_4\beta_1$/VCAM-1), directional locomotion towards the eosinophil chemotactic C-C chemokines (eotaxin, eotaxin-2, RANTES, MCP-3 and MCP-4), prolonged survival (delayed apoptosis) under the influence of IL-5, IL-3 and GM-CSF, and local differentiation of tissue-infiltrating eosinophil precursors induced by IL-5[58].

Allergic inflammation may also involve release of neuropeptides from nerve cells by the action of nerve growth factor (NGF), brain-derived neurotrophic factor (BDNF) and neurotrophin-3 (NT-3)[59,60]. These neurotrophins are secreted by many cell types including macrophages, T cells, eosinophils and mast cells[60]. Neuropeptides, particularly substance P, calcitonin gene-related peptide and neurokinin A (all located predominantly in sensory neurones, but also in inflammatory cells cause characteristic features of allergic inflammation such as vasodilatation, increased vascular permeability and, in the lung, airway smooth muscle contraction and mucous hypersecretion[61]. Further amplification of chronic allergic reactions may be mediated by histamine releasing factors. They also release histamine from lung mast cells[62]. Tryptase can also trigger nerve cells to release neuropeptides by binding to protease-activated receptors[63]. Pathways leading to acute and chronic allergic reactions are shown in Figure 3.

Allergic diseases and their treatment

Allergic rhinitis

Allergic rhinitis is characterized by episodes of nasal obstruction, sneezing, itching and rhinorrhoea. Perennial allergic rhinitis should be distinguished from non-allergic, non-infectious forms of rhinitis such as idiopathic ('vasomotor') rhinitis, non-allergic rhinitis with eosinophilia syndrome (NARES), hormonal rhinitis, drug-induced rhinitis, food-induced rhinitis and rhinitis due to emotional factors.

The basis of the treatment of allergic rhinitis and other allergic diseases consists of avoidance of the allergen (where possible and practicable), anti-allergic medication and specific allergen immunotherapy – also called hyposensitization or desensitization. The importance and usefulness of environmental control to limit the burden of allergen exposure is discussed by Woodcock and Custovic (p 1071). Currently, the drugs usually used for treating allergic rhinitis are antihistamines and anticholinergic agents (for relief of symptoms) and topical corticosteroids for suppression of allergic inflammation. Histamine H_1 receptor antagonists such as loratadine, cetirizine and fexofenadine are less sedative and more pharmacologically

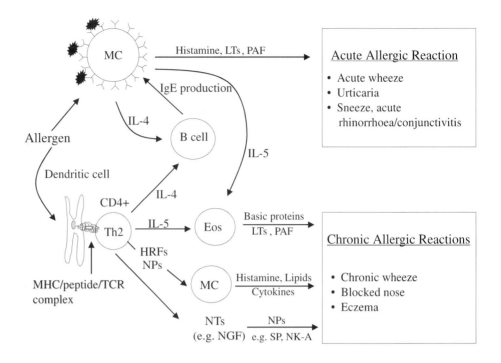

Fig. 3 Pathways leading to acute and chronic allergic reactions. Acute allergic reactions are due to the antigen-induced release of histamine and lipid mediators from mast cells. Chronic allergic reactions, included the late-phase response, may depend on a combination of pathways including eosinophil recruitment, liberation of mast cell products by histamine releasing factors[105] and neurogenic inflammation involving neurotrophins and neuropeptides. In the skin and upper airways basophils (not shown) may also participate in allergic tissue reactions.

selective than older antihistamines. Some H_1 blockers such as cetirizine are claimed to have the additional property of inhibiting allergen-induced tissue eosinophilia, an effect which may be H_1 receptor independent[64].

Specific immunotherapy, which has been used in the treatment of allergic disease for nearly 100 years, consists of administering increasing concentrations of allergenic extracts over long periods of time. In seasonal allergic rhinitis, and to a lesser extent perennial rhinitis, specific immunotherapy is extremely effective and long-lasting, especially when treatment is maintained for several years[65]. Unfortunately, all patients receiving conventional specific immunotherapy are at risk of developing general, and potentially fatal, anaphylaxis, particularly during the induction phase. Attempts to minimize systemic reactions include pretreatment of allergen extracts with agents like formaldehyde (resulting in the formation of so-called allergoids). However this results in reduced immunogenicity as well as a decrease in IgE binding.

The mode of action of specific immunotherapy is complex. IgG blocking antibodies that compete with IgE for allergen may prevent aggregation of FcεRI IgE complexes on mast cells through steric hindrance as well as interfering with antigen trapping by IgE bound to antigen presenting cells[66]. Several studies have shown that specific immunotherapy inhibits the release of pharmacological mediators from mast cells and basophils, prevents infiltration of allergic lesions by inflammatory cells[67] and decreases the number of tissue mast cells[68]. Central to these effects is the influence of specific immunotherapy on T lymphocyte function. There is evidence that specific immunotherapy induces a shift from a Th2 to a Th1 cytokine profile[69]: production of IL-4 and IL-5 decreases and the output of IFN-γ and IL-12 increases[66]. These changes can explain the marked inhibition of the late-phase allergic reaction caused by immunotherapy. After several months or years of treatment the early, immediate weal and flare reaction and total serum IgE concentration are also reduced[66].

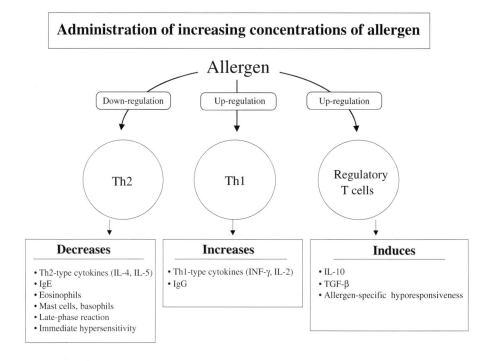

Fig. 4 Proposed mechanisms of specific immunotherapy (hyposensitization or desensitization). Specific immunotherapy is associated with a down-regulation of Th2 cells, immune deviation to Th1 cells and the induction of regulatory T cells (*e.g.* Tr1/Th3). This in turn leads to inhibition of allergic inflammation, increases in cytokines that control IgE production (IFN-γ, IL-12), 'blocking antibodies' (IgG), and cytokines involved in allergen-specific hyporesponsiveness (*i.e.* IL-10 and TGF-β).

In successful bee venom specific immunotherapy, induction of IL-10 secreting cells appears to be critical[70], but the role of this cytokine in desensitization against aero-allergens has yet to be established. IL-10 has a wide range of inhibitory effects on allergy, including the induction of long-term anergy in allergen-specific CD4+ cells, decreases the number of mast cells and inhibition of eosinophilopoiesis[71]. It has been proposed that SIT, as with other forms of immune modulation, may involve situations in which non-responsiveness induced (*e.g.* by IL-10) to one epitope of a molecule confers tolerance either to: (i) the whole molecule (linked suppression); (ii) other molecules being presented by the same, or adjacent, antigen presenting cells (bystander tolerance); or (iii) is passed to the next generation of naive T cells (infectious tolerance)[72]. Proposed mechanisms of specific immunotherapy are diagrammatically summarised in Figure 4.

Asthma

Asthma comprises episodes of wheezy breathlessness due to airway narrowing which are partially, or totally, reversible. Airway hyper-responsiveness is an almost invariable accompanying feature. The aetiology of asthma, as with other allergic diseases, is multifactorial, and appears to depend on the interplay between genetic factors, the environment and several specific and non-specific triggers (Fig. 2). Nevertheless, most asthmatics are atopic, although a minority have intrinsic, non-atopic disease which is often of later onset and runs a more protracted course. Recent studies indicate that there are more similarities than differences in the airway molecular immunopathology of atopic and non-atopic asthma[73]. Both variants are characterized by tissue infiltration of eosinophils and activated T cells and enhanced expression of IL-4, IL-5, IL-13 and C-C chemokines. Interestingly, there were also comparable numbers of bronchial mucosal cells mRNA+ for the ε germ-line transcript (Iε) and ε heavy chain of IgE (Cε)[73]. This indicates that intrinsic asthma may be associated with local production of specific IgE antibody directed against unknown antigens, possibly viral or autoimmune, and that immunological triggers may play a role in non-atopic as well as atopic disease.

Treatment of asthma consists of allergen avoidance (which in individuals sensitive to house dust mite and domestic animals is useful), broncho-dilators for relief and corticosteroids for prevention. Inhaled corticosteroids, when administered correctly, are highly effective and virtually free from side effects. However, a minority of chronic asthmatics are 'corticosteroid-dependent' and require oral medication to control their symptoms. In these situations, adverse effects are a problem and may present substantial difficulties in management. The effectiveness of corticosteroids in inhibiting allergic inflammation results from their ability to suppress multiple genes including those encoding Th2-type cytokines, inflammatory enzymes, adhesion molecules and inflammatory mediator receptors. Inflammation is regulated by several transcription factors including activator protein-1 (AP-1), NF-κB and nuclear factor of activated T cells (NF-AT) through a process which involves inhibition of core-histone acetylation[74]. Complexes formed by binding of corticosteroids to their cytosolic glucocorticosteroid receptor directly inhibit these transcription factors (*trans*-repression). The systemic side effects of corticosteroids are largely through DNA binding of the steroid/receptor complex (*trans*-activation). This may have important therapeutic implication because dissociated corticosteroids which *trans*-repress rather than *trans*-activate may retain anti-inflammatory properties but be free of side effects[75].

Ongoing corticosteroid-dependent severe asthma is associated with chronically activated T cells[76]. Several studies have shown that these patients respond well to relatively low doses of cyclosporin A and that this agent can also reduce the requirement for steroids[77]. Furthermore, a single injection of an anti-CD4 primatized monoclonal antibody to chronic severe asthmatics improved lung function for up to 2 weeks[78].

Other therapeutic options in asthma include theophylline, cromones and anti-leukotriene agents. Immunotherapy is generally less effective in chronic asthma than rhinitis. However mild asthma triggered predominantly by a single allergen, such as cat, can respond well to this form of treatment[79].

Anaphylaxis

Anaphylaxis is a severe systemic allergic reaction due to the massive release of histamine. It consists of a constellation of symptoms of which the most serious are laryngeal oedema or asthma (or both) and hypotension. The common causes of anaphylaxis are IgE-mediated sensitivity to foods (*e.g.* peanuts, tree nuts, fish, shellfish and dairy products), bee and wasp stings, drugs (*e.g.* penicillin and anaesthetic agents) and latex rubber. Food anaphylaxis is described in detail in the chapter by Sampson (p 925). Treatment of general anaphylaxis includes prompt administration of adrenaline, repeated if necessary, as this reverses the actions of histamine within minutes. This can be followed by an H_1 receptor antagonist antihistamine and corticosteroids. Prevention of anaphylaxis involves identification and avoidance of the cause. Preloaded adrenaline syringes are available for self-administration.

Specific immunotherapy with venom is highly effective in bee and wasp hypersensitivity. At present, specific immunotherapy has no place in the treatment of food anaphylaxis since severe reactions have been reported and there is no evidence of efficacy. However, modification of food allergens can reduce allergenicity indicating that such strategies may have therapeutic potential (see Sampson). For example, 10 IgE-binding epitopes were identified in the major peanut allergen, Ara h 2. Mutational analysis of the epitopes indicated that single amino acid changes resulted in loss of IgE binding and reduced skin test reactivity in peanut allergic individuals[80]. A different approach to immunotherapy, so far developed only in mice, is oral immunization with a plasmid vector containing DNA encoding Ara h 2. The DNA was protected from digestion by complexing it with the polysaccharide, chitosan[81]. This reduced allergen-induced anaphylaxis, lowered levels of IgE, and induced the production of protective secretory IgA and IgG_2a.

Atopic eczema

Atopic eczema affects 10–20% of children in Western populations. It is characterized by a red itchy rash, consisting of tiny papules, sometimes with an urticarial component, which may form confluent red sheets. Acute exacerbations may be weepy and crusted, usually signifying superinfection with *Staphylococci*. Chronic excoriated lesions are often thickened and lichenified. Total serum IgE concentrations may be markedly elevated and frequently there are high levels of IgE antibodies against aero-allergens and food allergens. Following cutaneous challenge with allergen there is an initial local response consisting of IL-4 and IL-5 (Th2-type cytokine response) followed by a mixed pattern (IFN-γ, IL-4 and IL-5; Th0)[82]. Allergen avoidance, with the possible exception of certain foods in children (Sampson) (particularly egg, peanut and milk) and exposure to the house dust mite[83], is disappointing in treating this condition. The mainstay of therapy is topical corticosteroids and antibiotics for bacterial superinfection. Notably, superantigens derived from *Staph. aureus* may cause polyclonal T cell proliferation in this disorder and treatment with low dose cyclosporin A can be highly beneficial. These observations suggest a role for the T lymphocyte in atopic eczema. More recently, topical tacrolimus (FK-506), which has a similar mode of action to cyclosporin A, has also been shown to be useful in severe disease and avoids the need for systemic immunosuppressants[84].

Urticaria and angioedema

Urticaria (widespread itchy weals or hives) and angioedema (deep muco-cutaneous swelling) often occur together. Acute urticaria is associated with sensitivity to foods, certain drugs and latex. The condition is often

IgE-mediated and the treatment is avoidance of the allergen. Chronic urticaria includes the physical urticarias and urticarial vasculitis; allergic causes of chronic urticaria are rarely identified. Some cases of chronic urticaria have been associated with circulating IgG auto-antibodies against FcεR1α[85] and sometimes auto-antibodies against IgE[86]. Uncharacterized non-immunoglobulin, low molecular weight histamine-releasing factors, have also been identified. A cause and effect relationship between levels of auto-antibodies and histamine-releasing factors and the clinical manifestations of chronic urticaria is yet to be established. However, severe cases often respond dramatically to plasmapheresis, consistent with a role for auto-antibodies or circulating histamine-releasing factors[87]. Hereditary angioedema is a rare autosomal dominant disorder caused by absence of the inhibitor of the first component of complement.

New approaches to the treatment of allergic diseases

As discussed by Larché (p 1019), allergen-specific immunotherapy, unlike anti-allergic drugs, promises to attenuate symptoms for several years after discontinuation of the therapy[65]. However, the safety of this treatment, particularly the threat of anaphylaxis, and the use of relatively crude allergen extracts limit its usefulness. To overcome these problems, newer approaches have been established in experimental animals or are undergoing clinical evaluation. Naturally occurring allergen isoforms from plants and trees have been shown to have a reduced capacity to bind IgE due to amino acid substitutions or deletions[88]. These hypo-allergenic isoforms may minimize the risk of anaphylaxis. The use of recombinant allergens should circumvent the problem of standardization of crude extracts by allowing production and purification of many of the major allergens in ways that eliminate batch variation and yield uniform products[89].

T cell peptide epitope immunotherapy involves the administration of short synthetic allergen-derived peptides which, on the one hand, induce T cell anergy or tolerance, but on the other are unable to cross-link IgE and induce anaphylaxis. Early clinical trials in patients with cat allergy, showed that a course of T cell peptides gave limited protection against allergic symptoms following exposure to cats[90]. Mixtures of allergen-specific peptides selected on the basis of their binding to common MHC class II molecules have potential for greater efficacy since they will be recognized by T cells of most individuals within a population[50,91]).

DNA vaccines also hold promise in the treatment of allergic diseases. Approaches include the use of CpG motifs such as GACGTC, which induce strong Th1 responses, administered either alone or in combination with allergen proteins[92]. Plasmid vectors containing allergen genes have been injected into animals, either before or after allergen challenge, and were shown to markedly abrogate Th2 and enhance Th1 responses and to suppress the allergic response. Virus-like particles, such as the yeast-derived Ty can also induce IFN-γ producing CD8[+] cells, rather than a Th2-type response, in a construct expressing a Der p 1 peptide[93].

Other therapeutic approaches under evaluation includes strategies to block IgE or IgE synthesis and to interrupt the Th2-dependent allergic cascade. For example, a humanized anti-IgE monoclonal antibody (rhuMAB-E25) virtually eliminated circulating IgE and markedly decreased expression of FcεRI on basophils[94]. Although E25 (omalizumab, Xolair®) neutralized IgE in blood and inhibited IgE production by B-cells, it did not activate mast cells, basophils or monocytes (*i.e.* was non-anaphylactogenic). MAB-E25 was shown to reduce symptoms of allergic rhinitis[95] and corticosteroid requirements in chronic asthma[96]. It also inhibited the allergen-induced early- and late-phase asthmatic reactions as shown by tests of lung function[97].

The recent description of the crystal structure of the complex between IgE and FcεRI[98] opens the way for the first structure-based design of small molecule inhibitors.

Several ways of inhibiting IL-4 are currently under investigation. For example, soluble recombinant IL-4 receptor was shown to improve moderately severe atopic asthma in a placebo-controlled trial[99]. Other approaches for functionally inhibiting IL-4R include anti-IL-4R antibodies and mutant IL-4 proteins[100]. Transcription factors involved in IL-4 signalling such as STAT-6 and c-maf are also attractive molecular therapeutic targets. Interference with FcεRI function, by for instance designing peptides that block IgE/FcεRIα chain interactions or inhibitors of Syk (required for intracellular signalling through FcεRIα) are therapeutic options for the future (see Stirling and Chung, p 1037).

In theory, chronic allergic inflammation should be controlled by targeting IL-5. In non-human primates, an anti-IL-5 monoclonal antibody almost completely abrogated eosinophilia and airway hyper-responsiveness (AHR) in an ascaris model of asthma[101]. Recent preliminary studies in patients with mild asthma have shown that a high affinity humanized IgG$_1$ anti-IL-5 monoclonal antibody abolished blood eosinophils and reduced sputum eosinophils but, surprisingly, had no apparent effect on the allergen-induced late-phase asthmatic reaction or non-specific airway hyper-responsiveness[102]. Long-term studies, in which total inhibition of tissue eosinophilia is achieved, will be required to establish conclusively the role of eosinophils and IL-5 in chronic atopic allergic disease and asthma. Other strategies for reducing eosinophil numbers include inhibition of $\alpha_4\beta_1$ (VLA-4) or CCR3, the receptor on eosinophils which binds to eotaxin and other eosinophil chemotactic C-C chemokines[103]. Wardlaw and colleagues (p 985) have reviewed the role of eosinophils in asthma and other allergic diseases and conclude that, even if they are only bystander cells, they remain clinically important as markers of disease severity.

Conclusions

IgE-mediated atopic allergic diseases are a major socio-economic problem caused by complex interactions between genes and the environment. In general, the production of IgE and allergic inflammation results from overexpression of Th2-type cytokines. Future approaches to controlling allergic diseases include improvements in the environment, safe and effective specific immunotherapy and inhibition of novel molecular targets in the allergic inflammatory cascade.

Acknowledgements

ABK is grateful to Drs Mark Larché, Douglas Robinson, Paul Cullinan, William Oldfield and Professor William Cookson for reviewing the manuscript. This chapter is based on *Allergy and Allergic Disease* by A.B. Kay (*N Engl J Med* 2001; **343**: 4 Jan (Part I), 11 Jan (Part II).

References

1   Aberg N, Hesselmar B, Aberg B, Eriksson B. Increase of asthma, allergic rhinitis and eczema in Swedish schoolchildren. *Clin Exp Allergy* 1995; **25**: 815–9
2   Smith DH, Malone DC, Lawson KA, Ikamoto LJ, Battista C, Saunders WB. A national estimate of the economic costs of asthma. *Am J Respir Crit Care Med* 1997; **156**: 787–93
3   von Pirquet C. Allergie. *Münch med Wochenstr* 1906; **30**: 1457 (Translated from the German by Prausnitz C. In: Gell PGH, Coombs RRA. (eds) *Clinical Aspects of Immunology*. Oxford: Blackwell Scientific, 1963)
4   Kemeny DM, Urbanek R, Ewan P *et al*. The subclass of IgG antibody in allergic disease: II. The IgG subclass of antibodies produced following natural exposure to dust mite and grass pollen in atopic and non-atopic individuals. *Clin Exp Allergy* 1989; **19**: 545–9
5   Romagnani S. Human TH1 and TH2 subsets: doubt no more. *Immunol Today* 1991; **12**: 256–7
6   Ebner C, Schenk S, Najafian N *et al*. Nonallergic individuals recognize the same T cell epitopes of Bet v 1, the major birch pollen allergen, as atopic patients. *J Immunol* 1995; **154**: 1932–40
7   Till S, Durham S, Dickason R *et al*. IL-13 production by allergen-stimulated T cells is increased in allergic disease and associated with IL-5 but not IFN-gamma expression. *Immunology* 1997; **91**: 53–7
8   Byron KA, O'Brien RM, Varigos GA, Wootton AM. *Dermatophagoides pteronyssinus* II-induced interleukin-4 and interferon-gamma expression by freshly isolated lymphocytes of atopic individuals. *Clin Exp Allergy* 1994; **24**: 878–83
9   Wierenga EA, Snoek M, Jansen HM, Bos JD, van Lier RA, Kapsenberg ML. Human atopen-specific types 1 and 2 T helper cell clones. *J Immunol* 1991; **147**: 2942–9.
10 Kay AB, Ying S, Varney V *et al*. Messenger RNA expression of the cytokine gene cluster, IL-3, IL-4, IL-5 and GM-CSF in allergen-induced late-phase cutaneous reactions in atopic subjects. *J Exp Med* 1991; **173**: 775–8

11 Robinson DS, Hamid Q, Ying S *et al*. Predominant T_{H2}-type bronchoalveolar lavage T-lymphocyte population in atopic asthma. *N Engl J Med* 1992; **326**: 298–304

12 Durham SR, Ying S, Varney VA *et al*. Cytokine messenger RNA expression for IL-3, IL-4, IL-5 and GM-CSF in the nasal mucosa after local allergen provocation: relationship to tissue eosinophilia. *J Immunol* 1992; **148**: 2390–4

13 Prescott S, Macaubas C, Holt BJ *et al*. Transplacental priming of the human immune system to environmental allergens: universal skewing of initial T cell responses towards the Th2 cytokine profile. *J Immunol* 1998; **160**: 4730–7

14 Holt PG, Macaubas C, Stumbles PA, Sly PD. The role of allergy in the development of asthma. *Nature* 1999; **402 (Suppl)**: B12–7

15 Constant SL, Bottomly K. Induction of Th1 and Th2 CD4⁺ T cell responses: the alternative approaches. *Annu Rev Immunol* 1997; **15**: 297–322

16 Rogers PR, Croft M. Peptide dose, affinity, and time of differentiation can contribute to the Th1/Th2 cytokine balance. *J Immunol* 1999; **163**: 1205–13

17 von Mutius E, Martinez FD, Fritzsch C, Nicolai T, Reitmeir P, Thiemann HH. Differences in the prevalence of asthma and atopic sensitisation between East and West Germany. *Am J Respir Crit Care Med* 1994; **149**: 358–64

18 von Mutius E, Weiland S, Fritzsch C, Duhme H, Keil U. Increasing prevalence of hay fever and atopy among children in Leipzig, East Germany. *Lancet* 1998; **351**: 862–6

19 Rook GA, Stanford JL. Give us this day our daily germs. *Immunol Today* 1998; **19**: 113–6

20 Sepp E, Julge K, Vasar M, Naaber P, Bjorksten B, Mikkelsaar M. Intestinal microflora of Estonian and Swedish infants. *Acta Pediatr* 1997; **86**: 956–61

21 Bjorksten B, Naaber P, Sepp E, Mikelsaar M. The intestinal microflora in allergic Estonian and Swedish 2-year-old children. *Clin Exp Allergy* 1999; **29**: 342–6

22 Braun-Fahrländer Ch, Gassner M, Grize L *et al* and the SCARPOL team. Prevalence of hay fever and allergic sensitization in farmers children and their peers living in the same rural community. *Clin Exp Allergy* 1999; **29**: 28–34

23 Cookson W. The alliance of genes and environment in asthma and allergy. *Nature* 1999; **402 (Suppl)**: B5–11.

24 Openshaw PJM, Hewitt CR. Protective and harmful effects of viral infections in childhood on wheezing disorders and asthma. *Am J Respir Crit Care Med* 2000; **162**: S40–3

25 Ball TM, Castro-Rodriguez JA, Griffith KA, Holberg CJ, Martinez FD, Wright AL. Siblings, day-care attendance, and the risk of asthma and wheezing during childhood. *N Engl J Med* 2000; **343**: 538–43

26 Schwartz J, Gold D, Dockery DW, Weiss ST, Speizer FE. Predictors of asthma and persistent wheeze in a national sample of children in the United States. Association with social class, perinatal events, and race. *Am Rev Respir Dis* 1990; **142**: 555–62

27 Call RS, Smith TF, Morris E, Chapman MD, Platts-Mills TA. Risk factors for asthma in inner city children. *J Pediatr* 1992; **121**: 862–6

28 Holgate ST. The epidemic of allergy and asthma. *Nature* 1999; **402 (Suppl)**: B2–4.

29 Burks W, Sampson HA, Bannon GA. Peanut allergens. *Allergy* 1998; **53**: 725–30

30 Marsh DG, Hsu SH, Roebber M *et al*. HLA-Dw2: a genetic marker for human immune response to short ragweed pollen allergen Ra 5. I. Response resulting primarily from natural antigenic exposure. *J Exp Med* 1982; **155**: 1439–51

31 Hill MR, Cookson WOCM. A new variant of the β subunit of the high-affinity receptor for immunoglobulin E (FcεRI-β E237G): association with measure of atopy and bronchial hyper-responsiveness. *Hum Mol Genet* 1996; **5**: 959–62

32 Marsh DG, Neely JD, Breazeale DR *et al*. Linkage analysis of IL-4 and other chromosome 5q31.1 markers and total serum immunoglobulin E concentrations. *Science* 1994; **264**: 1152–5

33 Moffatt ME, Cookson WOCM. Tumour necrosis factor haplotypes and asthma. *Hum Mol Genet* 1997; **6**: 551–4

34 Baldini M, Lohman IC, Halonen M, Erickson RP, Holt PG, Martinez FD. A polymorphism in the 5'-flanking region of the CD14 gene is associated with circulating soluble CD14 levels with total serum IgE. *Am J Respir Cell Mol Biol* 1999; **20**: 976–83

35 Sanak M, Simon HU, Szczeklik A. Leukotriene C_4 synthase promoter polymorphism and risk of aspirin-induced asthma. *Lancet* 1997; **350**: 1599–600

36 Kinet JP. The high affinity IgE receptor (Fc-epsilon RI): from physiology to pathology. *Annu Rev Immunol* 1999; **17**: 931–72

37 Stingl G, Maurer D. IgE-mediated allergen presentation via FcεRI on antigen-presenting cells. *Int Arch Allergy Immunol* 1997; **113**: 24–9

38 Smith SJ, Ying S, Meng Q *et al*. Blood eosinophils from atopic donors express mRNA for the α, β and γ subunits of the high affinity IgE receptor (FcεRI) and intracellular, but not cell surface, α subunit protein. *J Allergy Clin Immunol* 2000; **105**: 309–317

39 Corry DB, Kheradmand F. Induction and regulation of the IgE response. *Nature* 1999; **402 (Suppl)**: B18–23

40 Robinson D, Shibuya K, Mui A *et al*. IGIF does not drive Th1 development but synergizes with IL 12 for interferon-γ production and activates IRAK and NFκB. *Immunity* 1997; **7**: 1–20

41 Yoshimoto T, Nagai N, Ohkusu K, Ueda H, Okamura H, Nakanishi K. LPS-stimulated SJL macrophages produce IL-12 and IL-18 that inhibits IgE production *in vitro* by induction of IFN-gamma production from CD3intIL-2Rβ⁺ T cells. *J Immunol* 1998; **161**: 1483–92

42 Squire CM, Studer EJ, Lees A, Finkelman FD, Conrad DH. Antigen presentation is enhanced by targeting antigen to the FcεRII by antigen-anti-FcεRII conjugates. *J Immunol* 1994; **152**: 4388–96

43 Gustavsson S, Hjulstrom S, Liu T, Heyman B. CD23/IgE-mediated regulation of the specific antibody response *in vivo*. *J Immunol* 1994; **152**: 4793–800

44 Drazen JM, Israel E, O'Byrne PM. Drug therapy: treatment of asthma with drugs modifying the leukotriene pathway. *N Engl J Med* 1999; **340**: 197–206

45 Ying S, Robinson DS, Meng Q *et al*. C-C chemokines in allergen-induced late-phase cutaneous responses in atopic subjects: association of eotaxin with early 6-hour eosinophils, and eotaxin-2 and MCP-4 with the later 24-hour tissue eosinophilia, and relationship to basophils and other C-C chemokines (MCP-3 and RANTES). *J Immunol* 1999; **163**: 3976–84

46 Robinson DS, Hamid Q, Bentley A, Ying S, Kay AB, Durham SR. Activation of CD4⁺ T cells, increased Th2-type cytokine mRNA expression, and eosinophil recruitment in bronchoalveolar lavage after allergen inhalation challenge in atopic asthmatics. *J Allergy Clin Immunol* 1993; **92**: 313–24

47 Durham SR, Ying S, Varney VA *et al*. Cytokine messenger RNA expression for IL-3, IL-4, IL-5 and GM-CSF in the nasal mucosa after local allergen provocation: relationship to tissue eosinophilia. *J Immunol* 1992; **148**: 2390–4

48 Macfarlane AJ, Kon OM, Smith SJ *et al*. Basophils, eosinophils and mast cells in atopic and non-atopic asthma and in late-phase allergic reactions in the lung and skin. *J Allergy Clin Immunol* 2000; **105**: 99–107

49 Dolovich J, Hargreave FE, Chalmers R, Shier KJ, Gauldie J, Bienenstock J. Late cutaneous allergic responses in isolated IgE-dependent reactions. *J Allergy Clin Immunol* 1973; **52**: 38–46

50 Haselden BM, Kay AB, Larché M. IgE-independent MHC-restricted T cell peptide epitope-induced late asthmatic reactions. *J Exp Med* 1999; **189**: 1885–94

51 Larché M, Till S, Haselden BM *et al*. Costimulation through CD86 is involved in airway antigen-presenting cell and T cell responses to allergen in atopic asthmatics. *J Immunol* 1998; **161**: 6375–82

52 Wills-Karp M, Luyimbazi J, Xu X *et al*. Interleukin-13: central mediator of allergic asthma. *Science* 1998; **282**: 2258–63

53 Adamko DJ, Yost BL, Gleich GJ, Fryer AD, Jacoby DB. Ovalbumin sensitization changes the inflammatory response to subsequent parainfluenza infection. Eosinophils mediate airway hyperresponsiveness, m(2) muscarinic receptor dysfunction, and antiviral effects. *J Exp Med* 1999; **190**: 1465–78

54 Levi-Schaffer F, Garbuzenko E, Rubin A *et al*. Human eosinophils regulate human lung- and skin-derived fibroblast properties *in vitro*: a role for transforming growth factor beta (TGF-β). *Proc Natl Acad Sci USA* 1999; **96**: 9660–5

55 Palframan RT, Collins PD, Severs NJ, Rothery S, Williams TJ, Rankin SM. Mechanisms of acute eosinophil mobilization from the bone marrow stimulated by interleukin-5: the role of specific adhesion molecules and phosphatidylinositol 3-kinase. *J Exp Med* 1998; **118**: 1–12

56 Tavernier J, Van der Heyden J, Verhee A *et al*. Interleukin 5 regulates the isoform expression of its own receptor α-subunit. *Blood* 2000; **95**: 1600–1607

57 Clutterbuck EJ, Hirst EM, Sanderson CJ. Human interleukin-5 (IL-5) regulates the production of eosinophils in human bone marrow cultures: comparison and interaction with IL-1, IL-3, IL-6 and GM-CSF. *Blood* 1989; **73**: 1504–12

58 Denburg JA. Hemopoietic progenitors and cytokines in allergic inflammation. *Allergy* 1998; **53 (Suppl 45)**: 22–6

59 Bonini S, Lambiase A, Bonini S, Levi-Schaffer F, Aloe L. Nerve growth factor: an important molecule in allergic inflammation and tissue remodelling. *Int Arch Allergy Immunol* 1999; **118**: 159–62

60 Braun A, Lommatzch M, Renz H. The role of neurotrophins in allergic bronchial asthma. *Clin Exp Allergy* 2000; **30**: 178–86

61 Belvisi MG, Fox AJ. Neuropeptides. In: Kay AB. (ed) *Allergy and Allergic Diseases*, vol 1. Oxford: Blackwell Scientific, 1997; 447–80

62 Forsythe P, McGarvey LPA, Heaney LG, Macmahon J, Ennis M. Sensory neuropeptides induce histamine release from bronchoalveolar lavage cells in both nonasthmatic coughers and cough variant asthmatics. *Clin Exp Allergy* 2000; **30**: 225–32

63 Steinhoff M, Vergnolle N, Young SH *et al.* Agonists of proteinase-activated receptor 2 induce inflammation by a neurogenic mechanism. *Nat Med* 2000; **6**: 151–8

64 Slater JW, Zechnich AD, Haxby DG. Second generation antihistamines: a comparative review. *Drugs* 1999; **57**: 31–47

65 Durham SR, Walker SM, Varga EM *et al.* Long-term clinical efficacy of grass-pollen immunotherapy. *N Engl J Med* 1999; **341**: 468–75

66 Durham SR, Till SJ. Immunologic changes associated with allergen immunotherapy. *J Allergy Clin Immunol* 1998; **102**: 157–64

67 Creticos PS, Adkinson Jr NF, Kagey-Sobotka A *et al.* Nasal challenge with ragweed pollen in hay fever patients. Effect of immunotherapy. *J Clin Invest* 1985; **76**: 2247–53

68 Durham SR, Varney VA, Gaga M *et al.* Grass pollen immunotherapy decreases the number of mast cells in the skin. *Clin Exp Allergy* 1999; **29**: 1490–6

69 Varney VA, Hamid QA, Gaga M *et al.* Influence of grass pollen immunotherapy on cellular infiltration and cytokine mRNA expression during allergen-induced late-phase cutaneous responses. *J Clin Invest* 1993; **92**: 644–51

70 Akdis CA, Blesken T, Akdis M, Wüthrich B, Blaser K. Role of interleukin 10 in specific immunotherapy. *J Clin Invest* 1998; **102**: 98–106

71 Borish L. IL-10: evolving concepts. *J Allergy Clin Immunol* 1998; **101**: 293–7

72 Larché M. Allergen isoforms for immunotherapy: diversity, degeneracy and promiscuity. *Clin Exp Allergy* 1999; **29**: 1588–90

73 Humbert M, Menz G, Ying S *et al.* Viewpoint: the immunopathology of extrinsic (atopic) and intrinsic (non-atopic) asthma: more similarities than differences. *Immunol Today* 1999; **20**: 528–33

74 Barnes PJ. Therapeutic strategies for allergic diseases. *Nature* 1999; **402 (Suppl)**: B31–8

75 Vayssiere BM, Dupont S, Choquart A *et al.* Synthetic glucocorticoids that dissociate transactivation and AP-1 transpression exhibit anti-inflammatory activity *in vivo*. *Mol Endocrinol* 1997; **11**: 1245–55

76 Corrigan CJ, Kay AB. CD4 T-lymphocyte activation in acute severe asthma: relationship to disease severity and atopic status. *Am Rev Respir Dis* 1990; **141**: 970–7

77 Lock SH, Kay AB, Barnes NC. Double-blind, placebo-controlled study of cyclosporin A as a corticosteroid-sparing agent in corticosteroid-dependent asthma. *Am J Respir Crit Care Med* 1996; **153**: 509–14

78 Kon OM, Sihra BS, Compton CH, Leonard T, Kay AB, Barnes NC. Randomised, dose-ranging, placebo controlled study of a chimeric antibody to CD4 (keliximab) in chronic severe asthma. *Lancet* 1998; **352**: 1109–13

79 Varney VA, Edwards J, Tabbah K, Brewster H, Mavroleon G, Frew AJ. Clinical efficacy of specific immunotherapy to cat dander: a double-blind placebo-controlled trial. *Clin Exp Allergy* 1997; **27**: 860–7

80 Stanley JS, King N, Burks AW *et al.* Identification and mutational analysis of the immunodominant IgE binding epitopes of the major peanut allergen Ara h 2. *Arch Biochem Biophys* 1997; **342**: 244–53

81 Roy K, Mao HQ, Huang SK, Leong KW. Oral gene delivery with chitosan-DNA nanoparticles generates immunologic protection in a murine model of peanut allergy. *Nat Med* 1999; **5**: 387–91

82 Grewe M, Bruijnzeel-Koomen CA, Schopf E *et al.* A role for Th1 and Th2 cells in the immunopathogenesis of atopic dermatitis. *Immunol Today* 1998; **19**: 359–61

83 Tan BB, Weald D, Strickland I, Friedmann PS. Double-blind controlled trial of house dust mite allergen avoidance in atopic dermatitis. *Lancet* 1996; **347**: 15–8

84 Lipper GM, Arndt KA, Dover JS. Recent therapeutic advances in dermatology. *JAMA* 2000; **283**: 175–7

85 Hide M, Francis DM, Grattan CEH, Hakimi J, Kochan JP, Greaves MW. Autoantibodies against the high-affinity IgE receptor as a cause of histamine release in chronic urticaria. *N Engl J Med* 1993; **328**: 1599–604

86 Sabroe RA, Seed PT, Francis DM, Barr RM, Black AK, Greaves MW. Chronic idiopathic urticaria: comparison of the clinical features of patients with and without anti-FcεRI or anti-IgE autoantibodies. *J Am Acad Dermatol* 1999; **40**: 443–50

87 Grattan CEH, Francis DM, Slater NGP, Barlow RJ, Greaves MW. Plasmapheresis for severe unremitting chronic urticaria. *Lancet* 1992; **339**: 1078–80

88 Ferreira F, Hirtenlehner K, Jilek A *et al.* Dissection of immunoglobulin E and T lymphocyte reactivity of isoforms of the major birch pollen allergen Bet v 1: potential use of hypoallergenic isoforms for immunotherapy. *J Exp Med* 1996; **183**: 599–609

89 Breiteneder H, Ferreira F, Hoffmann-Sommergruber K *et al.* Four recombinant isoforms of Cor a I, the major allergen of hazel pollen, show different IgE-binding properties. *Eur J Biochem* 1993; **212**: 355–62

90 Norman PS, Ohman Jr JL, Long AA *et al.* Treatment of cat allergy with T-cell reactive peptides. *Am J Respir Crit Care Med* 1996; **154**: 1623–8

91 Texier C, Pouvelle S, Busson M *et al.* HLA-DR restricted peptide candidates for bee venom immunotherapy. *J Immunol* 2000; **164**: 3177–84

92 Tighe H, Corr M, Roman M, Raz E. Gene vaccination: plasmid DNA is more than just a blueprint. *Immunol Today* 1998; **19**: 89–97

93 Allsopp CE, Plebanski M, Gilbert S *et al.* Comparison of numerous delivery systems for the induction of cytotoxic T lymphocytes by immunization. *Eur J Immunol* 1996; **26**:1951–9

94 MacGlashan Jr DW, Bochner BS, Adelman DC *et al.* Down-regulation of FcεRI expression on human basophils during in vivo treatment of atopic patients with anti-IgE antibody. *J Immunol* 1997; **158**: 1438–45

95 Casale TB, Bernstein IL, Busse WW *et al.* Use of an anti-IgE humanized monoclonal antibody in ragweed-induced allergic rhinitis. *J Allergy Clin Immunol* 1997; **100**: 110–21

96 Milgrom H, Fick RB, Su JQ *et al.* Treatment of allergic asthma with monoclonal anti-IgE antibody. *N Engl J Med* 1999; **341**: 1966–73

97 Fahy JV, Fleming HE, Wong HH *et al.* The effect of an anti-IgE monoclonal antibody on the early- and late-phase response to allergen inhalation in asthmatic subjects. *Am J Respir Crit Care Med* 1997; **155**: 1828–34

98 Garman SC, Wurzburg BA, Tarchevskaya SS, Kinet JP, Jardetzky TS. Structure of the Fc fragment of human IgE bound to its high-affinity receptor FcεRIα. *Nature* 2000; **406**: 259–66

99 Borish L, Nelson HS, Lanz MJ *et al.* Interleukin-4 receptor in moderate atopic asthma. A phase I/II randomized, placebo-controlled trial. *Am J Respir Crit Care Med* 1999; **160**: 1816–23

100 Ryan JJ. Interleukin-4 and its receptor: essential mediators of the allergic response. *J Allergy Clin Immunol* 1997; **99**: 1–5

101 Mauser PJ, Pitman AM, Fernandez X *et al.* Effects of an antibody to interleukin-5 in a monkey model of asthma. *Am J Respir Crit Care Med* 1995; **152**: 467–72

102 Leckie MJ, ten Brinke A, Khan J *et al.* Effects of an interleukin-5 blocking monoclonal antibody on eosinophils, airway hyper-responsiveness, and the late asthmatic response. *Lancet* 2000; **356**: 2144–8

103 Heath H, Qin S, Rao P *et al.* Chemokine receptor usage by human eosinophils. The importance of CCR3 demonstrated using an antagonistic monoclonal antibody. *J Clin Invest* 1997; **99**: 178–84

104 Caramori G, Lim S, Ciaccia A, Fabbri LM, Barnes PJ, Adcock IM. GATA transcription factor expression in T cells, monocytes and bronchial biopsies of normal and asthmatic subjects. *Am J Respir Crit Care Med* 1999; **157**: A908

105 MacDonald SM, Rafnar T, Langdon J, Lichtenstein LM. Molecular identification of an IgE-dependent histamine-releasing factor. *Science* 1995; **269**: 688–90

The role of environmental factors in asthma

David P Strachan

Department of Public Health Sciences, St George's Hospital Medical School, London, UK

Although the everyday experience of asthmatic patients provides ample anecdotal evidence that environmental exposures provoke bronchospasm, it has proved more difficult to assess the impact of air quality on the timing of asthma attacks and the prevalence of asthma in populations.

Spectacular 'asthma epidemic days' are sometimes attributable to exceptional outdoor aero-allergen exposures. By comparison, effects of inorganic particles and gaseous pollutants in outdoor air on the incidence of asthma attacks are subtle and poorly quantified.

Environmental tobacco smoke and mould growth are the indoor factors most consistently associated with respiratory morbidity, but their roles in initiating allergic asthma remain uncertain. Evidence relating asthma risk to fumes from gas cooking, and to allergens from dust mites and household pets remains confused and controversial.

It is unlikely that trends in either outdoor or indoor air pollution have contributed substantially to the rise in prevalence of asthma and allergic disease in recent decades.

The role of environmental factors in relation to asthma and allergy has become increasingly topical through the 1990s. There has been widespread public concern that changing patterns of outdoor air pollution underlie the rising burden of asthma, but the professionals are not so sure[1-5]. The indoor environment, in which people spend most of their time, has received less attention[6]. This chapter summarises current evidence linking both outdoor and indoor air quality to temporal, spatial and individual variations in asthma and allergic sensitisation. The discussion of the indoor environment will focus on domestic exposures, and readers seeking details on occupational causes of asthma are referred to specialised reviews of this field[7,8].

Confusion often arises because the links between environment and asthma may operate at various stages in the development of this disease[4,5]. It is, therefore, useful to distinguish clearly between two questions: (i) what initiates (or induces) the **asthmatic state**, a tendency to develop episodic airflow obstruction on exposure to a range of environmental and non-environmental stimuli? – part of this process may involve the development of atopic sensitisation to environmental allergens; and (ii) what triggers (or provokes) **attacks of asthma** among persons who already have the disease?

Correspondence to: Prof. David P Strachan, Professor of Epidemiology, Department of Public Health Sciences, St George's Hospital Medical School, Cranmer Terrace, London SW17 0RE, UK

Table 1 Possible effects of environmental facxtors on asthma

Temporal variations
    Changes in asthma prevalence from year-to-year
    Daily fluctuations in the incidence of asthma attacks
    Occurrence of exceptional 'asthma epidemic days'

Spatial variations
    International differences in asthma prevalence
    Urban–rural differences in prevalence
    Variations between individual households

The environmental factors which may provoke attacks of bronchospasm include irritant gases, inorganic particles, allergens and infections. These are often identified by patients as triggers of symptoms and may be demonstrated more objectively by chamber experiments. There has been a tendency to implicate the same factors in the initiation of the asthmatic state, but the epidemiological evidence suggests that this simplistic approach to 'the cause of asthma' is likely to be misleading. It is more appropriate to seek explanations or 'causes' at different levels as summarised in Table 1.

Short-term variations in the incidence of asthma attacks

The frequency of asthma attacks varies considerably from day-to-day, as indicated by numbers of hospital admissions or accident and emergency attendances for asthma. In many countries, including Britain, there is a predictable seasonal variation[9], with peak incidence during the early autumn, particularly in children[10]. These seasonal fluctuations are thought to be more closely related to the timing of school holidays[11] and circulation of respiratory virus infections[12], than to seasonal variations in air quality or aero-allergen exposure[9].

Superimposed upon the seasonal pattern there are day-to-day variations in attack frequency which have attracted considerable interest in recent years as possible evidence of the adverse effects of outdoor air pollution levels. However, perhaps the most convincing evidence of an environmental influence on the incidence of asthma attacks arises from occasional 'asthma epidemic days'. Most of the patients affected in these documented epidemics are atopic asthmatics, and unusual aero-allergen exposures have been implicated in several instances.

Asthma epidemic days

There have been relatively few reports of noticeable 'epidemics' of asthma attacks lasting for 1–2 days, although retrospective analysis of hospital activity has revealed several epidemics which were not apparent at the time[13]. A striking example occurred on the night of 24–25 June 1994 when a thunderstorm over southern and eastern England was followed by a 10-fold increase in acute asthma attacks presenting to accident and emergency departments[14]. Levels of conventionally measured air pollutants were not unusual at the time[15]. There were earlier reports of thunderstorm-related asthma outbreaks from Melbourne[16,17] and Birmingham, UK[18], and a systematic time-series analysis suggested that a typical English thunderstorm is associated with a 25% relative increase in asthma admissions on the following day[19]. This excess is greater following periods of high grass pollen counts, and many of the affected patients were sensitised to grass pollen[14]. Osmotic rupture or physical disruption of pollen grains during the thunderstorm releases submicroscopic starch granules which carry allergens such as *Lol pIX* and are of a size which could be inhaled into the smaller airways[17,20]. Thus, these thunderstorm-related epidemics were probably due to 'aero-allergen pollution'.

Only one-third of asthma epidemic days in England during 1987–1994 were related to thunderstorms[13], and the cause of the remainder remains elusive. Nevertheless, the concept of mass outbreaks attributable to unusual aero-allergen exposures is supported by observations of repeated outbreaks of asthma recorded in Barcelona during the 1980s[21]. Air pollution levels and airborne pollen and spore counts on the epidemic days were below average for the city but subsequent investigation implicated the unloading of soybeans in the harbour as the cause[22]. Patients affected on epidemic days were found to have circulating soybean-specific IgE[23], and no further epidemics have occurred since modifications were made to the procedures for unloading soybeans.

Asthma epidemic days were a recognised phenomenon in New Orleans during the 1950s and 1960s[24]. Air pollution, possibly related to burning of rubbish dumps, was suspected initially, but the epidemics continued despite cessation of this seasonal activity[24]. The patients involved in epidemics were predominantly atopic asthmatics, with positive skin prick tests to many common aero-allergens[25]. Detailed investigations of airborne pollens and fungal spores failed to identify a specific allergen that might be responsible, but it was noted that autumn epidemic days tended to be associated with high total spore and pollen counts[25]. In this regard, it may be relevant that certain fungal spores, such as *Didymella exitialis* and *Sporobolomyces* are released during summer thunderstorms[18]. Some patients with late summer asthma may be allergic to *Didymella* spores[26], but in general, the role of outdoor fungal allergens as triggers of asthma attacks remains uncertain.

Daily fluctuations in air pollution and asthma

Although inorganic air pollution has not been implicated as a cause of exceptional asthma epidemic days, many studies have examined daily counts of asthma admissions or emergency room visits in relation to short-term fluctuations in measured pollutants. These time-series studies have used increasingly sophisticated statistical methods which can detect subtle daily variations in asthma attack incidence which are far too small to qualify as an 'epidemic'.

The global literature was comprehensively reviewed by the author in 1995[27], and subsequently by the author and colleagues in 1998[28]. Only a minority of the studies published evidence in a form which permitted an estimation of the dose-response relationship to individual pollutants. Quantitative estimates are rarely quoted when no significant correlation was observed between asthma incidence and pollutant levels. Thus, the results of overviews and meta-analyses tend to preferentially include 'positive' associations and may overestimate the dose-response gradient. With this cautionary proviso, the following conclusions may be drawn.

Associations between single pollutants and a health outcome such as asthma are often inconsistent. In our 1998 review of 16 'methodologically sound' studies[28], ozone, sulphur dioxide and particles were identified as significant correlates of daily asthma attack rates in no more than half of the reports, and one-quarter or less found a significant effect of particulate or nitrogen dioxide levels. Thus, effects of single pollutants should not be interpreted narrowly, but rather as indicative of complex pollutant mixtures, which may vary by location.

For instance, there is fairly consistent evidence that the type of 'summer haze' affecting southern Canada and the eastern US is associated with a modest short-term increase in the incidence of asthma attacks[29–32]. The causal agent, however, remains in doubt. Ozone is a possible candidate[33], but on the western coast of North America, ozone levels were either uncorrelated with asthma incidence (as in Vancouver[34] and Seattle[35]) or inversely correlated with daily asthma attack rates (as in Los Angeles[36]). In London, ozone levels were positively associated with asthma admissions in summer (possibly indicative of the 'summer haze' mixture) but inversely associated in winter (possibly due to scavenging of ozone by nitrogen oxides in vehicle exhausts)[28].

Acid aerosol was considered as a possible agent in southern Ontario, but direct measurements of airborne acid in New York[31] were no more closely correlated with asthma admissions than were ozone or sulphate levels. Airborne sulphates form a major part of the fine particulate fraction in Northeast US and it has been suggested that the effects of summer haze may be mainly attributable to these respirable particles[37]. However, the only summer haze study to measure fine particles directly[30] found no relationship between PM_{10} levels and the timing of asthma attacks.

In general, the evidence is less consistent with regard to winter pollutants[28]. This may reflect different emission sources, pollutant 'cocktails' and particle composition in different areas, or a correlation of outdoor conditions with indoor pollutant exposure which varies according to the fuel used for domestic heating. Where winter pollutant effects have been evaluated for different age groups, as in London[28] and Vancouver[34], the more significant findings are for the older age groups. This may be partly due to diagnostic confusion with other forms of chronic obstructive airways disease.

In December 1991, an episode of unusually high particulate and nitrogen dioxide pollution, mainly from vehicular sources, occurred in London. During the episode week, there was a small (3%) and statistically non-significant increase in asthma admissions in the capital, by comparison with previous years and the surrounding regions[38]. Other respiratory outcomes, notably chronic bronchitis and emphysema among the elderly, were affected to a greater extent than asthma admissions.

Temporary closure of a steel mill in Utah Valley during 1986–1987 offered an unusual opportunity to study the effects of changing levels of 'winter pollutants' on respiratory health at the community level[39,40]. Although there was no statistically significant reduction in asthma admission rates for all age groups, asthma and bronchitis admissions (combined) among preschool children were halved during the year of the mill closure, suggesting a reduction in 'wheezy bronchitis' rather than 'allergic asthma'.

Outdoor aero-allergen levels and asthma

Fewer studies have applied the time-series approach to study the relationship between asthma attacks and aero-allergen levels on a daily basis. However, apart from the special circumstances associated with thunderstorms, it seems that asthma admissions are not associated with daily variations in airborne counts of grass pollen[19,28,41], or tree pollens[13,28]. Thus, pollen levels are unlikely to be major confounders in studies of spring and summer air pollutants.

Allergic sensitisation to mould extracts occurs in a minority of asthmatic patients of all ages, although usually in association with other aero-allergens such as pollen, house dust mites and animal danders[42]. Sensitisation to the outdoor mould *Alternaria alternata* has been implicated as a major risk factor for fatal asthma attacks in Chicago, USA[43]. This may simply reflect a common association with severe asthma, but in Chicago, asthma deaths at ages 5–34 years occur about twice as commonly on days with a high total mould spore count (>1000 spores/m^3) as on days with lower spore counts[44]. Panel studies of asthmatic patients report inconsistent findings relating symptom severity to mould spore concentrations in outdoor air[45–49], but there has been a suggestion that fungal spores may be implicated in some asthma epidemic days[18,25].

Chamber experiments have suggested a synergistic interaction between prior exposure to a variety of gaseous air pollutants and bronchial responsiveness to allergen challenges[50–53]. The interaction between ozone and pollen exposure is perhaps the most relevant to the outdoor environment, but in the only time-series study to specifically address this combination, there was no evidence of a synergistic effect in relation to asthma admissions in the London area[28].

Outdoor air pollution and the prevalence of asthma

Whereas daily time-series offer some insights into the acute effects of outdoor air quality on asthma attacks, the more fundamental concern is whether long-term exposure to air pollution influences the prevalence of asthma[4,5]. This has been addressed by area-level studies comparing asthma prevalence in whole towns or cities with differing levels or mixtures of pollution, and by individual or household studies, relating asthma risk to proximity to roads or to other indices of traffic exposure.

Comparisons of areas of high and low pollution

The pollutants which have been most often measured in geographical comparisons relating the prevalence of wheezing illness to air pollution are sulphur dioxide and airborne particles. The evidence relating each of these to asthma and wheezing at the area level is inconsistent[54]. Comparisons within eastern Europe (often at high levels of smoke and SO_2) generally support an association with life-time prevalence of wheezing in children, whereas similar studies in elsewhere (often at lower levels of SO_2 and particulate pollution) present a mixed picture[55].

Fewer studies have addressed possible hazards due to 'newer' pollutants (nitrogen oxides and ozone). In general, NO_2 levels are correlated with SO_2 and particulate concentrations in area comparisons and it is difficult to distinguish their independent effects. Two equally competent studies of wheeze among non-smoking adults yield conflicting findings in relation to photochemical pollutants. In the Swiss SAPALDIA study[56], no associations were found between the prevalence of wheezing or current asthma and the annual mean concentrations of particles, ozone or nitrogen dioxide at 8 study centres. However, cough, phlegm and breathlessness were positively associated with particulate pollution among never smokers. Among

Seventh Day Adventists in California[57], the incidence of adult-onset asthma diagnosed by physician was significantly and positively associated with cumulative outdoor exposure to particulate air pollution. Unfortunately, ambient particle concentrations were highly correlated with ozone levels so it was not possible to discriminate with certainty the independent effects of each pollutant[57].

An unusual opportunity to study the effects of air pollution on health arose from the re-unification of Germany, but comparisons of symptoms related to asthma are complicated by a large difference in prevalence of allergy between East and West Germany[58]. A consistent finding was a lower prevalence of positive skin prick responses in the polluted areas of East Germany than in West German cities[59,60]. There appeared to be an excess of irritant symptoms (including 'bronchitis') in the most heavily polluted areas of the former GDR, balanced by a reduced prevalence of 'allergic asthma'[61].

Small area variations and exposure to traffic

Although the differences in prevalence of asthma and allergy between East and West Germany could not be explained on the basis of hazards from 'old-fashioned' smoke and sulphur dioxide pollution, exposure to 'modern' pollutants derived from vehicle exhaust was higher in West Germany. Concern that traffic exposure might increase the risk of asthma was raised by several population surveys from Germany and The Netherlands which found a higher prevalence of asthma and allergic disease among children living close to busy roads or heavy truck traffic[62–65]. The variations in prevalence across extremes of traffic exposure in these studies were generally between 25–50% in relative terms, but some of this may reflect reporting bias, particularly in studies which rely on self-reporting of traffic exposure.

British studies are based on larger numbers of asthma cases but yield less consistent findings. Within London, no association was found between proximity to major roads and asthma diagnosis, treatment or hospital admissions[66,67]. However, in Birmingham, young children were more likely to be admitted with asthma from heavily trafficked areas[68]. A study from Stockholm also found an association of modelled traffic exposure with 'wheezing bronchitis' in infancy[69], but it is likely that most of the cases in these studies were 'viral associated wheezing' rather than 'allergic asthma'.

Not only is the published evidence inconsistent, but there is also considerable uncertainty whether any 'positive' associations could be due to air pollution from vehicle emissions[70]. Place of residence is an imperfect indicator of personal activity patterns, and although mean nitrogen oxide concentrations decrease with distance from the kerbside, the decline beyond 20 m is small[71]. No correlation between traffic density and ambient NO_2 concentrations was found within Münich[62], although carbon monoxide, benzene and toluene (vehicle-related pollutants which are not implicated in asthma) were more concentrated in areas of higher traffic flow. Higher traffic density was **inversely** correlated with levels of ozone[62], which is formed at some distance from emission sources, and 'scavenged' in city centres by NO from vehicles. Personal exposure to NO_2 and particles is influenced to a small degree by distance from major roads, but to a much larger extent by indoor sources (cooking and heating fuels, and environmental tobacco smoke)[72]. It is, therefore, appropriate to turn our attention now to the influence of indoor air quality on asthma.

Indoor air quality and the prevalence and severity of asthma

Gas cooking and indoor nitrogen dioxide

Nitrogen dioxide has been widely used in studies of outdoor air quality as a marker of pollution related to vehicle emissions. However, the most important source of personal NO_2 exposure is unvented gas appliances, particularly gas cookers[6,73]. Comparison of disease prevalence between homes with and without gas cookers, therefore, offers a simple method of evaluating whether long-term exposure to NO_2 specifically (but not other motor vehicle emissions) induces the asthmatic state. However, because indoor NO_2 levels are influenced by house design and ventilation, use of a gas cooker is arguably a better marker of **peak** NO_2 exposure than **average** levels[73].

An early meta-analysis of epidemiological studies suggested a pooled relative risk of 1.2 (relative excess of 20%) for a range of respiratory illnesses among children exposed to gas cooking in the home[74]. Many of these studies did not specifically report results for asthma or wheezing. More recent large studies from Europe and North America, among both children and adults, have reported conflicting evidence: some showing up to a 2-fold increase in asthma prevalence in gas cooking homes[75,76], others finding no differences[77–79]. International differences in the strength and direction of the association are apparent even when the survey techniques were similar[80], and it remains unresolved whether the inconsistencies can be explained by variations in cooker design, use or other factors[81].

Two studies of adults find no association between gas cooking and allergic sensitisation[78,80] and atopic asthmatics do not appear to have more severe symptoms or an adverse prognosis if exposed to gas cooking[78]. A causal relationship between nitrogen dioxide exposure and asthma severity has not been disproved, but the balance of evidence suggest it is unlikely.

Environmental tobacco smoke

Many asthmatic patients identify other people's tobacco smoke as an environmental trigger for their symptoms, but there is a surprisingly sparse literature documenting effects of passive smoking on either the prevalence or severity of asthma in adults[82]. Perhaps the most convincing studies are those of lifelong non-smoking Seventh Day Adventists in California[57], showing a 50% relative increase in the incidence of doctor-diagnosed asthma over 10 years among adults exposed to environmental tobacco smoke.

The literature relating parental smoking to asthma, wheezing and allergic disease in children is much more extensive and has recently been reviewed both qualitatively and quantitatively by the author and colleagues[83–87]. The results are complex and require careful interpretation, distinguishing between the various wheezing syndromes which may present in childhood.

The most consistent results relate to lower respiratory illnesses in infancy[83]. Smoking by either parent, and particularly by the mother, increases the risk of both wheezing and non-wheezing chest illnesses up to 2 years of age by about 50% (relative risk 1.5), independent of other factors. The medium-term prognosis of these early wheezing episodes is less favourable in smoking households, but as the child grows through adolescence, remission is more likely if the mother smokes[86].

At school ages there is a higher prevalence of asthmatic symptoms (relative risk about 1.3) among children whose parents smoke[84], and among children with asthma, markers of disease severity are generally worse in those exposed to smoking in the home[86]. In contrast, allergic sensitisation, at least as measured by skin prick tests, is no more common in the offspring of smoking parents[85], and the association of wheeze with passive smoke exposure appears stronger among non-atopic children[86].

One interpretation is that passive smoking is related more closely to transient 'wheezy bronchitis' than to 'allergic asthma'. Its association with symptom prevalence and asthma severity in school age children thus reflects a role predominantly as a trigger of symptomatic episodes (alone, or in combination with viral infection), rather than as a factor initiating the development of allergic sensitisation or atopic asthma[87].

Dampness and indoor moulds

An association of asthma with 'damp houses and fenny countries' was observed three centuries ago by Sir John Floyer[88]. Studies of the relationship between home dampness or domestic mould growth and asthma have generally used questionnaire reports of wheeze and dampness/mould to characterise disease and exposure, and most have concentrated on children in order to discount the confounding effects of active smoking, occupation, and selection into different types of housing. The results are fairly consistent, finding that wheeze is about twice as likely to occur in homes reported to be mouldy[89-94].

Fewer studies have attempted objective or independent assessment of housing conditions or allergic symptomatology. Those that have been reported generally show little relationship with mould[95-98], raising the possibility that at least some of the association in questionnaire data is due to reports of symptoms being increased by awareness of mould in the home (or *vice versa*)[99]. However, one recent study reported an association between asthma severity and independent assessments by surveyor of dampness and mould growth in the patients' homes[100].

A large number of potentially allergenic mould species have been isolated from homes and indoor humidity is an important determinant of fungal growth. However, in most cases, the same species of fungi occur in the homes of both affected and unaffected people, often in the same proportions[97,98]. Allergic sensitisation to indoor moulds is uncommon, even among asthmatic patients[42]. It is, therefore, difficult to attribute the difference in the prevalence of symptoms between mouldy and non-mouldy homes to fungal allergy. A more likely interpretation is that variations in the levels of other airborne allergens, especially from house dust mites, underlie the relationship between damp, mouldy housing and asthma. Cockroach allergen may be a contributory factor in some areas, particularly in the US[101].

House dust mite allergens

The role of house dust mites in the induction and provocation of asthma has been the subject of a number of international workshops and systematic reviews[102-104], but the importance of mite allergen exposure in determining the prevalence and severity of asthma remains contro-versial[105,106]. The evidence needs to be considered at various levels.

There is consistent evidence for a correlation between level of exposure and degree of sensitisation to mite allergen in both children and adults[102-106]. It is now considered unlikely that there is a threshold level below which sensitisation does not occur, as had been suggested by a WHO workshop in 1987[102]. However, the **total** prevalence of allergic sensitisation is not greatly influenced by mite allergen levels[107], and by no means all people with demonstrable mite sensitisation have clinical allergic disease. Thus studies of sensitisation in relation to allergen exposure provide only indirect evidence of a health risk.

International variations in the prevalence of asthma[108,109] do not bear any obvious relationship to the local mite prevalence. Within Australia, widely varying climatic conditions give rise to large regional variations in mite allergen levels, but the prevalence of childhood asthma is similar throughout the country.[107,108] Mite allergen levels are generally similar in the homes of asthmatic and non-asthmatic subjects,[106] although some studies have reported an association between domestic mite allergen exposure and severity of asthma[105]. A concern in these cross-sectional and case-control studies is that causal associations may have been diluted because of allergen avoidance measures by families of allergic or asthmatic patients. This bias can be reduced, but not totally avoided, by longitudinal studies relating allergen exposure in infancy to subsequent incidence of asthma. So far, few long-term follow-up studies have been published[110,111], so the relative importance of perinatal and later exposure remains uncertain.

Intervention studies may offer a more direct evaluation of the importance of current house dust mite exposure. The evidence is reviewed in greater detail elsewhere in this issue. Unfortunately, attempts at mite allergen avoidance have generally been disappointing in terms of their efficacy (reduction in allergen exposure). It remains unresolved whether the more efficacious interventions are clinically effective (in terms of improving asthma symptoms) or of prophylactic value (for primary prevention of asthma)[112-114].

Household pets

Studies of mite allergen exposure in large population samples are expensive and time-consuming, but a simpler model for the hypothesis that allergen exposure induces asthma would relate to pet danders. Presence of a cat or dog in the home is a powerful determinant of exposure to the relevant allergens (*Fel d1* and *Can f1*, respectively), and this can be demonstrated in both dust samples and air samples[115]. However, pet avoidance by allergic families is a potential bias which needs to be addressed in observational studies[116].

Several large studies have found either no association between asthma and pet ownership[77], or an inverse relationship, particularly with early dog ownership[117]. On the other hand, inconsistent results emerged from two case-control studies of asthma among teenage children which adjusted for pet avoidance[118], one showing an association of early pet ownership with more severe asthmatic symptoms, the other finding less asthma and, paradoxically, less cat allergy among children exposed to cats in infancy[119].

Recent observations of a reduced prevalence of allergic diseases among children of farmers[120] raise the possibility that animal exposure may reduce the tendency to allergic sensitisation through other mechanisms, perhaps related to infection[121]. Thus, whereas animal dander may exacerbate asthmatic symptoms among sensitised individuals[122], pet ownership in a more general sense may have relatively little effect on the prevalence of pet allergy or associated allergic asthma.

Bedding

For many years, asthmatic patients have been advised to avoid feather bedding on the premise that allergen exposure (from both house dust mites and feathers themselves) would thereby be reduced. More recently, this assumption has been challenged by both exposure measurements and epidemiological studies.

Contrary to expectation, mite allergen levels in dust samples from feather pillows are 5–10 times lower than in dust from synthetic pillows[123–125], possibly due to the more tightly woven covers required for feather pillows acting as a barrier to allergen release. Two case-control studies of wheezy children in south London, from 1978 and 1991, found that use of a feather pillow (rather than a synthetic one) was associated with a reduced risk of asthmatic symptoms, even after allowance for deliberate changes to the child's bedding as a result of asthma or allergy[126]. Two further studies of British children confirm a strong inverse association of feather pillow use with both mild and severe asthma[118,127]. Taken together, these four studies suggest that asthma is about twice as common in children using synthetic pillows as those sleeping on feather ones, with a dose-response gradient in relation to symptom severity.

Conclusions

A look to the past

The prevalence of asthma and other allergic diseases has been rising in many Westernised countries over the past few decades, at a time when exposure to most measured air pollutants has declined[54]. Although the epidemiological evidence does not exclude a relatively weak relationship between outdoor air pollution and asthma prevalence, a strong association is unlikely. It is also apparent that indoor air quality is often a more important determinant of personal pollution exposure. For these reasons, it is unlikely that changes in the levels or composition of outdoor air pollution have been a major factor underlying the trends in asthma prevalence in most countries, including Britain[1–4].

Few studies have compared measures of indoor air quality over a similar period of time. The sparse evidence in relation to mite allergen levels suggests little change between 1979 and 1989, at least in southern England[110]. Comparison of two studies in south London in 1978 and 1991[126] found that changes in pet ownership, parental smoking habits, domestic central heating and cooking fuel could not explain the rise in prevalence of wheezing among 8-year-old children over this period. Indeed, the increase in use of non-feather pillows from 44% to 67% over the 13-year period was the only indoor environmental factor studied which potentially explained any substantial part of the increase in prevalence of wheezing from 1978 to 1991[126].

A view to the future

Asthma is a disease characterised by variability of airflow obstruction and episodic occurrence of symptoms in individual patients ('attacks'). It is also a disease which varies in prevalence and severity within populations, between countries, and over time. The environment, defined narrowly as in this chapter, in terms of chemical and biological air pollutants, is much more clearly related to the provocation of asthma **attacks** and to asthma **severity** than it is to the induction of the asthmatic **state** and the **prevalence** of asthma[4,5].

Variations in indoor or outdoor air quality and allergen exposure account for neither the large international variations in asthma prevalence, nor the long-term time trends. In seeking to explain these, and ultimately to prevent asthma, a much broader definition of 'environment' is required. Areas which are currently topical include the intra-uterine environment[128] and the microbial environment, including commensal bowel flora[129]. These, in turn, may interface with components of life-style (*e.g.* infant feeding and dietary habits) or medical care (*e.g.* obstetric care and antibiotic prescribing). The need for a broad perspective in asthma research during the 21st century is as important today as when it was first suggested 15 years ago[130].

References

1 Bousquet J, Burney PGJ. Evidence for an increase in atopic disease and possible causes. *Clin Exp Allergy* 1993; **23**: 484–92

2 Peat JK. The rising trend in allergic illness: which environmental factors are important? *Clin Exp Allergy* 1994; **24**: 797–800

3 Seaton A, Godden DJ, Brown K. Increase in asthma: a more toxic environment or a more susceptible population? *Thorax* 1994; **49**: 171–4

4 Department of Health Committee on the Medical Effects of Air Pollutants. *Asthma and Outdoor Air Pollution*. Chapter 1. Executive summary. London: HMSO, 1995; 1–2

5 Burr ML. Pollution – does it cause asthma? *Arch Dis Child* 1995; **72**: 377–9

6 Samet JM, Marbury MC, Spengler JD. Health effects and sources of indoor air pollution. *Am Rev Respir Dis* 1987; **136**: 1486–508 and 1988; **137**: 221–42

7 Chan-Yeung M, Malo JC. Epidemiology of occupational asthma. In: Busse W, Holgate ST. (eds) *Mechanisms in Asthma and Rhinitis: Implications for Diagnosis and Treatment*. Oxford: Blackwell Scientific, 1994; 44–57

8 Cullinan P, Newman Taylor AJ. Occupational asthma: a model for asthma acquired outside the workplace? In: Holgate ST, Boushey HA, Fabri LM. (eds) *Difficult Asthma*. London: Martin Dunitz, 1999; 113–26

9 Department of Health Committee on the Medical Effects of Air Pollutants. *Asthma and Outdoor Air Pollution*. Chapter 7. Asthma, allergy and air pollution in Great Britain: time trends and geographical variations. London: HMSO, 1995; 85–129

10 Khot A, Burn R, Evans N, Lenney C, Lenney W. Seasonal variation and time trends in childhood asthma in England and Wales 1975–1981. *BMJ* 1984; **289**: 235–7

11 Storr J. Lenney W. School holidays and admission with asthma. *Arch Dis Child* 1989; **64**: 103–7

12 Johnston SL, Pattemore PK, Sanderson G *et al*. Community study of the role of viral infections in exacerbations of asthma in 9–11 year old children. *BMJ* 1995; **310**: 1225–9

13 Newson R, Strachan D, Archibald E, Emberlin J, Hardaker P, Collier C. Acute asthma epidemics and their predictors in England, 1987–94. *Eur Respir J* 1998; **11**: 694–701

14 Venables KM, Allitt U, Collier CG *et al*. Thunderstorm-related asthma – the epidemic of 24/25 June 1994. *Clin Exp Allergy* 1997; **27**: 725–36

15 Anderson HR, Atkinson R, Limb ES, Strachan DP. Epidemic of asthma was not associated with episode of air pollution. *BMJ* 1996; **312**: 1606–7

16 Bellomo R, Gigliotti P, Treloar A *et al*. Two consecutive thunderstorm associated epidemics of asthma in the city of Melbourne. The possible role of rye grass pollen. *Med J Aust* 1992; **156**: 834–7

17 Knox RB. Grass pollen, thunderstorms and asthma. *Clin Exp Allergy* 1993; **23**: 354–9

18 Packe GE, Ayres JG. Asthma outbreak during a thunderstorm. *Lancet* 1985; **ii**: 199–204

19 Newson R, Strachan D, Archibald E, Emberlin J, Hardaker P, Collier C. The effect of thunderstorms and airborne grass pollen on acute asthma incidence in England, 1990–94. *Thorax* 1997; **52**: 680–5

20 Suphioglu C, Singh MB, Taylor P *et al*. Mechanism of grass-pollen-induced asthma. *Lancet* 1992; **339**: 569–72

21 Anto JM, Sunyer J, Asthma Collaborative Group of Barcelona. A point source asthma outbreak. *Lancet* 1986; **i**: 900–3

22 Anto JM, Sunyer J, Rodriguez-Roisin R, Suarez-Cervera M, Vazquez L. Community outbreaks of asthma associated with inhalation of soybean dust. *N Engl J Med* 1989; **320**: 1097–102

23 Sunyer J, Anto JM, Rodrigo MJ, Morell F. Case-control study of serum immunoglobulin-E antibodies reactive with soybean in epidemic asthma. *Lancet* 1989; **i**: 179–82

24 Carroll RE. Environmental epidemiology. V. Epidemiology of New Orleans epidemic asthma. *Am J Public Health* 1968; **58**: 1677–83

25 Salvaggio J, Kawai T, Seabury J. New Orleans epidemic asthma: semiquantitative aerometric sampling, epidemiologic and immunologic studies. *Chest* 1973; **63** (Suppl): 14S–5S

26 Harries MG, Lacey J, Tee RD, Cayley GR, Newman-Taylor AJ. *Didymella exitialis* and late summer asthma. *Lancet* 1985; **i**: 1063–6

27 Department of Health Committee on the Medical Effects of Air Pollutants. *Asthma and Outdoor Air Pollution*. Chapter 8. Air pollution and the timing of asthma attacks: population studies. London: HMSO, 1995; 131–52

28 Anderson HR, Ponce de Leon A, Bland JM, Bower JS, Emberlin J, Strachan DP. Air pollution, pollens and daily admissions for asthma in London. *Thorax* 1998; **53**: 842–8

29 Bates DV, Sizto R. Air pollution and hospital admissions in Southern Ontario: the acid summer haze effect. *Environ Res* 1987; **43**: 317–31

30 Cody RP, Weisel CP, Birnbaum G, Lioy PJ. The effect of ozone associated with summertime photochemical smog on the frequency of asthma visits to hospital emergency departments. *Environ Res* 1992; **58**: 184–94

31 Thurston GD, Ito K, Kinney PL, Lippmann M. A multi-year study of air pollution and respiratory hospital admissions in three New York State metropolitan areas: results for 1988 and 1989 summers. *J Exp Anal Environ Epidemiol* 1992; **2**: 429–50

32 Delfino RJ, Becklake MR, Hanley JA. The relationship of urgent hospital admissions for respiratory illnesses to photochemical air pollution levels in Montreal. *Environ Res* 1994; **67**: 1–19

33 Bates DV, Sizto R. The Ontario air pollution study: identification of the causal agent. *Environ Health Perspect* 1989; **79**: 69–72

34 Bates DV, Baker-Anderson M, Sizto R. Asthma attack periodicity: a study of hospital emergency visits in Vancouver. *Environ Res* 1990; **51**: 51–70

35 Schwartz J, Slater D, Larson TV, Pierson WE, Koenig JQ. Particulate air pollution and hospital emergency room visits for asthma in Seattle. *Am Rev Respir Dis* 1993; **147**: 826–31

36 Richards W, Azen SP, Weiss J, Stocking S, Church J. Los Angeles air pollution and asthma in children. *Ann Allergy* 1981; **47**: 348–54

37 Dockery DW, Pope CA. Acute respiratory effects of particulate pollution. *Annu Rev Public Health* 1994; **15**: 107–32

38 Anderson HR, Limb ES, Bland JM, Ponce de Leon A, Strachan DP, Bower JS. The health effects of an air pollution episode in London, December 1991. *Thorax* 1995; **50**: 1188–93

39 Pope CA. Respiratory disease associated with community air pollution and a steel mill, Utah Valley. *Am J Public Health* 1989; **79**: 623–8

40 Pope CA. Respiratory hospital admissions associated with PM_{10} pollution in Utah, Salt Lake and Cache Valleys. *Arch Environ Health* 1991; **46**: 90–7

41 Rossi OVJ, Kinnula VL, Tienari J *et al.* Association of severe asthma attacks with weather, pollen and air pollutants. *Thorax* 1993; **48**: 244–8

42 Hendrick DJ, Davies RJ, D'Souza MF, Pepys J. An analysis of skin prick reactions in 656 asthmatic patients. *Thorax* 1975; **30**: 2–8

43 O'Halloren MT, Yuninger JW, Offord KP *et al.* Exposure to an aeroallergen as a possible precipitating factor in respiratory arrest in young patients with asthma. *N Engl J Med* 1991; **325**: 206–8

44 Targonski PV, Persky VW, Ramekrishnan V. Effect of environmental moulds on risk of death from asthma during the pollen season. *J Allergy Clin Immunol* 1995; **95**: 955–61

45 Malling HJ. Diagnosis and immunotherapy of mould allergy. IV: Relation between asthma symptoms, spore counts and diagnostic tests. *Allergy* 1986; **41**: 342–50

46 Beaumont F, Kauffman HF, Sluiter HJ, de Vries K. Sequential sampling of fungal air spores inside and outside the homes of mould-sensitive asthmatic patients: a search for a relationship to obstructive reactions. *Ann Allergy* 1985; **55**: 740–6

47 Epton MJ, Martin IR, Graham P *et al.* Climate and aeroallergen levels in asthma: a 12 month prospective study. *Thorax* 1997; **52**: 528–34

48 Delfino RJ, Zeiger RS, Seltzer JM *et al.* The effect of outdoor fungal spore concentrations on daily asthma severity. *Environ Health Perspect* 1997; **105**: 622–35

49 Delfino RJ. Daily asthma severity in relation to personal ozone exposure and outdoor fungal spores. *Am J Respir Crit Care Med* 1996; **154**: 633–41

50 Molfino NA, Wright SC, Katz I *et al.* Effect of low concentrations of ozone on inhaled allergen responses in asthmatic subjects. *Lancet* 1991; **338**: 199–203

51 Jörres R, Nowak D, Magnussen H. The effect of ozone exposure on allergen responsiveness in subjects with asthma or rhinitis. *Am J Respir Crit Care Med* 1996; **153**: 56–64

52 Tunnicliffe WS, Burge PS, Ayres JG. Effect of domestic concentrations of nitrogen dioxide on airway responses to inhaled allergen in asthmatic patients. *Lancet* 1994; **44**: 1733–6

53 Devalia JL, Rusnak C, Herdman MJ *et al.* Effect of nitrogen dioxide and sulphur dioxide on airway response of mild asthmatic patients to allergen inhalation. *Lancet* 1994; **344**: 1668–71

54 Department of Health Committee on the Medical Effects of Air Pollutants. *Asthma and Outdoor Air Pollution*, Chapter 9. Air pollution and the prevalence of asthma: population studies. London: HMSO, 1995; 153–76

55 Colley JRT, Brasser LJ. *Chronic respiratory disease in children in relation to air pollution: report on a WHO study*. Copenhagen: WHO, 1980

56 Zemp E, Elsasser S, Schindler C *et al.* Long-term ambient air pollution and respiratory symptoms in adults (SAPALDIA study). *Am J Respir Crit Care Med* 1999; **159**: 1257–66

57 Abbey DE, Petersen F, Mills PK, Beeson WL. Long-term ambient concentrations of total suspended particulates, ozone and sulfur dioxide and respiratory symptoms in a non-smoking population. *Arch Environ Health* 1993; **48**: 33–47

58 Magnussen H, Jörres R, Nowak D. Effect of air pollution on the prevalence of asthma and allergy: lessons from the German reunification. *Thorax* 1993; **48**: 879–81

59 von Mutius E, Martinez FD, Fritzsch C, Nicolai T, Roell G, Thiemann HH. Prevalence of asthma and atopy in two areas of West and East Germany. *Am J Respir Crit Care Med* 1994; **149**: 358–64

60 Nowak D, Heinrich J, Jörres R *et al.* Prevalence of respiratory symptoms, bronchial hyper-responsiveness and atopy among adults: West and East Germany. *Eur Respir J* 1996; **9**: 2541–52

61 von Mutius E, Fritsch C, Weiland SK, Röll G, Magnussen H. Prevalence of asthma and allergic disorders among children in the united Germany: a descriptive comparison. *BMJ* 1992; **305**: 1395–9

62 Wjst M, Reitmar P, Dold S *et al.* Road traffic and adverse effects on respiratory health in children. *BMJ* 1993; **307**: 596–600

63 Weiland SK, Mundt KA, Rückmann A, Keil U. Self-reported wheezing and allergic rhinitis in children and traffic density on street of residence. *Ann Epidemiol* 1994; **4**: 79–83

64 Oosterlee A, Drijver M, Lebret E, Brunekreef B. Chronic respiratory symptoms in children and adults living along streets with high traffic density. *Occup Environ Med* 1996; **53**: 241–7

65 van Vliet P, Knape M, de Hartog J, Janssen N, Harssema H, Brunekreef B. Motor vehicle exhaust and chronic respiratory symptoms in children living near freeways. *Environ Res* 1997; **74**: 122–32

66 Livingstone AE, Shaddick G, Grundy C, Elliott P. Do people living near inner city main roads have more asthma requiring treatment? A case control study using routine general practice data. *BMJ* 1996; **312**: 676–7

67 Wilkinson P, Elliott P, Grundy C *et al.* Case-control study of hospital admission with asthma in children aged 5-14 years: relation with road traffic in north west London. *Thorax* 1999; **54**: 1070–4

68 Edwards J, Walters S, Griffiths RK. Hospital admissions for asthma in preschool children: relationship to major roads in Birmingham, United Kingdom. *Arch Environ Health* 1994; **49**: 223–7

69 Pershagen G, Rylander E, Norberg S, Eriksson M, Nordvall SL. Air pollution involving nitrogen dioxide exposure and wheezing bronchitis in children. *Int J Epidemiol* 1995; **24**: 1147–53

70 Strachan DP. Traffic exposure and asthma: problems of interpretation. *BMJ* 1996; **312**: 677

71 Nitta H, Sato T, Nakai S, Maeda K, Aoko S, Ono M. Respiratory health associated with exposure to automobile exhaust. I. Results of cross-sectional studies in 1979, 1982 and 1983. *Arch Environ Health* 1993; **48**: 53–8

72 Ono M, Hirano S, Murakami M, Nitta H, Nakai S, Maeda K. Measurements of particle and NO_2 concentrations in homes along the major arterial roads in Tokyo. *J Jpn Soc Air Pollut* 1989; **24**: 90–9

73 Fuhlbrigge A, Weiss S. Domestic gas appliances and lung disease. *Thorax* 1997; **52** (Suppl 3): S58–62

74 Hassleblad V, Eddy DM, Kotchmar DJ. Synthesis of environmental evidence: nitrogen dioxide epidemiology studies. *J Air Waste Management Assoc* 1992; **42**: 662–71

75 Dekker C, Dales R, Bartlett S, Brunekreef B, Zwanenburg H. Childhood asthma and the indoor environment. *Chest* 1991; **100**: 922–6

76 Jarvis D, Chinn S, Luczynska C, Burney P. Association of respiratory symptoms and lung function in young adults with use of domestic gas appliances. *Lancet* 1996; **347**: 426–31

77 Burr ML, Anderson HR, Austin JB, Harkins L, Kaur B, Strachan DP, Warner JO. Respiratory symptoms and the home environment in children: a national survey. *Thorax* 1999; **54**: 27–32

78 Moran SE, Strachan DP, Johnston IDA, Anderson HR. Effects of exposure to gas cooking in childhood and adulthood on respiratory symptoms, allergic sensitization and lung function in young adults. *Clin Exp Allergy* 1999; **29**: 1033–41

79 Dow L, Phelps L, Fowler L, Waters K, Cogoon D, Holgate ST. Respiratory symptoms in older people and use of domestic gas appliances. *Thorax* 1999; **54**: 1104–6

80 Jarvis D, Chinn S, Sterne J, Luczynska C, Burney P, on behalf of the European Community Respiratory Health Survey. The association of respiratory symptoms and lung function with the use of gas for cooking. *Eur Respir J* 1998; **11**: 651–8

81 Jarvis D. Gas cooking and respiratory disease. *Thorax* 1999; **54**: 1054

82 Coultas DB. Passive smoking and risk of adult asthma and COPD: an update. *Thorax* 1998; **53**: 381–7

83 Strachan DP, Cook DG. Parental smoking and lower respiratory illness in infancy and early childhood. *Thorax* 1997; **52**: 905–14

84 Cook DG, Strachan DP. Parental smoking and prevalence of respiratory symptoms and asthma in school age children. *Thorax* 1997; **52**: 1081–94

85 Strachan DP, Cook DG. Parental smoking and allergic sensitisation in children. *Thorax* 1998; **53**: 117–23

86 Strachan DP, Cook DG. Parental smoking and childhood asthma: longitudinal and case-control studies. *Thorax* 1998; **53**: 204–12

87 Cook DG, Strachan DP. Summary of effects of parental smoking on the respiratory health of children and implications for research. *Thorax* 1999; **54**: 357–66

88 Sakula A. Sir John Floyer's *A Treatise of the Asthma* (1698). *Thorax* 1984; **39**: 248–54

89 Strachan DP. Damp housing and childhood asthma: validation of reporting of symptoms. *BMJ* 1988; **297**: 1223–6

90 Dales RE, Zwanenburg H, Burnett R, Frankin CA. Respiratory effects of home dampness and moulds among Canadian children. *Am J Epidemiol* 1991; **134**: 196–203

91 Dales RE, Burnett R, Zwanenburg H. Adverse health effects among adults exposed to home dampness and molds. *Am Rev Respir Dis* 1991; **143**: 505–9

92 Brunekreef B. Associations between questionnaire reports of home dampness and childhood respiratory symptoms. *Sci Total Environ* 1992; **127**: 79–89

93 Brunekreef B. Damp housing and adult respiratory symptoms. *Allergy* 1992; **47**: 498–502

94 Jaakkola JJK, Jaakkola N, Ruotsalainen R. Home dampness and molds as determinants of respiratory symptoms and asthma in pre-school children. *J Exp Anal Environ Epidemiol* 1993; **3**: 129–42

95 Platt S, Martin C, Hunt S, Lewis C. Damp housing, mould growth and symptomatic health state. *BMJ* 1997; **298**: 1673–8

96 Waegemaekers M, van Wageningen N, Brunekreef B, Boleij JSM. Respiratory symptoms in damp homes. *Allergy* 1989; **44**: 192–8

97 Strachan DP, Flannigan B, McCabe EM, McGarry F. Quantification of airborne moulds in the homes of children with and without wheeze. *Thorax* 1990; **45**: 382–7

98 Verhoeff AP, van Wijnen JH, van Reene-Hoekstra ES *et al.* Fungal propagules in house dust, II: relation with residential characteristics and respiratory symptoms. *Allergy* 1994; **49**: 540–7

99 Strachan DP. Damp housing, mould allergy and childhood asthma. *Proc R Coll Physicians Edinb* 1991; **21**: 140–6

100 Williamson IJ, Martin CJ, McGill G, Monie RDH, Fennerty AG. Damp housing and asthma: a case-control study. *Thorax* 1997; **52**: 229–34

101 Rosenstreich DL, Eggleston P, Kattan M *et al.* The role of cockroach allergy and exposure to cockroach allergen in causing morbidity among inner-city children with asthma. *N Engl J Med* 1997; **337**: 1356–63

102 Platts-Mills TAE, de Weck AL. Dust mite allergens and asthma - a worldwide problem. *J Allergy Clin Immunol* 1989; **83**: 416–27

103 Platts-Mills TAE, Thomas W, Aalberse RC, Vervloet D, Chapman MD. Dust mite allergens and asthma: report of a second international workshop. *J Allergy Clin Immunol* 1992; **89**: 1046–60

104 Platts Mills TAE, Vervloet D, Thomas WR, Aalberse RC, Chapman MD. Indoor allergens and asthma: report of the third international workshop. *J Allergy Clin Immunol* 1997; **100** (6 pt 1): S2–24

105 Custovic A, Smith A, Woodcock A. Indoor allergens are a primary cause of asthma. *Eur Respir Rev* 1998; **53**: 155–8

106 Pearce N, Douwes J, Beasley R. Is allergen exposure the major primary cause of asthma? *Thorax* 2000; **55**: 424–31

107 Peat JK, Tovey E, Toelle BG *et al.* House dust mite allergens. A major risk factor for childhood asthma in Australia. *Am J Respir Crit Care Med* 1996; **153**: 141–6

108 The International Study of Asthma and Allergies in Childhood (ISAAC) Steering Committee. Worldwide variations in prevalence of asthma symptoms: the International Study of Asthma and Allergies in Childhood (ISAAC). *Eur Respir J* 1998; **12**: 315–35

109 European Community Respiratory Health Survey (ECRHS). Variations in the prevalence of respiratory symptoms, self-reported asthma attacks, and use of asthma medication in the European Community Respiratory Health Survey (ECRHS). *Eur Respir J* 1996; **9**: 695-7

110 Sporik R, Holgate ST, Platts-mills TAE, Cogswell JJ. Exposure to house-dust mite allergen (*Der pI*) and the development of asthma in childhood. *N Engl J Med* 1990; **323**: 502–7

111 Burr ML, Limb ES, Maguire MJ *et al.* Infant feeding, wheezing and allergy: a prospective study. *Arch Dis Child* 1993; **68**: 724–8

112 Custovic A, Simpson A, Chapman MD, Woodcock A. Allergen avoidance in the treatment of asthma and atopic disorders. *Thorax* 1998; **53**: 63–72

113 Goetzche PC Hammarqvist C, Burr M. House dust mite control measures in the management of asthma: meta-analysis. *BMJ* 1998; **317**: 1105–10

114 Strachan DP. House dust mite allergen avoidance in asthma. *BMJ* 1998; **317**: 1096–7

115 Custovic A, Smith A, Pahdi H, Green RM, Chapman MD, Woodcock A. Distribution, aerodynamic characteristics and removal of the major cat allergen *Fel d1* in British homes. *Thorax* 1998; **53**: 33–8

116 Brunekreef B, Groot B, Hoek G. Pets, allergy and respiratory symptoms in children. *Int J Epidemiol* 1992; **21**: 338–42

117 Svanes C, Jarvis D, Chinn S *et al.* Childhood environment and adult atopy: results from the European Community Respiratory Health Survey. *J Allergy Clin Immunol* 1999; **103**: 415–20

118 Strachan DP, Carey IM. The home environment and severe asthma in adolescence: a population based case-control study. *BMJ* 1995; **311**: 1053–6

119 Hesslemar B, Åberg N, Åberg B *et al.* Does early exposure to cat or dog protect against later allergy development? *Clin Exp Allergy* 1999; **29**: 611–7

120 Lewis S. Animals and allergy. *Clin Exp Allergy* 2000; **30**: 153–7

121 Strachan DP. Family size, infection and atopy: the first decade of the 'hygiene hypothesis'. *Thorax* 2000: **55**(Suppl 1): S2–S10

122 Noertjojo K, Dimich-Ward H, Obata H, Manfreda J, Chan-Yeung M. Exposure and sensitization to cat dander: asthma and asthma-like symptoms among adults. *J Allergy Clin Immunol* 1999; **103**: 60–5

123 Kemp TJ, Siebers RW, Fishwick D, O'Grady GB, Fitzharris P, Crane J. House dust mite allergen in pillows. *BMJ* 1996; **313**: 916

124 Rains N, Siebers RW, Crane J, Fitzharris P. House dust mite allergen (*Der pI*) accumulation on new synthetic and feather pillows. *Clin Exp Allergy* 1999; **29**: 182–5

125 Hallam C, Custovic A, Simpson B, Houghton N, Woodcock A. House dust mite allergen in feather and synthetic pillows. *Allergy* 1999; **54**: 407–8

126 Butland BK, Strachan DP, Anderson HR. The home environment and asthma symptoms in childhood: two population based case-control studies 13 years apart. *Thorax* 1997; **52**: 618–24

127 Strachan DP, Carey IM. Reduced risk of wheezing in children using feather pillows is confirmed. *BMJ* 1997; **314**: 518

128 Björkstén B. The intrauterine and postnatal environments. *J Allergy Clin Immunol* 1999; **104**: 1119–27

129 Martinez FD, Holt PG. Role of microbial burden in the aetiology of allergy and asthma. *Lancet* 1999; **354** (Suppl II): 12–5

130 Gregg I. Epidemiological research in asthma: the need for a broad perspective. *Clin Allergy* 1986; **16**: 17–23

Early life events in allergic sensitisation

Jill A Warner and **John O Warner**

Allergy and Inflammation Sciences Division (Child Health) University of Southampton, Southampton, UK

The timing of events leading to allergic sensitisation has become a very important area in the attempt to halt the dramatic increase in the prevalence of diseases such as asthma, eczema and hay fever. Recent research has demonstrated that events taking place during the gestational period may well play a role in determining whether or not a genetic susceptibility becomes translated into disease processes. Maternal atopy seems to have an important effect on the developing immune response of the infant and increases the chances of the child developing allergy in later life. Maternal IgE, IgG and amniotic fluid cytokines, combined with the presence of allergen in the feto–maternal environment are all possible factors involved in the ultimate outcome in terms of infant Th-1/Th-2 responses to common environmental antigens. Immune modulation at this stage of development may, in the future, be a way forward in the prevention of allergy.

The dramatic increase in the incidence of allergic disease has highlighted the need for effective preventative strategies. However, before these can be put in place it is necessary to define the time course of events that lead to allergic sensitisation and identify predictive markers that can distinguish susceptible individuals.

Up until relatively recently, it was considered that the neonate was immunologically naïve and the development of specific immune responses was restricted to the period after birth. However, it is now recognised that infants are born with the capacity to mount an immune response, that can only have developed *in utero*, to common environmental antigens. A number of studies have shown that peripheral blood mononuclear cell sensitivity to allergens exists at birth[1–3] and, by studying the peripheral blood mononuclear cell responses from fetuses through gestation, it has been possible to establish that specific allergen induced responses can occur from as early as 22 weeks' gestation[4]. That these responses are modified by events after birth is not in question, and allergens[5], infections[6], diet[7], and microbial gut flora[8] have all been implicated in the development, or not, of subsequent allergy. However, the mechanisms put in place during gestation may well be the starting point for eventual disease.

Correspondence to:
Dr Jill A Warner,
Allergy and Inflammation
Sciences Division (Child
Health), Level G, Centre
Block, Southampton
General Hospital,
Tremona Road,
Southampton
SO16 6YD, UK

When preventative strategies are considered there are three levels at which they can be implemented: primary (before sensitisation); secondary (after sensitisation, but before disease); and tertiary (treatment of disease). Those most likely to be effective in the short-term are those which can be applied at more than one level, but it must be remembered that the factors which have caused the increase in allergic disease may not, necessarily be the triggers for symptoms in already sensitised individuals.

The gestational period

It is surprising that fetal sensitisation has been ignored for so long. Stem cells are present in the human yoke sac at 21 days of gestation with a first lymphocyte seen in the thymus at the end of the 9th week of gestation. B lymphocytes can be seen in a range of organs including the lungs and gut from 14 weeks and by 19–20 weeks, circulating B cells have detectable surface IgM[9]. This implies that the full sensitisation process must have occurred from antigen presentation through T-cell proliferation to B-cell stimulation and antibody production.

However, there remains a belief that the neonate is immunologically naïve[10]. Evidence would now suggest that this is not true immunological naiveté due to lack of sensitisation, but more to a late gestation suppression of immune responses. Indeed, one study has been able to demonstrate that birch and timothy grass pollen exposure via the mother only sensitises fetuses if it takes place in the first 6 months of pregnancy. Exposure in later pregnancy appears to result in either immune suppression or tolerance[11].

It has been shown by several groups that responses set up during pregnancy can be predictive of subsequent allergic disease[1,12,13]. During one of those studies, the workers were able to show that under certain laboratory conditions over 70% of babies were able to demonstrate proliferative responses to the major house dust mite allergen[12].

So, while there is wide-spread priming to environmental antigens occurring before birth, in those infants destined to be allergic and develop diseases such as asthma, the responsiveness is altered. A small percentage of infants destined to have allergic disease already have raised cord blood total and specific IgE. This has proved to be a highly specific but very insensitive marker of later disease[14-18]. Other studies have demonstrated differences in cytokine profiles from allergen and mitogen stimulated peripheral blood mononuclear cells in neonates who subsequently become allergic[1,13-19]. All of these studies suggest that there is a disturbance of the balance between cytokines that suppress an allergic response as characterised by T helper 1 (Th-1) phenotypic responses compared with allergy promoting Th-2 responses. In the former, the characteristic cytokines are interleukin-12 (IL-12) and interferon-gamma (IFN-γ), and in the latter IL-4, IL-5, IL-10 and IL-13.

Materno–fetal interactions during pregnancy

There appears to be a powerful maternal and placental influence on the developing fetal immune response. Animal models have shown that during pregnancy the maternal immune response becomes heavily biased towards Th-2 phenotype, with increasing IL-4 and IL-10 during gestation being detected in the murine system[20]. IL-4 has been shown to be produced in the human amnion epithelium in both the first and third trimesters of pregnancy[21]. IL-13 has been shown to be produced by the placenta during the second trimester of pregnancy[22], and the concentration of IL-10 is higher in the amniotic fluid of atopic women than non-atopic women in the second trimester[23].

Clinically, a picture of reduced cell mediated immunity has been described in pregnancy[24]. The benefit of this loss of cell mediated immunity may be reduction in NK cell activity. These cells have been shown to have a role in spontaneous abortion and may attack the trophoblast[25]. Additionally, IFN-γ is an abortifactant, whose effect may be mediated through the activation of NK cells by this cytokine[26]. Clearly Th-1 type cell mediated immune responses are undesirable for maintenance of pregnancy.

The concentration of IFN-γ is highest in fetal plasma in the first trimester of pregnancy[27]; however, PBMCs from most fetuses spontaneously release IFN-γ during the 2nd and 3rd trimesters of pregnancy, but there are some which do not release this Th-1 cytokine even when stimulated with PHA.

The role of non-specific fetal PBMC IFN-γ production may be to counteract the effects of the Th-2 environment produced by the placenta and/or mother. A mechanism such as this would be essential to prevent an allergic (Th-2) phenotype in all newborns. Failure of this mechanism may underlie the development of atopy.

Fetal allergen exposure

The cytokines generated by decidual tissues are present in significant quantities in amniotic fluid[28]. Furthermore, we have also found significant levels of IgE proportionate to maternal IgE levels in amniotic fluid. Thus, those mothers with higher levels who are themselves atopic, expose their fetuses to higher quantities of IgE through the amniotic fluid even though this IgE does not cross the placenta into the fetal circulation[29]. Very recently, we have detected the allergens *Der p 1* of house dust mite and ovalbumin from hen's egg in some amniotic fluids. The protein turnover in amniotic fluid occurs at a rate of 70% each day with much of this removal being via fetal swallowing[30]. The fetus also aspirates amniotic fluid into the respiratory tract and, in addition, has a highly permeable skin through which direct exposure might occur. The fetal gut has been established as containing the most mature immune active tissues during gestation. We have found many HLA-DR positive cells including macrophages, B-cells and dendritic cells in lymphoid follicles of the rudimentary Peyer's patches from fetuses very early in the second trimester of pregnancy. Surface markers on these cells suggest that they have all the necessary co-stimulatory signals available to facilitate antigen presentation to T lymphocytes, which can also be detected from as early as 16 weeks' gestation. The antigen presenting cells also have high and low affinity IgE as well as IgG receptors. Therefore, there is the potential not only for sensitisation to occur but also for IgE to facilitate this process to occur by so-called antigen focusing which allows sensitisation to remarkably low concentrations of allergen[31].

The role of maternal IgG

A number of studies have suggested that IgG may have a role in modulating the fetal immune response to allergen. We have shown that proliferative responses to house dust mite by cord blood peripheral mononuclear cells is inversely correlated with the level of cord blood house dust mite specific IgG[23]. High levels of cord blood IgG antibodies to cat dander and the major allergen of birch pollen were associated with less atopic symptoms in children during the first 8 years of life. There was an inverse relationship between cat IgE antibodies in children and their levels of IgG cat antibodies at birth[32]. The levels of IgG in the cord blood clearly are a reflection of maternal IgG, which in turn is likely to reflect maternal allergen exposure. Thus high exposure will increase the IgG levels. Children of mothers who have undergone rye grass immunotherapy during pregnancy and consequently have high IgG antibody levels, compared with children born to untreated mothers, have been followed postnatally and had fewer positive skin tests to the grass 3–12 years later[33]. This would also be consistent with the observation that birch pollen exposure during the last 2–3 months of pregnancy, when IgG transfer across the placenta is maximal, is associated with much less birch pollen reactivity of the offspring than occurs if the exposure was between 3 and 6 months' gestation[11]. Several studies have shown an increased risk for allergy to seasonal allergens in children born shortly before the relevant pollen season. Birth at this time of year would be associated with the lowest maternal and thus, fetal, levels of IgG antibody[32].

Maternal diet during pregnancy

There has been some discussion about the possible role of the declining consumption of fresh fruit and vegetables, particularly in the UK, in the increase in allergic disease[34]. The hypothesis is that such foods are associated with antioxidant activity and could, therefore, prevent the development of inflammation, particularly the IL-4 dependent IgE production by B-cells. On the basis of the above discussions this could have a role during pregnancy, but as yet, there is no supporting evidence for the genesis of disease, only for the severity of disease once it is established[35].

The other nutrients which have been shown to have some influence on established asthma, namely fatty acids, may also have an effect in the genesis of disease. There has been an increased consumption of poly-unsaturated fatty acids (PUFA) in recent decades. Diets rich in linolenic acid promote prostaglandin E_2 production that, in turn, promotes IL-4 production[35]. It is well-established that fish oil supplementation produces a decrease in production of pro-inflammatory mediators such as tumour necrosis factor–α and leukotrienes[36]. The effects on clinical features of the condition are modest or non-existent[37]. Under such circumstances, one might consider that fatty acid dietary supplementation would have a greater impact if introduced at an early stage in the evolution of the disease.

Events after birth

The areas currently most discussed in relation to the influences on the developing immune response in early life are: (i) the hygiene hypothesis; (ii) gut microbial flora; and (iii) allergen exposure. It seems likely that they may all have a role to play in determining whether the events set up during pregnancy result in the development of allergic disease and they will be considered in turn.

The hygiene hypothesis

In 1989, Strachan demonstrated an inverse relationship between birth order in families and the prevalence of hay fever. He proposed that infections in early infancy brought home by older siblings might prevent sensitisation[38]. There is clearly a highly credible biological explanation to support this hypothesis. Early infection, whether with viruses or bacteria, will tend to stimulate a Th-1 immune response, which, if early enough postnatally, will switch any Th-2 biased allergic immune responses to common allergens to a Th-1 immunising pattern[39]. These observations have promoted research into the development of Th-1 immuno-adjuvants as a treatment for allergic disease. BCG and heat killed *Listeria monocytogenes* are currently the main focuses of work, though in the longer term DNA vaccines may prove to be more effective[40]. It must, however, be noted that there are some anomalies to this theory, in that some infections, for example respiratory syncytial virus, are actually associated with more, rather than less, allergy[41], and immunisation with altered organisms does not have the same effect as active infection[42,43]. There are clearly still issues to be addressed in this area.

Gut microbial flora

It has been reported that allergic children are more likely to have a low colonisation of *Lactobacilli* in their gut than non-allergic children. Also, children in Estonia, where the prevalence of allergies is low, have a very different gut flora to those in Sweden where the prevalence of allergy is higher[44]. Allergic children tended to have higher counts of aerobic micro-organisms such as coliforms and *Staphylococcus aureus*. A number of groups have questioned whether this might explain the remarkable observation that there is a much lower risk of asthma amongst children of farmers who have been born on farms. Ingestion of higher quantities of raw and sometimes unpasteurised milk containing a higher microbial load, particularly of *Lactobacilli*, may well have been protective[45,46]. This observation may, however, also be explained by a greater exposure to infecting organisms and particularly their products such as lipopolysaccharide (LPS) which would be consistent with the earlier hygiene hypothesis[47]. LPS-induced immune responses are primarily mediated via the receptor CD14. It is likely that the early switch from Th-2 to Th-1 biased response postnatally is a consequence of postnatal microbial exposure as described above. Those infants with an intact response to microbial antigens such as LPS will have a very rapid switch orchestrated through the CD14 molecule once the gut becomes colonised with organisms. Those infants with abnormalities in this response and those who have already had significant over-commitment to a Th-2 response as a result of antenatal factors, will not be so easily switched and have a higher probability of having a persistent response going on to atopic disease.

Allergen exposure

There is a good correlation between early high level exposure to house dust mite and the subsequent increase in prevalence and severity of asthma[5]. Similar associations have been found in relation to cockroach exposure[48]. Indeed, high level exposure to a number of indoor allergens is strongly associated with sensitisation in the first 3 years[49] and early sensitisation is associated with greater probability of persistence of bronchial hyper-responsiveness and symptoms of asthma in late childhood and adolescence[50].

The main difficulty in employing allergen avoidance strategies is that techniques to reduce exposure to the commonest allergen, the house dust mite, are far from satisfactory. Indeed, a recent heavily criticised meta-analysis of trials suggested that it was not likely to be effective[51]. The studies that have attempted allergen avoidance in high risk infants with or without pre-existing evidence of sensitisation but not yet disease have yielded very disappointing outcomes. Some interventions have even commenced antenatally. The attitude to antenatal dietary avoidance has been formed on the basis of one study where elimination of egg, milk, fish and nuts from the maternal diet in the last trimester of pregnancy had no impact on outcome in relation to disease. Furthermore, the mothers gained less weight during pregnancy as a consequence of the diet[52]. However, one might argue that the intervention was started too late, as we now have evidence that sensitisation might have occurred at an earlier stage in the pregnancy. Nevertheless, it also sounds a note of warning about potential adverse nutritional consequences of antenatal dietary manipulation.

Postnatal avoidance has again tended to focus on diet with promotion of breast feeding. Many studies have been performed with very diverse results extending from reduced prevalence of food associated atopic disease, through no effect, to some studies showing a higher prevalence of atopy in intervention groups. Importantly, however, only one of many studies has demonstrated any long-term effects of early dietary manipulation on the prevalence of asthma[53]. Most studies, if they have demonstrated any benefits at all, have been to reduce period prevalence of food associated atopic disease in infancy but with no long-term impact on any atopic problems and certainly not on asthma[54,55]. The latter study also employed house dust mite avoidance measures. However, the degree of reduction in house dust mite levels was probably not enough to achieve any meaningful benefits. A number of trials are now in progress to attempt to reduce aero-allergen exposure to a far greater extent from early in pregnancy and it remains to be seen whether these strategies will be truly effective in reducing prevalence of disease.

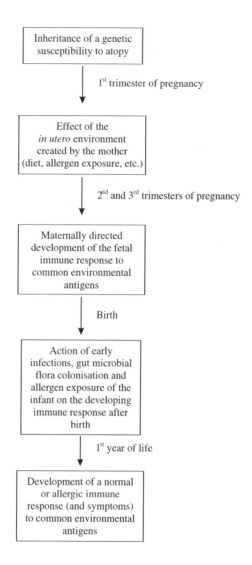

Fig. 1 The influences on the developing immune response of an infant during pregnancy and the first year of life which dictate whether a normal or allergic response to common environmental antigens is established.

The flow chart contains the following boxes connected by downward arrows:

Inheritance of a genetic susceptibility to atopy

→ 1st trimester of pregnancy

Effect of the *in utero* environment created by the mother (diet, allergen exposure, etc.)

→ 2nd and 3rd trimesters of pregnancy

Maternally directed development of the fetal immune response to common environmental antigens

→ Birth

Action of early infections, gut microbial flora colonisation and allergen exposure of the infant on the developing immune response after birth

→ 1st year of life

Development of a normal or allergic immune response (and symptoms) to common environmental antigens

Conclusions

It has become clear that factors acting during the gestational period play a role in directing the developing immune response of a fetus. There is an interaction between inherited genetic characteristics of both mother and father and the *in utero* environment created by the mother. The presence of maternal IgG and IgE antibodies may influence the type of response elicited in the fetus to antigens present in the amniotic fluid and in the maternal plasma. There is a complex inter-relationship between maternal, placental and fetal cytokine production which normally works to prevent rejection of the fetus, but which can, if unbalanced, result in a persistent Th-2 type response in the newborn infant, instead of the transient Th-2 response to antigens seen in all infants at birth. Modulation of these interactions may be a future means to preventing the primary sensitisation leading to subsequent allergic reactions. The responses set up during pregnancy are acted upon by external factors after birth, which are likely to determine whether disease develops. These factors include infection, diet and allergen exposure and manipulation of these may be a means whereby a susceptible infant can be prevented from going on to manifest allergic symptoms. Figure 1 demonstrates the time course of events, which may dictate whether normal or allergic responses to common antigens are established.

Acknowledgements

We would like to thank Dr Catherine Jones, Dr Judith Holloway and Dr Gillian Vance for their roles in producing some of the findings ascribed to our own laboratory and described in this chapter.

References

1 Warner JA, Miles EA, Jones AC et al. Is deficiency of interferon-gamma production by allergen triggered cord blood cells a predictor of atopic eczema? Clin Exp Allergy 1994; 24: 423–30

2 Prescott SL, Macaubas C, Holt BJ et al. Transplacental priming of the human immune system to environmental allergens: Universal skewing of initial T cell responses towards the Th-2 cytokine profile. J Immunol 1998; 160: 4730–7

3 Kondo N, Cubiyashi Y, Shinoda S et al. Cord blood lymphocyte responses to food antigens for the prediction of allergic disease. Arch Dis Child 1992; 67: 1003–7

4 Jones AC, Miles EA, Warner JO et al. Fetal peripheral blood mononuclear cell proliferative responses to mitogenic and allergenic stimuli during gestation. Pediatr Allergy Immunol 1996; 7: 109–16

5 Sporik R, Holgate ST, Platt-Mills TAE et al. Exposure to house dust mite allergen (Der p 1) and the development of asthma in childhood. N Engl J Med 1990; 323: 502–7

6 Strachan DP. Hay fever, hygiene, and household size. BMJ 1989; 299: 1259–60

7 Seaton A, Godden DJ, Brown KM. Increase in asthma: a more toxic environment or a more susceptible population? Thorax 1994; 49: 171–4

8 Bjorksten B, Naaber P, Sepp E, Mikelsaar N. The intestinal microflora in allergic Estonian and Swedish 2-year-old children. Clin Exp Allergy 1999; 39: 342–6

9 Hayward AR. Development of lymphocyte responses and interactions in the human fetus and newborn. Immunol Rev 1981; 57: 39–60

10 Hayward AR. Ontogeny of the immune system. In: Ulijaszek SJ, Johnston FE, Preece MA. (eds) The Cambridge Encyclopaedia of Growth and Development. Cambridge: Cambridge University Press, 1998; 166–9

11 Van Duren-Schmidt K, Pichler J, Ebner C et al. Prenatal contact with inhalant allergens. Pediatr Res 1997; 41: 128–31

12 Prescott SL, Macaubas C, Holt BJ et al. Transplacental priming of the human immune system to environmental allergens: universal skewing of initial T cell responses towards the Th-2 cytokine profile. J Immunol 1998; 160: 4730–7

13 Kondo N, Cubiyashi Y, Shinoda S et al. Cord blood lymphocyte responses to food antigens for the prediction of allergic disease. Arch Dis Child 1992; 67: 1003–7

14   Michel FB, Bousquet J, Greillier P *et al*. Comparison of cord blood immunoglobulin E and maternal allergy for the prediction of atopic diseases in infancy. *J Allergy Clin Immunol* 1980; **65**: 422–30

15   Croner S, Kjellman N-IM. Development of atopic disease in relation to family history and cord blood IgE levels – 11 year follow-up in 1,654 children. *Pediatr Allergy Immunol* 1990; **1**: 14–21

16   Edenharter G, Burgmann RL, Burgmann KE *et al*. Cord blood IgE as risk factor and predictor of atopic diseases. *Clin Exp Allergy* 1998; **28**: 671–8

17   Ruiz RGG, Richards D, Kemeny DM, Price JF. Neonatal IgE: a poor screen for atopic disease. *Clin Exp Allergy* 1991; **21**: 467–72

18   Hide DW, Arshad SH, Twiselton R, Stevens M. Cord serum IgE: an insensitive method for prediction of atopy. *Clin Exp Allergy* 1991; **21**: 739–43

19   Tang MLK, Kemp AS, Thorburn J, Hildy J. Reduced IFN-γ and subsequent atopy. *Lancet* 1994; **344**: 983–5

20   Wegmann T, Lin H, Guilbert L, Mosmann T. Bi-directional cytokine interactions in the maternal fetal relationship: is successful pregnancy a Th-2-like phenomenon? *Immunol Today* 1993; **14**: 353–6

21   Jones CA, Williams KA, Finlay-Jones JF, Hart HA, Harty PH. Interleukin-4 production by human amnion epithelial cells and regulation of its activity by glycosa amino glycan binding. *Biol Reprod* 1995; **52**: 839–47

22   Williams TJ, Jones CA, Miles EA, Warner JO, Warner JA. Fetal and neonatal interleukin-13 production during pregnancy and at birth and subsequent development of atopic symptoms. *J Allergy Clin Immunol* 2000; **105**: 951–59

23   Warner JA, Jones CA, Jones AC, Miles EA, Francis T, Warner JO. Immune responses during pregnancy and the development of allergic disease. *Pediatr Allergy Immunol* 1997; **8**: 5–14

24   Weinberg ED. Pregnancy-associated depression of cell-mediated immunity. *Rev Infect Dis* 1984; **6**: 814–31

25   Gendron RL, Baines MG. Infiltrating decidual natural killer cells are associated with spontaneous abortion in mice. *Cell Immunol* 1988; **113**: 261–7

26   Robertson SA, Mayrhofer G, Seamark RF. Uterine epithelial cells synthesise granulocyte-macrophage colony-stimulating factor (GM-CSF) and interleukin-6 (IL-6) in pregnant and non-pregnant mice. *Biol Reprod* 1992; **46**: 1064–79

27   Abbas A, Thiliginathan B, Buggins AGS *et al*. Fetal plasma IFN-γ concentration in normal pregnancy. *Am J Obstet Gynecol* 1993; **168**: 1414–6

28   Jones CA, Holloway JA, Warner JO. Does atopic disease start in foetal life? *Allergy* 2000; **55**: 2–10

29   Jones CA, Warner JA, Warner JO. Fetal swallowing of IgE. *Lancet* 1998; **351**: 1859

30   Bloomfield FH, Harding JE. Experimental aspects of nutrition and fetal growth. *Fetal Mat Med Rev* 1998; **10**: 91–107

31   Warner JO, Jones CA. Fetal origins of lung disease. In: Barker DJP. (ed) *Fetal Origins of Cardiovascular Lung Diseases*. Monographs from Lung Biology and Health and Disease. National Heart Lung & Blood Institute. New York: Marcel Dekker, 2000; 297–321

32   Jenmalm MC, Bjorksten B. Cord blood levels of immunoglobulin G subclass antibodies to food and inhalant allergens in relation to maternal atopy and the development of atopic disease during the first 8 years of life. *Clin Exp Allergy* 2000; **30**: 34–40

33   Glovsky MM, Ghekiere L, Rejzek E. Effect of maternal immunotherapy on immediate skin test reactivity, specific rye IgG and IgE antibody and total IgE of the children. *Ann Allergy* 1991; **67**: 21–4

34   Butland BK, Strachan DP, Anderson HR. Fresh fruit intake and asthma symptoms in young British adults: confounding or effect modification by smoking. *Eur Respir J* 1999; **13**: 744–50

35   Langley-Evans S. Fetal programming of immune function and respiratory disease. *Clin Exp Allergy* 1997; **27**: 1377–9

36   Arm JP, Horton CE, Spurr BW *et al*. The effects of dietary supplementation with fish oil lipids on the airways response to inhaled allergen in bronchial asthma. *Am Rev Respir Dis* 1989; **139**: 1395–400

37   Hodge L, Salome CM, Hughes JM *et al*. Effect of dietary intake of omega-3 and omega-6 fatty acids on severity of asthma in children. *Eur Respir J* 1998; **11**: 361–5

38 Strachan DP. Hay fever, hygiene, and household size. *BMJ* 1989; **299**: 1259–60
39 Folkerts G, Walzl G, Openshaw PJM. Do childhood infections teach the immune system not to be allergic? *Immunol Today* 2000; **21**: 118–20
40 Wills-Karp M. Potential use of Th-1 promoting immunoadjuvants in the treatment of allergic disorders (Proceedings). *Postgrad Syllabus Am Acad Allergy, Asthma Immunol* 1999: 107–25
41 Sigurs N, Bjarnason R, Sigurbergsson F *et al*. Asthma and immunoglobulin E antibodies after respiratory syncytial virus bronchiolitis: a prospective cohort study with matched controls. *Pediatrics* 1995; **95**: 500–5
42 Alm JS, Lilja G, Pershagen G, Scheynius A. Early BCG vaccination and development of atopy. *Lancet* 1997; **350**: 400–3
43 Golding J. Immunisations. In: Butler N, Golding J. (eds) *From Birth to Five. A study of the health and behaviour of Britain's five year olds*. Oxford: Pergamon, 1986; 295–319
44 Bjorksten B, Naaber P, Sepp E, Mikelsaar. The intestinal microflora in allergic Estonian and Swedish 2-year-old children. *Clin Exp Allergy* 1999; **39**: 342–6
45 Von Ehrenstein OS, Von Mutius E, Illi S, Baumann L, Bohm O, Von Kries R. Reduced risk of hay fever and asthma among children of farmers. *Clin Exp Allergy* 2000; **30**: 187–93
46 Riedler J, Eder W, Oberfeld G, Schreuer M. Austrian children living on a farm have less hay fever, asthma and allergic sensitisation. *Clin Exp Allergy* 2000; **30**: 194–200
47 Kilpelainen M, Terho EO, Helenius H, Koskenvuo M. Farm environment in childhood prevents the development of allergies. *Clin Exp Allergy* 2000; **30**: 201–8
48 Platts-Mills TAE, Vervloet D, Thomas WR *et al*. Indoor allergens and asthma. Report of the Third International Workshop. *J Allergy Clin Immunol* 1997; **100**: S1–24
49 Wahn U, Lau S, Bergmann R *et al*. Indoor allergen exposure is a risk factor for sensitisation during the first 3 years of life. *J Allergy Clin Immunol* 1997; **99**: 763–9
50 Peat JK, Salome CM, Woolcock AJ. Longitudinal changes in atopy during a 4-year period. *J Allergy Clin Immunol* 1990; **85**: 65–74
51 Gotzsche PC, Hammarquist C, Burr M. House dust mite control measures in the management of asthma: meta-analysis. *BMJ* 1998; **317**: 1105–10
52 Falth-Magnusson K, Kjellman N-IM. Allergy prevention by maternal elimination diet during late pregnancy – a 5-year follow-up of a randomised study. *J Allergy Clin Immunol* 1992; **89**: 709–11
53 Saarinen UM, Kajosaari M. Breastfeeding as prophylaxis against atopic disease: prospective follow-up study until 17 years. *Lancet* 1995; **346**: 1065–9
54 Zeiger RS, Heller S, Mellon MH, Halsey JF, Hamburger RN, Sampson HA. Genetic and environmental factors affecting the development of atopy through age 4 in children of atopic parents: a prospective randomised study of food allergen avoidance. *Pediatr Allergy Immunol* 1992; **3**: 110–27
55 Hide DW, Matthews S, Tariq S, Arshad SH. Allergen avoidance in infancy and allergy at 4 years of age. *Allergy* 1996; **51**: 89–93

Genetics of allergic disease

Marlies Feijen*†, Jorrit Gerritsen† and Dirkje S Postma‡

*Department of Pulmonary Rehabilitation, Beatrixoord Rehabilitation Centre, Haren, The Netherlands, †Department of Pediatric Pulmonology, Beatrix Children's Clinic, The Netherlands, ‡Department of Pulmonology, University Hospital Groningen, The Netherlands

Atopy can express itself as asthma, rhinitis and eczema. The presence of atopy can be assessed by increased levels of total serum IgE and specific IgE to common allergens, skin test positivity and increased numbers of peripheral blood eosinophils. Genetic studies indicate that multiple genes are involved in the pathogenesis of atopy and that different genes regulate the presence of increased levels of serum total IgE and specific IgE. Linkage of these traits to chromosomal regions likely to contain atopic susceptibility genes has been replicated in several studies. Genome-wide screens have identified several new chromosomal locations that are likely to contain atopic genes. These regions also contain candidate genes. Moreover, the available literature suggests that multiple, yet different genes may be involved in the translation of atopy to a distinct clinical phenotype. We anticipate that understanding of the genetic basis of atopy will lead to new therapeutic interventions and early diagnosis.

It has now been widely accepted that atopy constitutes a genetic disease, yet the exact genes and their loci have not been established so far. More than one gene is most likely involved in the expression of atopy and their

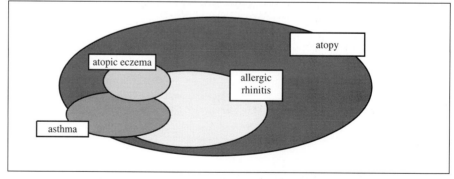

Fig. 1 The phenotypic heterogeneity of atopy. The outer box represents a general population: approximately 40% is atopic as defined by skin test positivity. Allergic rhinitis has a population prevalence of 20%. There is a considerable overlap between asthma and rhinitis; however, not all asthmatics are atopic. Atopic eczema has also an overlap with asthma and allergic rhinitis. Please note that figures are estimations for a population of children and adults.

*Correspondence to:
Prof. Dr Dirkje S Postma,
Department of
Pulmonology, University
Hospital Groningen,
PO Box 30.001, 9700 RB
Groningen,
The Netherlands*

interaction may result in different disease expressions such as asthma, rhinitis or atopic dermatitis (Fig. 1).

The prevalence of atopy, asthma, rhinitis and atopic eczema in childhood are 40%, 10–20%, 20% and 10–20%, respectively. It has been well established that the prevalence of atopic diseases is increasing[1]. This rise in prevalence of atopy can not simply be explained by genetic factors alone, because it has occurred within one or two generations. Thus the clinical expression of the atopic trait has to be also dependent on environmental factors. Important environmental factors in the development of atopic diseases are allergen exposure, (maternal) smoking, breast feeding, Western life-style and possibly lack of infections or hygiene[2].

Phenotypes of atopy

Atopy can be defined as a prolonged increased production of IgE as a response on exposure to common allergens. Atopy can be assessed by increased levels of total serum IgE and specific IgE to common allergens and by skin test positivity to inhalant or food allergens. Furthermore, it can be suggested that atopy is present when increased levels of peripheral blood eosinophils exist. The clinical expression of atopy includes asthma, rhinitis and dermatitis. Asthma has been defined as a chronic inflammatory disease in the airways of the lung, characterised by variable airway obstruction and airway hyper-responsiveness accompanied by symptoms such as wheeze, breathlessness or cough. Asthma generally develops in childhood, but symptoms occasionally start in adulthood. Allergic rhinitis can be defined as a recurrent or persistent inflammation of the nostrils with one or more of the following symptoms: nasal congestion, rhinorrhoea, sneezing and itching. The most common form of allergic rhinitis, *i.e.* hay fever, starts around the age of 7 years, but the onset can also be earlier or later in life. Atopic dermatitis is a disease most prominent in early childhood, it is characterised by an itchy red rash that has an easily broken surface.

The genetic basis of atopic disease

Family studies

It has long been known that asthma clusters in families. Until recently the route of inheritance was not known. Familial aggregation studies are the logical first step to determine the mode of inheritance. This can either be performed by twin studies or in families ascertained by a proband with the phenotype under study. Significant aggregation of asthma and atopic phenotypes in families screened by an asthmatic proband has been described[3].

Twin studies

Twin studies are especially important to estimate both the genetic and environmental contribution to complex traits. Monozygotic (MZ) and dizygotic (DZ) twins are compared for similarities and differences between these twin types. MZ twins share 100% of their genetic information and DZ twins share 50% on average. Thus, MZ twins should resemble each other to a greater extent than DZ twins if a trait is influenced by genetic factors. The major assumptions of twin studies are that the twins are samples of the same gene pool, that they are representative of the general population, that self-reported zygosity is correct in questionnaire-based studies and that the environment for both MZ and DZ twins is similar.

Twin studies have provided evidence of a considerable genetic component of asthma, hay fever and eczema[4-6]. Atopic phenotypes such as elevated serum total IgE and positive skin tests were studied by Hopp and co-workers and genetic contribution to both of the phenotypes was suggested[7].

Table 1 provides an overview on atopic twin studies and shows that atopy itself (IgE and positive skin test) is genetically determined as well as asthma, rhinitis and eczema (modified table, references from review article by Los *et al.*[8]). Heritability lies in general between 0.60 and 0.70 and monozygotic twins have always a higher concordance of the trait under study than dizygotic twins.

Segregation analyses

Segregation analyses are used to model inheritance patterns in families. The distribution of a disease is studied in families and the observed frequency of the disorder in offspring and siblings is compared to the expected distribution using different genetic models of inheritance (*e.g.* dominant, co-dominant, recessive or polygenic).

Different genetic models have been found for total serum IgE. Several explanations may be given for these different findings. The first explanation may be the variable definition of atopy between studies. Secondly, the ascertainment of families for segregation studies may play a role. In families screened for asthma, estimates on frequencies of alleles regulating total serum IgE are expected to be higher than in families sampled randomly from the general population. A final explanation may

Table 1 Twin studies of atopic traits

Phenotype	First author	Population	Number of twin pairs	MZ correl-ation	DZ correl-ation	Probandwise concordance MZ/DZ	H	Comments
Total IgE	Hopp	US, A and B	107	0.82	0.52*		0.61	
	Hanson	US apart, A	70	0.64	0.49*			Twins raised apart
		US together, A	61	0.42	0.26			Twins raised together
		Finland, A	158	0.56	0.37*			Twins raised together
Specific IgE	Hanson	US apart, A	26			0.50/0		Twins raised apart
		US together, A	14			0.50/0.33		Twins raised apart
Skin test	Hopp	US, B and C	107	0.82	0.46*		0.72	
	Hanson	US apart, A	39			0.55/0.50		
		US together, A	41			0.70/0.28		
Asthma	Edfors-Lubbs	Sweden, A	6996	0.65	0.25*	0.19#/0.05#*		Population study, self-reported asthma
	Hopp	US, B and C	107			0.50#/0.33#	0.72	Questionnaire
	Duffy	Australia, A	3808	0.65	0.24*		0.60–0.75	Population study, self-reported asthma
	Nieminen	Finland, A	13.888	0.43~	0.25~*	0.13/0.07	0.36	Population study, doctor's diagnosis of asthma
	Lichtenstein	Sweden, C	434 M			0.62/0.26*	0.76	Questionnaire
			456 F			0.41/0.18*	0.62	
	Harris	Norway, B	2559	0.75	0.21	0.45/0.12*	0.75	Population study
	Laitinen	Finland, B	1713	0.76	0.45	0.42/0.19*	0.79	Parental/twin design
	Skadhauge	Denmark,	11.688				0.73	Population study, self-reported asthma
		B	1929 M	0.76	0.36	0.48/0.19*		
			2131 F	0.71	0.47	0.42/0.26*		
		A	1867 M	0.81	0.37	0.51/0.16*		
			2110 F	0.65	0.15	0.38/0.09*		
Hayfever	Edfors-Lubbs	Sweden, A	6996	0.45~	0.25~*	21.4#/13.6#*		Population study, self-reported hayfever
	Duffy	Australia, A	3808	0.61	0.25*		0.60–0.75	Population study, self-reported hayfever
	Lichtenstein	Sweden, C	434 M			0.60/0.43*	0.33	Questionnaire
			456 F			0.59/0.34*	0.70	
Eczema	Edfors-Lubbs	Sweden, C	6996			15.4#/4.5#*		Population study, self-reported eczema
	Lichtenstein	Sweden, C	434 M			0.54/0.35*	0.74	Questionnaire
			456 F			0.73/0.40*	0.71	
Urticaria	Lichtenstein	Sweden, C	434 M			0.52/0.33*	0.54	Questionnaire
			456 F			0.68/0.38*	0.60	

*Statistically significant differences between monozygous (MZ) and dizygous pairs. A, adults; B, young adults; C, children; M, male; F, female. ~Correlation is calculated by Duffy et al[6]. #Concordance: pairwise concordance. H: heritability.

be genetic heterogeneity. This means that in different populations, separate genes act in the regulation of these phenotypes. To date, this cannot be investigated since the exact locations of these genes are still unknown.

Using a single locus approach, the best fitting models for high serum IgE levels were the models of a major Mendelian gene, either co-dominant, recessive, mixed model of recessive inheritance, dominant, or in two other studies of polygenic inheritance. In a study of 243 Australian nuclear families, evidence for recessive inheritance of total serum IgE and significant residual familial correlations were found[9]. However, these correlations were not significant when the presence of the specific immune response was accounted for in the analysis. Therefore, it suggests that regulation of total serum IgE is genetically independent from the regulation of allergen specific IgE. A two locus model on IgE in 92 Dutch families screened through a proband with asthma provided a significantly better fit of the data than a one-locus model[10]. In addition, evidence was presented for two unlinked loci regulating total serum IgE in these families. The first locus alone explained 50.6% of the variance of the level of total serum IgE, the second 19%. Considered jointly, the two loci accounted for 78.4% of the variability of total serum IgE. No data on the segregation of skin test positivity or specific IgE levels to allergens as a representative for atopy have been presented so far.

In the European Community Respiratory Health Survey of 13,963 asthma patients, the complex segregation analysis of the asthma pheno-type provides evidence for a two-allele gene with co-dominant inherit-ance[11]. Other studies on aggregation of asthma and wheeze in families are summarised in Table 2 (for references see the review article by Los *et al.*[8]). The segregation of asthma in these families appears to be predominantly consistent with the action of multiple genes with a small effect.

In summary, segregation analyses of asthma or atopy, when expressed as total serum IgE, confirms a genetic trait, but the mode of inheritance is yet uncertain as are the number of genes involved. There are no data available on eczema and rhinitis.

Linkage

Linkage analysis is used to determine a chromosomal region which co-segregates with a certain trait within families. The likelihood that a trait co-segregates with a marker is expressed as a LOD score, *i.e.* the log of the ratio of the likelihood of linkage and the likelihood of no linkage. A value of +3 is traditionally taken as evidence for linkage and a value of −2 is considered evidence against linkage. Linkage analysis requires pedigree data as opposed to association studies in which unrelated cases

Table 2 Segregation analyses of atopic traits

Phenotype	First author	Year	Number of families/ population	Genetic model	Hertitability	Comments
Total IgE	Gerrard	1973	173 USA	Model major gene Dominant allele suppresses high levels of IgE	0.43	Selected population for ragweed allergy
	Blumenthal	1981	3 USA	Major gene with polygenic transmission	0.43	Extended families selected for ragweed allergy
	Meyers	1982	23 USA	Mendelian co-dominant model		No selection for allergy. Amish in-bred
	Hasstedt	1983	5 USA	No major gene, polygenetic inheritance		Selected population for ragweed allergy
	Meyers	1987	42 USA	Mixed model with recessive inheritance of high IgE levels	0.36	No selection for allergy
	Martinez	1994	291 USA	Major gene, co-dominant inheritance for high IgE levels		Hispanic and non-Hispanic No selection for allergy
	Lawrence	1994	131 UK	Polygenic model		Random population sample
	Xu	1995	92 The Netherlands	Two locus recessive model with epistasis		Families ascertained through a proband with asthma
	Dizier	1995	234 Australia	Recessive major gene controlling high IgE levels		No selection for allergy
	Panhuysen	1996	92 The Netherlands	Two-locus recessive model		Families ascertained through a proband with asthma
Asthma	Lawrence	1994	131 UK	Mixed model, two-locus model	0.28–0.63	Common genes of small effect Questionnaire, population-based sample
	Holberg	1996	906 USA	Polygenetic or oligogenetic model, not a single two-allele gene		Questionnaire, physician diagnosed asthma
	ECRHSG	1997	13.963 Europe	Two-allele gene with co-dominant inheritance		Questionnaire, self-reported asthma
	Jenkins	1997	7,394 Australia	Oligogenetic model		Questionnaire, population of school children
	Chen	1998	309 USA	Single locus model Contribution of polygenes and environment		Questionnaire, self-reported wheeze

and controls are needed. To study linkage using the LOD score approach, a genetic model has to be specified for different parameters such as mode of inheritance, allele frequencies and penetrance. Sometimes these parameters can be estimated from segregation analyses, which is preferable; but, in most cases, the parameters are not known. No specification of a genetic model is needed in non-parametric approaches such as the sibling pair analysis and affected relative pair analysis. These methods test whether the inheritance of a chromosomal region is not consistent with random segregation. If this is the case, affected relatives inherit identical copies of alleles in this region more often than would be expected by chance[12]. The observed and expected distributions of alleles can be tested with a χ^2-test.

In general, evidence for linkage is assumed to be present when the reviewed linkage from one study has been replicated by others.

Identifying atopic disease genes

In identifying genes there are two general approaches. In the genome-wide screen all chromosomes are searched until the approximate location of the gene is discovered. The localisation of the gene is progressively refined until the gene itself is isolated by linking the inheritance of specific chromosomal regions with the inheritance of disease. This approach is often referred to as positional cloning. The candidate gene approach is used when a gene is a plausible candidate for being the disease gene because of its function. The strategy is to find polymorphisms in a known gene and to compare the frequency of alleles in cases and controls. The finding of a positive association of an allele and a trait can be interpreted in three ways[12]: (i) the allele of interest is the relevant mutation in the disease gene; (ii) the allele is in linkage disequilibrium, which means that it is physically very close to the gene; or (iii) the association is a result of population admixture. This occurs if a certain trait has a higher prevalence in an ethnic subgroup within a mixed population. Any allele with a higher frequency within this subgroup will show association with the trait.

Genome-wide search

Recently, genome-wide searches have contributed significantly to the mapping of atopic genes by conducting searches in different human populations. Families were recruited in Western Australia, Sweden, Germany, The Netherlands and from the US (both African Americans, Caucasians, Hispanics and Hutterites)[3,13].

Table 3 Replication of linkage of atopic traits

Chromosome	Atopy broadly defined	IgE	Specific IgE	Skin prick test	Eosinophilia	Asthma	Eczema
1				X			
2						X	
3							
4		X					
5		X				X	
6		X			X		
7		X					
8							
9							
10							
11	X	X		X			
12		X					
13							
14							
15							
16							
17							
18							
19							
20							
21							
22							

Evidence for linkage to multiple chromosomal regions was reported in each study. Linkage by multiple groups were found on chromosomes 1, 2q, 3, 4, 5q, 6p, 7, 9, 11q, 12q, 13q, 14, 16 and 17q. 'Novel' regions of interest are 17p, 19 and 21 because they were only observed in one study.

Linkage and association of atopy

Table 3 shows the replicated linkages on the different atopic traits. Genome-wide screens show many regions of interest, but just a few linkages have been replicated.

Atopy

Linkage for atopy (broadly defined) was found on chromosome 5, 6, 11, 13. Only the linkage to chromosome 11 has been replicated. Cookson and co-workers reported linkage of a broadly defined atopic phenotype to markers on chromosome 11q[14]. Seven families were studied, and most of the LOD score was contributed by one single family using an autosomal dominant mode of inheritance. The investigators confirmed their findings in other samples. In addition, other studies from The Netherlands,

Germany, Japan and Australia found evidence for linkage between an atopic phenotype and markers on chromosome 11q[8]. Sequence variants in the high-affinity IgE receptor (FcεR) gene on chromosome 11 may increase the risk for development of atopy[3]. Linkage of chromosome 11q to atopy and asthma remains controversial due to multiple failures to replicate the linkage in several other populations. Subsequent work of Cookson et al. suggested that the linkage in other studies may have been obscured by maternal inheritance[15]. Possible explanations for maternal inheritance of atopy are paternal imprinting (a process by which a particular gene is differentially activated or silenced, depending on the sex of the parent from whom it was inherited) or maternal modification of the developing immune response.

Total serum IgE

Linkage of total serum IgE to chromosomes 1, 2, 4, 5, 6, 7, 9, 11, 12, 13, 14, 15 and 16 has been found by several research groups. Replication of significant linkage has been found to chromosomes 5, 11 and 12.

In 1994, Marsh et al. were the first to report linkage between serum total IgE levels and chromosome 5q in an American Amish population[16]. Meyers et al. replicated this finding in a study of Dutch families[17]. More studies have replicated linkages on chromosome 5 whereas others could not[8]. This can be due to different populations, definitions of phenotypes, founder effects, admixture, and possibly varying environmental influences.

Specific IgE

Linkage for specific IgE has been found to chromosomes 1, 2, 4, 6, 7, 9, and 12. There is only limited data available with regard to linkage of specific IgE to particular chromosomal regions. Most linkages are not significant, i.e. they do not reach the maximum LOD score of 3. Furthermore, significancies are very low. Summary of the available literature shows that the required replication of linkage to a chromosomal area is still not found.

Skin prick test

Linkage for skin prick tests was found on chromosomes 1, 3, 6, 9, 11 and 16. Replication of linkage of a positive skin prick test existed for chromosomes 1 and 11. Ober was the first to investigate skin prick tests as an atopic phenotype by itself[13]. Other investigators have always used a composite score of atopy, including skin prick test.

Peripheral blood eosinophilia

Linkage for peripheral blood eosinophilia was reported on chromosomes 1, 3, 4, 5, 6, 7, 11, 14 and 16. Linkage of eosinophilia to chromosome 6 is significant and has been replicated.

Asthma

Linkage for asthma was found on chromosomes 1, 2, 3, 5, 6, 9, 11-14, 17, 19 and 21. Evidence for linkage and association for both asthma and total IgE to chromosome 12q was reported in an Afro-Caribbean population[18]. Other studies confirmed a linkage for IgE or asthma on chromosome 12q. An interesting finding is that the chromosomal regions on 12q implicated in these studies are not exactly the same[3]. Further studies are needed to fine map this region and may answer the question whether one or more regions on 12q are implicated in asthma and atopy.

Several candidate genes map to this wide region such as interferon-gamma, IGF1 (promotes differentiation of both B and T lymphocytes), a mast cell growth factor and the β-subunit of nuclear factor-Y (possibly up-regulating transcription of both IL-4 and the HLA genes). For references, see Wiesch et al[3].

Atopic eczema

Linkage of atopic eczema (AE) has been reported on chromosome 5q31[19]. There are only a few genetic studies on atopic eczema. Shirwaka et al. confirmed the association between FcεRIβ on chromosome 11q13 and atopy underlying AE (for references see Tanaka and co-workers[20]). Significant association of AE and mast-cell chymase (MCC; a serine protease secreted by skin mast cells) on 14q11 has also been reported[21]. Recently, an association between AE and a functional mutation in the promoter region of the C-C chemokine RANTES was found in children from Germany[22].

Allergic rhinitis

No reports are available about linkage of allergic rhinitis.

Asthma and atopy genes

When reviewing the literature there are some interesting and promising polymorphisms in genes related to atopy, for instance the CD14 polymorphism, IL-4, IL-13 and β$_2$-receptor.

CD14

The CD14 gene is located on chromosome 5q31, expressed on the surface of macrophages and monocytes, and is also present in serum in a soluble form (sCD14). CD14 is an important high affinity receptor for lipopolysaccharide (LPS) and other bacterial wall products. LPS exposition by bacterial infections in infancy may shift the Th-1/Th-2 balance in favour of Th-1 type immune response, thereby suppressing the Th-2 response, which leads to atopy[23]. Binding of LPS to CD14 can provide activation signals for Th-1 maturation. IgE synthesis is controlled by inhibitory cytokines from Th-1 cells and by stimulatory cytokines provided by Th-2 cells[24].

Baldini *et al.* identified a C–T base change polymorphism in the 5' regulatory region of the CD14 gene that was associated with low levels of total serum IgE[24].

IL-4 and IL-13

There are many candidate genes for atopy on chromosome 5q, such as a cluster of cytokine genes IL-3, IL-4, IL-5, IL-9 and IL-13. These cytokines are mediators of inflammation in atopy; IL-4 is an important mediator in regulating the production of IgE and skewing the Th-1/Th-2 balance to Th-2. IL-13 acts on B-cells to produce IgE and there is increasing evidence that IL-13 is crucial in inducing asthma in animal models (for references see Shirakawa *et al.*[25]). Five variants have been reported in the IL-4 promoter region, four of them being very rare. Recently, two variants of IL-13 have been identified, a promoter polymorphism associated with increased risk of allergic asthma as well as a coding variant (gln110arg) of IL-13 that is associated with both atopic and non-atopic asthma in a British and a Japanese population[25]. IL-4 and IL-13 operate through the IL-4 and IL-13 receptor, both receptors share the IL-4Rα chain[25]. IL-4 binds to both types of receptors through the IL-4Rα chain, whereas IL-13 can bind only to the IL-13 receptor. The IL-4 receptor can be expressed on both B- and T-cells, the IL-13 receptor only on B-cells. Thus, IL-4 can stimulate both B- and T-cells, whereas IL-13 can activate B-cells only. Both receptors activate STAT6 (signal transducer and activator of transcription 6), the IL-4Rα–STAT6 interaction is essential for IL-4 and IL-13 signalling. STAT6 induces GATA3 activation and enables Th-2 cells to maintain their Th-2 characteristics, while inducing B-cells to produce IgE. Therefore, the observation that polymorphisms in these genes are associated with asthma has important implications for both the understanding of asthma and the possibility of devising new strategies for prevention or amelioration of the disease. Finally, a strong linkage has been found between atopy and flanking markers to IL-4R on chromosome 16p12.

β₂-Adrenergic receptor

β_2-Adrenergic receptors are localised on airway smooth muscle, epithelium and inflammatory cells (mast cells, macrophages, eosinophils and T-lymphocytes). β_2-Adrenergic receptor function is mainly regulated by circulating epinephrine and mediates most of the effects of β_2-agonists on airway function. The β_2-adrenergic receptor (β_2AR) gene is localised on chromosome 5q 31-32. This gene is intronless and has a coding block consisting of 1239 nucleic acids. Nine known polymorphisms varying within the normal population are situated in this region, and four polymorphisms result in amino acids variations on positions 16, 27, 34, and 164. One polymorphism has been identified in the 5' leader cistron sequence, a peptide that modifies β_2AR translation. Although no differences in the polymorphism frequencies were found in asthmatics compared with non-asthmatic controls, cell and transgenic mouse studies have shown altered function or regulation of the β_2AR (for references see Liggett[26]).

Two variants may play a role in asthma treatment. The first is the gly16 variant which is a common polymorphism in the general population. Tan and co-workers reported that homozygous individuals with this variant showed reduced treatment response following either acute or chronic exposure to β_2–agonists. Secondly, ile164 is an example of a rare polymorphism, which may be important since *in vitro* functional studies have demonstrated that the ile164 receptor has an approximately 3-fold decreased affinity for β_2–agonists.

β_2AR polymorphisms can have a pharmacogenetic effect or act as disease-modifiers. For instance, β_2-adrenergic receptor associations have been found with nocturnal asthma, bronchial hyper-responsiveness, increased IgE levels, and asthma severity.

5-Lipoxygenase

The core promotor of the 5-lipoxygenase (ALOX5) gene is localised on chromosome 10q11.2[27]. The level of ALOX5 activity determines to a certain extent the level of bronchoconstrictor leukotrienes in the airways. This gene is the first to provide evidence that pharmacogenetics can be applied to asthma. One study showed that The ALOX5 locus contains 3–6 tandem repeats of the Sp1-binding motif GGGCGG. Asthma patients without the wild type (5 tandem repeats) allele do not improve or improve to a smaller extent when treated with a drug which mechanism of action is the inhibition of ALOX5. Thus treatment response is to a certain extent determined by genetic variants in the 5-lipoxygenase gene.

Implications of results of the available studies and future directions

Atopy has different disease expressions such as asthma, rhinitis and eczema which all have been shown to contain a significant genetic contribution. The available literature shows that linkage of the different measures of atopy are found on distinct chromosomes. Whereas replicated linkage exists on chromosome 11 for a broadly defined atopy phenotype, for total serum IgE and skin prick tests, this is not the case for specific IgE. Linkage of total serum IgE has been replicated for chromosomes 4–7, yet no linkage whatsoever or no replication has been found for specific IgE or skin prick test. Thus, either different genes are to be involved in the regulation of total IgE and allergen specific responses or one (or more) gene may interact with the environment or both. Furthermore, distinct combinations of genes may result in different disease expressions such as asthma, rhinitis and atopic dermatitis. For instance it is hypothetical, but not totally improbable, that genes for atopy and airway hyper-responsiveness are to be present in case of the clinical expression of asthma, yet the latter genes are not mandatory for eczema (or even rhinitis).

Several candidate genes have been identified, yet more atopic genes are to be discovered in the future. These genes will give us more insight of the pathophysiological mechanisms of atopic disease. It can be expected that this will lead to new and more effective therapeutic interventions, new methods for early diagnosis, development for disease prevention in susceptible individuals and more insight in the pharmacogenetics.

References

1   Aberg N, Hesselmar B, Aberg B, Eriksson B. Increase of asthma, allergic rhinitis and eczema in Swedish schoolchildren between 1979 and 1991. *Clin Exp Allergy* 1995; **25**: 815–9
2   Cogswell JJ. Influence of maternal atopy on atopy in the offspring. *Clin Exp Allergy* 2000; **30**: 1–3
3   Wiesch DG, Meyers DA, Bleecker ER. Genetics of asthma. *J Allergy Clin Immunol* 1999; **104**: 895–901
4   Koppelman GH, Los H, Postma DS. Genetics and environment in asthma: the answer of twin studies *Eur Respir J* 1999; **13**: 2–4
5   Edfors-Lubs ML. Allergy in 7000 twin pairs. *Acta Allergol* 1971; **26**: 249–85
6   Duffy DL, Martin NG, Battistutta D, Hopper JL, Mathews JD. Genetics of asthma and hayfever in Australian twins. *Am Rev Respir Dis* 1990; **142**: 1351–8

7   Hopp RJ, Bewtra AK, Watt GD, Nair NM, Towley RG. Genetic analysis of allergic disease in twins. *J Allergy Clin Immunol* 1984; **73**: 265–70

8   Los H, Koppelman GH, Postma DS. The importance of genetic influences in asthma. *Eur Respir J* 1999; **14**: 1210–27

9   Dizier MH, Hill M, James A *et al.* Detection of a recessive major gene for high IgE levels acting independently of specific response to allergens. *Genet Epidemiol* 1995; **12**: 93–105

10 Xu J, Levitt RC, Panhuysen CI *et al.* Evidence for two unlinked loci regulating total serum IgE levels. *Am J Hum Genet* 1995; **57**: 425–30

11 European Community Respiratory Health Survey Group. Genes for asthma? An analysis of the European Community Respiratory Health Survey. *Am J Respir Crit Care Med* 1997; **146**: 1773–80

12 Lander ES, Schork NJ. Genetic dissection of complex traits. *Science* 1994; **265**: 2037–48

13 Ober C, Tsalenko A, Willadsen S *et al.* Genome-wide screen for atopy susceptibility alleles in the Hutterites. *Clin Exp Allergy* 1999; **29** (Suppl 4): 11–5

14 Cookson WO, Sharp PA, Faux JA, Hopkin JM. Linkage between immunoglobulin E responses underlying asthma and rhinitis and chromosome 11q. *Lancet* 1989; **i**: 1292–5

15 Cookson WO, Young RP, Sandtford AJ *et al.* Maternal inheritance of atopic IgE responsiveness on chromosome 11q. *Lancet* 1992; **340**: 381–4

16 Marsh DG, Neely JD, Breazeale DR *et al.* Linkage analysis of IL-4 and other chromosome 5q31.1 markers and total serum IgE concentrations. *Science* 1994; **264**: 1152–6

17 Meyers DA, Postma DS, Panhuysen CI *et al.* Evidence for a locus regulating total serum IgE levels mapping to chromosome 5. *Genomics* 1994; **23**: 464–70

18 Barnes KC, Neely ND, Duffy DL *et al.* Linkage of asthma end total serum IgE concentration to markers on chromosome 12q: evidence from Afro-Caribbean and Caucasian population. *Genomics* 1996; **37**: 41–50

19 Forrest S, Dunn K, Eliott K *et al.* Identifying genes predisposing to atopic eczema. *J Allergy Clin Immunol* 1999; **104**: 1066–70

20 Tanaka K, Sugiura H, Uehara M, Sato H, Hashimoto-Tamaoki T, Furuyama J. Association between mast cell chymase genotype and atopic eczema: comparison between patients with atopic eczema alone and those with atopic eczema and atopic respiratory disease. *Clin Exp Allergy* 1999; **29**: 800–3

21 Mao XQ, Shirakawa T, Yoshikawa K *et al.* Association between genetic variants of mast-cell chymase and eczema. *Lancet* 1996; **384**: 581–3

22 Nickel RG, Casolaro V, Wahn U *et al.* Atopic dermatitis is associated with a functional mutation in the promoter of the C-C chemokine RANTES. *J Immunol* 2000; **164**: 1612–6

23 Holt PG, Sly PD, Bjorksten B. Atopic versus infectious diseases in childhood: a question of balance? *Pediatr Allergy Immunol* 1997; **8**: 53–8

24 Baldini M, Lohman IC, Halonen M, Erickson RP, Holt PG, Martinez FD. A polymorphism in the 5' flanking region of the CD14 gene is associated with circulating soluble CD14 levels and with total serum immunoglobulin E. *Am J Respir Cell Mol Biol* 1999; **20**: 976–83

25 Shirakawa T, Deichmann KA, Izuhara K, Mao XQ, Adra CN, Hopkin JM. Atopy and asthma: genetic variants of IL-4 and IL-13 signalling. *Immunol Today* 2000; **21**: 60–4

26 Liggett SB. β_2-Adrenergic receptor pharmacogenetics. *Am J Respir Crit Care Med* 2000; **161**: S197–201

27 Drazen JM, Yandava CN, Dubé L *et al.* Pharmacogenetic association between ALOX5 promotor genotype and the response to anti-asthma treatment. *Nat Genet* 1999; **22**: 168–70

IgE isotype determination: ε-germline gene transcription, DNA recombination and B-cell differentiation

Hannah J Gould*, Rebecca L Beavil* and **Donata Vercelli†**

*The Randall Centre for Molecular Mechanisms of Cell Function, King's College London, London, UK and †Respiratory Sciences Center, University of Arizona Health Sciences Center, Tucson, Arizona, USA

Immunoglobulin class switching is the process which determines whether a B-cell secretes antibodies of the IgM, IgG, IgA or IgE class (or isotype). IgE is the antibody that mediates the allergic response by sensitising mast cells to allergens at the mucosal barrier. Class switching proceeds by three successive steps, culminating in the synthesis and secretion of antibody: these are germline gene transcription, DNA recombination and B-cell differentiation. We review here the present state of knowledge concerning the mechanisms involved in each of these steps, with particular reference to IgE. Intervention in the mechanisms that specify the selection of IgE may offer a means to combat allergy.

Immunoglobulin class switching

Correspondence to:
Prof. Hannah J. Gould,
The Randall Centre for
Molecular Mechanisms of
Cell Function, King's
College London,
Guy's Campus,
London SE1 1UL, UK

Immunoglobulin (Ig) molecules are made up of two identical heavy (H)- and two identical light (L)-chains, each with a variable (V) and constant (C) region. Igs have three functional domains, a pair of Fab arms, bearing the antigen combining sites at their tips, and the Fc domain, through which the molecule attaches to cell surface receptors. Human antibodies fall into nine different classes (IgM, IgD, IgG1, IgG2, IgG3, IgG4, IgA1, IgA2 and IgE), differing in their heavy-chain 'constant' regions, which pair off in forming the Fc domain. Class-specific Fc receptors (FcR) are differentially distributed and differentially regulated across the broad range of cell types that mediate different effector functions. The effector function of an antibody, in other words, depends on its class and the location of its effector cells.

IgGs comprise the most abundant antibody classes in blood and lymph, while IgAs predominate in respiratory, digestive and urogenital secretions. IgE, which is the least abundant Ig in blood and lymph (1000 times less abundant than IgG), is sequestered in mucosal tissues by way of the high-affinity IgE receptor α-chain, FcεRIα, on the resident mast

---

cells and antigen-presenting cells. IgE sensitises mast cells to allergens in mucosal tissues to mediate the allergic response. (The only known beneficial effect is to provide protective immunity against parasites.) Crosslinking by allergen of the IgE–FcεRI complexes on mast cells results in the release of mediators of both the immediate and the late-phase responses.

The antigen specificity of an antibody is determined by intra-chromosomal recombination of variable (V, D and J, or collectively V) and constant (C) region sequences in the IgH- and IgL-chain genes of B-cell precursors in the bone marrow (Fig. 1A). The individual's antibody repertoire is continually renewed by the turnover of these cells. B-cells emerging from the bone marrow into the circulation express IgM and IgD on their plasma membranes (mIgM and mIgD). Cells migrate to secondary lymphoid organs, where the antigen specificity is fine-tuned by the process of somatic hypermutation of the V regions, and are then selected for high antigen affinity; unsuccessful B-cells undergo programmed cell death (apoptosis) and are replaced by the next cohort. Following antigen activation, the B-cells generally undergo class switching, with substitution of a new heavy-chain constant (CH) region. It is at this stage of B-cell differentiation that the antibody class is determined, and with it the commitment to IgE production.

Nine CH genes, Cμ, Cδ, Cγ3, Cγ1, Cα1, Cγ2, Cγ4, Cε and Cα2 defining, the nine antibody classes, lie in a tandem array on human chromosome 14 (Fig. 1A). Upstream of each CH gene are the associated intervening (I) and switch (S) regions, which play essential roles in class switching. Class switching involves DNA recombination between S regions, starting with Sμ, the furthest up-stream, as the donor, and proceeding directly or sequentially to the downstream S regions. The resulting hybrid S regions contain the 5′ donor and the 3′ acceptor sequences of the participating S regions. At each jump, the intervening DNA sequence is cut out to form a covalently closed circle. Then VDJ, linked to the new neighbouring CH, is transcribed into mRNA (Fig. 1B).

Class switching requires the stimulation of B-cell proliferation. In the T cell-dependent immune response *in vivo*, this is achieved by the interaction of B-cells and activated cognate T helper (Th) cells. Th cells can be activated by professional antigen-presenting cells or by B-cells. A B-cell can present a specific antigen through its antigen receptor or through a specific IgE antibody, bound to the low-affinity IgE receptor, CD23a. Th cell activation can be mimicked *in vitro* by exposure to anti-CD3 and anti-CD28, or to polyclonal T cell activating agents. The activity of Th cells on B-cells can be simulated *in vitro* by other B-cell mitogens, by membrane preparations from activated T cells, by a T cell membrane protein called CD40-ligand (CD40-L/CD154) or by anti-CD40.

Depending on local conditions, Th cells specialise to a greater or lesser extent in the secretion of one of two sets of cytokines[1,2]. Highly polarised Th-1 cells produce interleukin-2 (IL-2) and interferon-γ (IFN-γ), while Th-2 cells produce IL-3, IL-4, IL-5, IL-6, IL-9, IL-10 and IL-13. Human Th-1 cells stimulate class switching to IgG1, IgG2 and IgG3, Th-2 cells to IgG4, IgE or, in the presence of TGF-β, to IgA1 and IgA2. The

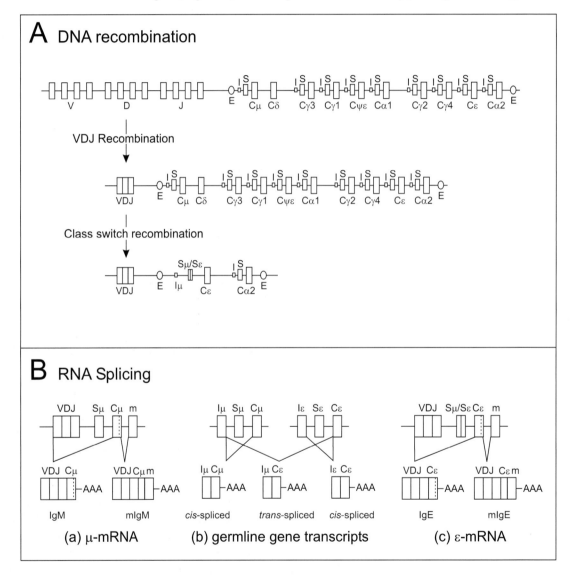

Fig. 1 Organisation of the human immunoglobulin heavy-chain gene locus and transcription products. (A) The heavy-chain gene locus on chromosome 14, showing the sequence of elements discussed in the text and the two somatic recombination events, VDJ recombination and class switch recombination (CSR), which occur during B-cell development. (B) RNA splicing to produce (a) mRNA for membrane-bound and secreted Ig μ-chains before CSR, (b) germline gene transcripts from Cμ and Cε, and (c) mRNA encoding the membrane and secreted ε-chains after CSR.

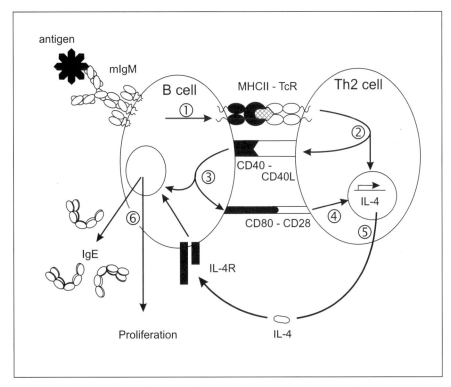

Fig. 2 Dynamics of Th cell–B-cell collaboration in heavy-chain switching to IgE. Numbers denote the sequence of events: (1) Presentation of antigen (hatched) to the Th cells. (2) Up-regulation of CD40-L on the Th cell and interaction of CD40-L with CD40 on the B-cell. (3) Up-regulation of CD80 on the B-cell and interaction of CD80 with CD28 on the Th cell, together with stimulation of B-cell proliferation. (4) Up-regulation of IL-4 synthesis in the Th cell. (5) Secretion of IL-4 and binding to the IL-4R on the B-cell. (6) Stimulation of class switching to IgE in the B-cell.

dynamics of the Th-2 cell-B-cell interaction, leading to class switching to IgE, are illustrated in Figure 2. The antigen (or allergen) is internalised and processed and the resulting peptide is presented to Th cells in the context of the major histocompatibility complex (MHC) class II antigen. The peptide-MHC class II antigen complex is recognised by the Th cell receptor (TcR) on cognate Th cells (step 1), resulting in transient expression of CD40-L on the Th cell (step 2). Interaction of CD40-L with constitutively expressed CD40 on the B-cell up-regulates CD80 on the B-cell and stimulates B-cell proliferation (step 3). The binding of CD80 to CD28 on the Th cell stimulates IL-4 synthesis (step 4) and secretion (step 5). Binding of IL-4 to the IL-4 receptor on the B-cell directs class switching to IgE and cell proliferation (step 6).

The initial action of the cytokines is to stimulate germline gene transcription from promoters in the 5′ flanking sequence of the I region, corresponding to the target CH gene. Transcription proceeds from the initiation sites through I, S and CH and terminates in the 3′ flanking region of CH; finally, the transcripts are polyadenylated. This germline gene transcript (GLT) is spliced from the 3′ end of the I region to the 5′ end of the CH gene, and the mature transcript thus contains an I exon unique for each antibody class. The I exon in the germline gene transcript occupies the position of the VDJ exon in mRNA, synthesised after class switch recombination (CSR; Fig. 1B).

After CSR the B-cell expresses the new mIg, which allows further affinity maturation and antigen presentation to Th cells, leading to cell death or clonal expansion. mIg may also be a signal for isotype selection, as described below (B-cell differentiation). B-cells must undergo a substantial phenotypic change into the terminally differentiated plasma cell if they are to synthesise and secrete Igs. The choice between membrane and secreted Ig is made at the level of RNA splicing (Fig. 1B). To form the message for mIg the cell uses a splice site within the RNA sequence encoding the terminal exon ($C\varepsilon4$) which defines the secreted form; this is spliced to a down-stream membrane exon (m). The splice donor site at which this occurs is inactive in plasma cells. The plasma cell has a highly developed endoplasmic reticulum and devotes up to 50% of its protein synthesis activity to the secreted Ig.

Molecular mechanism of class switching to IgE

We now consider in more depth the sequence of steps involved in class switching, focusing, as far as the evidence allows, on human IgE. Information in this area is derived from studies on transgenic mice or mice with engineered gene defects (knock-out mice), as well as from human and murine cell systems and recombinant proteins and DNA sequences *in vitro*. The evident similarity of the known aspects in mouse and man justifies extrapolation to the human system. For example, CD40-L is required for heavy-chain switching to any of the antibody classes; hence, patients with defects in this gene present with the X-linked hyper-IgM syndrome and CD40-L knock-out mice exhibit a similar condition. The IL-4 receptor (IL-4R) and CD40 signalling cascades require highly homologous proteins in the two species. We discuss in turn germline gene transcription, DNA recombination and B-cell differentiation.

Germline gene transcription

More comprehensive reviews and extensive references are cited else-where[3–8]. Activation of ε-germline gene transcription is an essential gateway to IgE expression (see below). Both IL-4 and IL-13 induce ε-germline gene transcription in human B-cells, especially in synergy with a second signal through CD40. The second signal is also required for DNA recombination to Sε, in common with other switch variants. Human ε-GLT synthesis is initiated at multiple start sites within 90 bp of the furthest 3′ start site. Transcription proceeds through Iε, Sε and Cε, terminates in the 3′ flanking sequence of Cε, and is followed by poly-adenylation of the RNA precursor. The Iε exon of ~0.5 kb is spliced to Cε in the RNA, with deletion of the 3.5 kb intervening sequence, to yield the 1.7 kb ε-germline gene transcript; the ε-chain mRNA by contrast is 2.2 kb. Iε, like other mouse and human I exons, contains stop codons in all three reading frames and ε-GLT cannot, therefore, be translated into a protein fragment containing Cε.

The role of IL-4 in the activation of ε-germline gene transcription is now understood in terms of the signalling pathway between IL-4R on the cell membrane and the ε-germline gene in the cell nucleus (Fig. 3). The mouse and human ε-GLT promoters are highly homologous and conserve many of the same regulatory sequences. One such is the IL-4 response element, which is also common to the ε- and other genes, including those for the MHC class II antigen, the FcεRIα-chain, CD23b and the IL-4 gene itself. (Co-ordinate control of these five and possibly even more genes may be essential for orchestrating the effector functions IgE, once it is present.) IL-4R is a heterodimer of an α- and a γ-chain; the γ-chain is common to several cytokine receptors (IL-2, IL-7, IL-9 and IL-15). The IL-13 receptor (IL-13R) contains the same α-chain and a ligand-specific chain in place of the γ-chain. Dimerisation of IL-4R, contingent on ligand binding, leads to activation by cross-phosphoryl-ation of Jak1, attached to the α-chain, and Jak3, attached to the γ-chain. The ligand-specific chain of the IL-13R binds Tyk2 instead of Jak3. JAKS (Janus kinases) are a family (comprising Jaks1, 2 and 3 and Tyk2)

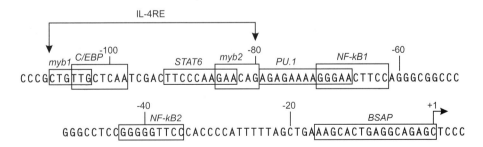

Fig. 3 The human ε-germline gene promoter. The 5′ flanking sequence of the template strand of the ε-germline gene, the Iε promoter sequence, with its various regulatory protein binding sites or response elements (REs) boxed. The response elements are identified in the text.

of tyrosine kinases involved in signal transduction through various cytokine receptors. The α-chain is then phosphorylated to generate docking sites for Stat6.

STATs (signal transducers and activators of transcription) are a family (comprising Stat1–6) of transcription factors. Tyrosine phosphorylation of the Stats allows them to form homodimeric or heterodimeric transcription factors, which migrate to the nucleus and there activate transcription from the IL-4 response elements. The sequence motif recognised by Stat6 is 5′-TTC($N_{3\ or\ 4}$)GAA-3′, where N can be any of the four bases. The different Stats recognise very similar sequences with subtle differences in affinity. Stat1 has a preference for N_3 and Stat6 for N_4. It may be significant that Stat6 binding sites, which will not bind other STAT proteins, are present in IL-4-inducible genes. The Stat6 site in the murine ε-germline gene does however bind the B-cell lymphoma (Bcl)-6 gene product, which may act to repress transcription in the absence of Stat6[7].

Full activation of the human Iε promoter in response to IL-4 and CD40 engagement requires a constellation of nuclear factors, which are either constitutively expressed or recruited to the promoter by specific activating signals (Fig. 3). The ε-germline promoter contains binding sites for endogenous myb proteins and a Stat6 element, partially overlapping the 3′ myb site. Because myb proteins are known to act as cell cycle sensors, the presence of myb binding sites may reflect a mechanism for the synchronisation of germline transcription, switch recombination and cell division in the cell cycle, as described below. Both Stat6 and myb interact with two proteins, p300 and CBP, which possess acetyltransferase activity and may, therefore, play a part in chromatin remodelling, as well as in the interaction with the basal transcription machinery, required for RNA chain initiation.

NF-κB binds to two distinct sites in the ε-germline gene promoter and co-operates with Stat6 in synergistic activation of transcription. In accordance with the well-known ability of CD40 signalling to induce NF-κB activation, the participation of these proteins may explain the CD40-dependent enhancement of IL-4-induced ε-germline gene transcription. NF-κB activity is at the same time essential for IL-4 responsiveness. Both effects most probably reflect the physical association between NF-κB/Rel proteins and Stat6[9,10]. Interaction with NF-κB appears to induce profound changes in the activity of Stat6: DNA binding affinity is substantially enhanced and most importantly *trans*-activating activity appears[10]. Activation of Stat6 or NF-κB requires no *de novo* protein synthesis, and both pass rapidly to the nucleus. More recently, a PU.1 binding site, overlapping with an NF-κB site further up-stream in the sequence of the promoter, has been found essential for activity of promoter constructs; This introduces another level of cell cycle regulation of ε-germline gene transcription[11].

Of special note is the binding site for the B-cell-specific activator protein (BSAP), which is expressed in a stage-dependent manner in the B-cell lineage from the pro-B to the mature B-cell, but not in plasma cells. BSAP binds to a highly conserved region immediately upstream of the major Iε transcription initiation site in murine and human B-cells. Overexpression of BSAP stimulates IgE and inhibits IgA expression in a mouse B-cell line[12]. Antisense-mediated down-regulation of BSAP inhibits cell proliferation, perhaps because BSAP represses transcription of the tumour suppressor gene, p53, and eliminates a block between the G1 and S phases of the cell cycle. TGF-β also inhibits transcription of the ε-germline gene and enhances transcription of the α-germline gene. IFN-γ secreted by Th-1 cells acts on bystander cells to inhibit ε-germline gene transcription by an unknown mechanism. The numerous regulatory elements in the ε-germline gene promoter may be needed to integrate the various signals reaching a B-cell at successive stages of its development and migration.

A different pathway is apparently required for the stimulation of B-cell proliferation by both IL-4 and IL-13. After phosphorylation of the α-chains by Jak 1 and Jak3, the insulin receptor substrates-1 and 2 (IRS-1 and IRS-2) are recruited to IL-4R and IL-13R, where they are phosphorylated by Fes and thus enabled to activate the phospho-inositol-3 (PI-3) kinase and the small ribosomal subunit protein, S6, kinase (p70^{S6K}) pathways, leading to cell proliferation. Increase in the B-cell clonal population is also promoted by the inhibition of apoptosis. Binding of SHIP, an inositol phosphatase, to IL-4R results in the phosphorylation of SHIP, and accompanying partial dephosphorylation of the products of PI-3 kinase; the latter activate the anti-apoptotic kinase, Akt. The negative regulation of these pathways has also been elucidated in great detail[8].

DNA recombination

More comprehensive reviews and extensive references are cited elsewhere[7,13–17]. The targets for class switch recombination (CSR) are the 1–10 kb S regions up-stream of all but one CH; the exception is Cδ, which is expressed by differential splicing of an mRNA precursor containing Cμ and Cδ. The S regions contain short (pentanucleotide) and long (20–80 bp) repeats, which show varying degrees of similarity to each other and to those in other S regions. Switch junctions can occur almost anywhere in the S regions, and to a lesser extent in the flanking sequences. They appear to be excluded from the I regions. No common sequences have been found at any fixed distance from or in the switch junctions, in contrast to the signal sequences in VDJ recombination sites[18–20].

Moreover, class switching occurs normally in mice deficient in the products of the recombination activating genes (Rag-1 and Rag-2), the nucleases responsible for site-specific DNA recognition and cleavage during VDJ recombination.

One peculiarity of S sequences is the presence of G-rich and C-rich runs, the latter concentrated in the template DNA strand. A possible function for these sequences is implied by the discovery of RNA loops (R-loops), formed by nascent germline gene transcripts following transcription of S region DNA *in vitro*[21]. An R-loop is an RNA–DNA hybrid, in which one strand of the DNA duplex is replaced by RNA complementary to the other strand of DNA (Fig. 4A). Such hybrids are a general feature of DNA transcription, persisting up to a length of 10–12 bp behind the last ribonucleotide to be added to the RNA chain. Beyond this length, as it reaches the trailing edge of the polymerase–protein complex the heteroduplex is actively dissociated to regenerate the double-stranded DNA template, with liberation of single-stranded RNA.

In switch regions, the nascent RNA–DNA hybrids may reach several hundred base pairs in length[21]. It is known that rG–dC polymers are more thermostable than the corresponding dG–dC polymers. As mentioned above, the template strand of S is rich in oligo-dC runs and this may well account for the unusual resistance of the RNA–DNA hybrid as RNA polymerase works through the S region. The R-loops formed by transcription of S regions *in vitro* can be cleaved by the nucleotide excision repair nucleases, XPF-ERCC1 and XPG[21], which function in general DNA repair processes. These may not be the nucleases that act during CSR *in vivo*.

For CSR to occur, two S regions, up to several megabases apart, must be cleaved on both strands with release of three DNA fragments, and the two outermost fragments must then be joined. How can chromosome 14 be cut into three fragments without falling apart? In VDJ recombination, this problem was in principle solved with the discovery of the 'synaptic complex' by Rag-1 and Rag-2 proteins, apposed at the two sites of recombination before and after DNA cleavage[22-25]. This mechanism is not available for CSR.

The fact that germline gene transcription always precedes CSR, and the conserved nature of the transcripts, both imply that germline gene transcripts are an essential feature of the CSR mechanism. It is now clear that transcription of the germline gene does not merely unfold the chromatin so that recombinases can gain access to the DNA[26]. Such a simple mechanism is at odds with several pieces of evidence: (i) when the I exon and its promoter are deleted from the mouse genome, no CSR occurs; (ii) when the I exon and its promoter are replaced by another promoter-gene construct, transcription ensues, but not necessarily CSR; (iii) if CSR is to occur, the replacement gene must contain an intron; and

(iv) removal of a 114 bp sequence containing the splice site from the replacement gene abrogates switching. It thus appears that transcription upstream of S and splicing of the RNA precursor are both required for CSR. The I exon of the germline gene transcript therefore plays more than a passive role in CSR.

A novel mechanism for tethering the fragments of chromosome 14 during CSR is based on the existence of hybrid germline gene transcripts (Fig. 1B)[27]. These contain an up-stream I spliced to a down-stream CH, but not the CH directly linked to I that can be merely one of several products of the splicing machinery at the site of germline gene transcription. Kinoshita and Honjo have suggested that the stalling of RNA polymerases in switch regions may allow random assembly of the donor and acceptor spliceosome components, leading to the generation of hybrid germline gene transcripts[28]. The volume within which this search proceeds would of course be limited by the length of DNA between the S regions. Ligation of the chromosome 14 fragments to breaks in other chromosomes, which could lead to oncogenic transformation of the B-cell (see Hiom et al.[29]), may thus be strictly contained.

The early stages of VDJ recombination are now well understood, thanks to the development of in vitro reconstitution systems. This approach is not yet available for the study of CSR. The late stages of VDJ recombination are less clear and may be similar in CSR. Both must occur by the process known as non-homologous recombination/end joining (NHEJ) or illegitimate recombination. Mammalian enzymes implicated in the NHEJ pathway fall into four complementation groups, XRCC4, XRCC5, XRCC6 and XRCC7[30-33]. XRCC4 associates with mammalian DNA ligase IV and may enhance its activity. The other three gene products are components of the DNA-activated protein kinase (DNA-PK)-Ku complex. DNA-PK is a member of the PI-3 kinase superfamily. Ku is a heterodimeric DNA end-binding protein that is the DNA-binding factor of the DNA-PK complex. XRCC5 and XRCC6 encode the 86 kDa and 70 kDa subunits of Ku, while XRCC7 encodes the kinase. Gene defects in any of the three loci block class switching, as well as VDJ recombination, and implicate these proteins in the repair mechanisms.

Even supposing that the 5'- and 3'-ends of the DNA are in random motion after scission of the two S regions involved in recombination, there may yet be a way for the two strands to unite without complementary base-pairing. Experiments with purified components in vitro showed that Ku was required for efficient ligation by DNA ligase IV under the stringent conditions (short or zero overlap, physiological salt and temperature) required for end-joining in cells[34]. Thus, while the formation of RNA-DNA hybrids and trans-splicing may tether the broken ends of the DNA, Ku may be required to bring them together (Figs 1B & 4B).

A R-loop

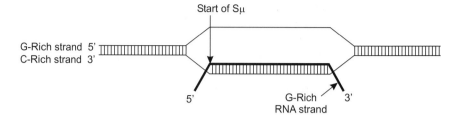

B Class switch recombination

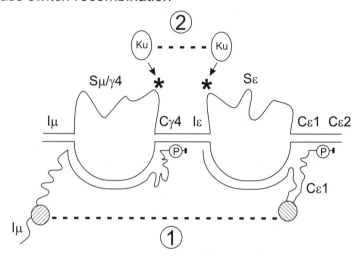

Fig. 4 Scheme for maintaining the continuity of chromosome 14 during CSR from IgG4 to IgE. (A) The RNA-loop (R-loop) generated by germline gene transcription through an S region[21]. (B) After formation of R-loops at Sμ and Sε, spliceosome subunits (hatched) bring the nascent RNAs into contact and catalyse splicing of Iμ to Cε (1). This is followed by cleavage of the DNA (*) and then non-homologous end-joining and repair facilitated by Ku (2). Stalled polymerases (P) may provide time for these events to occur.

VDJ and CSR recombination may occur following the recruitment of the DNA repair complex, termed MRN (comprising Mre11, Rad50 or Rad51 and Nbs1), to the broken DNA segments. Pieces of this puzzle have been assembled in the case of the more general double-strand break repair processes, *e.g.* X-irradiation-induced double-stranded breaks[35,36]. Histone 2AX (H2AX), a sub-type of histone 2A (H2A), associated with DNA in the region of double-stranded breaks, is found to be phosphorylated at a specific residue (ser139) in the C-terminal tail. (H2A is one of the four histones that make up the nucleosome structure of chromatin. The C-terminal tail is located near the linker region of DNA between nucleosomes, where it may affect the accessibility of the DNA.) Within several hours, H2AX recruits successively the breast cancer-related tumour suppressor gene, Brac1, product and the MRN complex. Mre11 acts as a 3′ to 5′ exonuclease and an endonuclease on single-stranded DNA and hairpin structures. Mre11 promotes the joining of non-complementary ends *in vitro* by pausing at sequences of short homology within the DNA sequences. Switch regions may thus be an ideal substrate for such activity. The Nijmegan breakage syndrome gene product (Nbs1) stimulates the unwinding of DNA duplexes and hairpin cleavage, while Rad50 is responsible for ATP binding by the MRN complex[37]. The participation of the MRN complex, and perhaps an error prone DNA polymerase, may account for the abundance of mutations, insertions and deletions observed in switch junctions.

A recent discovery by Honjo and colleagues promises to implicate yet another protein in CSR[38,39]. In their studies of class switching to IgA, induced by IL-4, TGF-β and anti-CD40 in the murine B lymphoma line, CH12F3-2B, they observed that the protein synthesis inhibitor, cycloheximide, inhibits CSR. They accordingly created a subtracted cDNA library, using mRNA from induced *versus* uninduced cells. This threw up a cDNA clone encoding a protein with homology to a family of cytidine deaminases. The closest homologue is APOBEC-1, which changes a C to a U in the mRNA for apolipoprotein, thus generating a termination codon. The resulting apolipoprotein mRNA codes for a truncated protein. The new protein from CH12F3-2B-cells is called activation-induced cytidine deaminase or AID.

Induction of AID begins in the CH12F3-2B-cells within 3 h, reaching a maximum at 48 h. Cycloheximide prevents the synthesis of AID, although germline gene transcription proceeds normally. Germline gene transcription depends on protein phosphorylation but not protein synthesis, as already mentioned. AID is expressed only in lymphoid tissue. It is up-regulated in mouse spleen by immunisation and appears during the period of class switching. AID knock-out mice exhibit a hyper-IgM syndrome, while overexpression of the protein leads to lymphoid hyperplasia, resembling that seen in human patients with the X-linked hyper-IgM syndrome (deficient in CD40-L; see above). A different group of patients with a hyper-IgM syndrome are now known to have lesions in the AID rather than the CD40-L gene[40]. The human AID gene has been mapped to chromosome 12[41]. The AID defect inhibits somatic hypermutation as well as CSR, but not VDJ recombination. The substrate of AID must be an RNA (ribozyme or mRNA) that participates in the first two processes only.

B-cell differentiation culminating in immunoglobulin synthesis and secretion

More comprehensive reviews and extensive references are cited elsewhere[42,43]. Class switching occurs in antigen (or surrogate antigen)-activated cells that are stimulated into cell cycle and proliferation. After a number of cell divisions, the cells may undergo one of three possible fates: they may die, or they may differentiate into memory B-cells or into plasma cells. Somewhere along the survival pathway they may switch to another antibody class. In the germinal centres of secondary lymphoid organs, on which most studies of somatic mutation, antibody affinity maturation and class switching have focused, cells mature along a defined pathway as they pass from one compartment to the next. Naïve B-cells are activated by specific antigen and cognate interaction with T cells outside of the germinal centres in the T cell-rich zone. Depending on the level of CD40 signalling, such B-cells differentiate into primary plasma cells secreting IgM or into founder B-cells, which enter the germinal centre reaction. After migrating into the dark zone of the germinal centre, the founder B-cells undergo rapid proliferation (6 h cycling time) and become centroblasts. Somatic hypermutation occurs at this stage. Migrating into the light zone as smaller centrocytes, the B-cells then compete for antigen, presented by follicular dendritic cells, and either die or progress into the extrafollicular T cell-rich zone. There they differentiate into memory B-cells or plasma cells. The different cell types are characterised by cell markers, on the basis of which separations can be achieved. Germline gene transcripts (GLTs) and switch circles are found only in centroblasts and centrocytes[44]: this fixes the time of class switching during B-cell development.

B-cell development has also been followed after stimulating the human B lymphoma line, CL-01, with IL-4, IL-10, IL-6 and CD40-L or anti-CD40 *in vitro*[45]. As before, GLTs and switch circles appear in the centroblast and centrocyte fractions. IL-6 is required for differentiation of the cells to plasmacytes, a process that is blocked by anti-IL-6. Anti-TGF-β inhibits the synthesis and secretion of IgA, while anti-IL-10 inhibits the synthesis of IgG (but not of Cγ CSR). Clearly then, despite the critical stages of germline gene transcription and DNA recombination, the fate of a B-cell is further determined, and IgE synthesis and secretion regulated, by post-CSR events accompanying cell differentiation.

Informative results have also emerged from studies on class switching in cytokine-stimulated B-cells as a function of cell cycle stage and the number of cell cycles completed. Hodgkin and co-workers separated murine B-cells, stimulated with IL-4 and anti-CD40, into populations which had divided from 1 to 10 times. Analysis of the antibodies produced by these cells showed that IgG appeared after about three rounds of replication and IgE after five[46]. These authors concluded that

CSR was a stochastic process with a probability determined by the number of cell divisions. *Trans*-splicing (Fig. 4B) could operate as a stochastic mechanism.

Other workers separated the B-cells at different stages of the cell cycle[47]. Germline gene transcripts were found only in cells that had progressed into cycle and had reached the G1/S boundary. Low numbers were found at the G2/M stage, when the DNA is replicated and the cells divide. If class switching involves DNA breakage and repair, this would make excellent sense, because genome integrity is required for viability during mitosis. This cell cycle connection may also shed light on the results of Hasbold and co-workers, mentioned above[46], as germline gene transcription is required for CSR and may need to be repeated in successive cycles for the chance event(s) to occur with sufficient frequency (Fig. 4B).

IL-4 does not uniquely specify IgE, for it also stimulates class switching to IgG and IgA. The probability of switching to IgE increases with the number of cell divisions, perhaps because the cell can switch to IgG or IgA1 before settling on IgE. Alternatively, the longer distance between the donor S and acceptor Sε may affect the probability of switching. Less obvious characteristics of the S region sequences, such as the length and conformation of single-stranded segments of the DNA, the nature and number of protein binding sites, the distribution of polymerase pausing sites and the existence of 'hot spots' for DNA cleavage, may also play a part.

Isotype selection at the post-CSR is a neglected subject. Some light is now beginning, however, to fall on this dark corner. We have dwelt on the synergism between IL-4R and CD40 in promoting ε-germline gene transcription. IL-4 also stimulates, by a less well-characterised pathway, changes in the cytoskeleton of B-cells, which engender the extrusion of microvilli and onset of motility[48]. IL-4 promotes homotypic association of B-cells and heterotypic association of B with T cells. These interactions may be important because the strength or duration of the B-cell-T cell contacts may govern the number of times the B-cell proliferates before differentiation into a plasma cell; this may determine whether CSR continues from IgG or IgA1 to IgE. Another Th-2 cell cytokine, IL-10, has different activities, and instead promotes the differentiation of cells that have undergone CSR at the Cγ1 or Cγ3 loci into IgG1- and IgG3-secreting plasma cells[49]. Premature differentiation may deprive the immature B-cells of the option to undergo a further switch to IgE. As B-cells proliferate and detach from the cell clusters, they must be exposed to autocrine and paracrine IL-6, which promotes cell differentiation.

IL-4 stimulates transcription of the gene for the low-affinity IgE receptor, CD23b, which first appears on the membranes of B-cells and is then proteolytically cleaved with release of a soluble fragment (sCD23). sCD23 induces B-cell differentiation into plasma cells and up-regulates

Bcl-2, thereby rescuing B-cells from apoptosis[50]. Bcl-2 may enable B-cells to complete a developmental programme without abortion. sCD23 has also been shown to stimulate class switching to IgE[51]. CD23 co-ligates sIgE and CD21 on the surface of B-cells (*see* Fig. 3 in Aubry *et al.*[52]). This provides a synergistic signal for the preferential growth of cells committed to IgE synthesis[53] and is thus a model for isotype-, as distinct from antigen affinity-based B-cell selection.

Conclusions

At the conclusion of Ig class switching, a B-cell secretes an antibody characterised by one of nine antibody classes and any one of an effectively infinite number of possible antigen specificities. The antigen specificity is fixed (except for somatic hypermutation), but class switching specifies the antibody class. Each of the three stages of this process – germline gene transcription, DNA recombination and B-cell differentiation – is biochemically complex, and the range of antibody classes that the B-cell may ultimately express is reduced at each stage. For IgE the activation of ε-germline gene transcription is essential, and the requirement for multiple rounds of cell division is critical for class switch recombination. At the final stage of B-cell differentiation, additional factors are involved in isotype determination, and IL-4 is once again required for IgE expression.

Acknowledgements

HJG thanks the Medical Research Council, The Wellcome Trust, The National Asthma Campaign and The British Lung Foundation for support. DV thanks the National Institutes of Health for support. We are grateful to Dr Martin Gellert, Dr Natalie McCloskey and Dr Walter Gratzer for helpful comments on the manuscript.

References

1 Rao A, Avni O. Molecular mechanisms of T-cell switching. *Br Med Bull* 2000; **56**: 969–984
2 Robinson DS. Th-2 cytokines in allergic disease. *Br Med Bull* 2000; **56**: 956–968
3 Agresti A, Vercelli, D. Regulation of ε-germline gene transcription: Q and A. In: Vercelli D. (ed) *IgE regulation*. Chichester: Wiley, 1997; 179–91
4 Chai SK, Rothman P. Cytokine signal transduction and its role in isotype class switching. In: Vercelli D. (ed) *IgE regulation*. Chichester: Wiley, 1997; 121–35
5 Bacharier LB, Jabara H, Geha RS. Molecular mechanisms of immunoglobulin E regulation. *Int Arch Allergy Immunol* 1998; **115**: 257–69
6 Oettgen HC, Geha RS. IgE in asthma and atopy: cellular and molecular connections. *J Clin Invest* 1999; **104**: 829–35

7   Oettgen HC. Regulation of the IgE isotype switch: new insights on cytokine signals and the functions of ε germline transcripts. *Curr Opin Immunol* 2000; **12**: 618–23

8   Jiang H, Harris M, Rothman P. IL-4/IL-13 signaling beyond JAK/STAT. *J Allergy Clin Immunol* 2000; **105**: 1063–70

9   Iciek LA, Delphin SA, Stavnezer J. CD40 cross-linking induces Igε germline transcripts in B-cells via activation of NF-κB: synergy with IL-4 induction. *J Immunol* 1997; **158**: 4769–79

10 Shen C-H, Stavnezer J. Interaction of Stat6 and NF-κB: direct association and synergistic activation of interleukin-4-induced transcription. *Mol Cell Biol* 1998; **18**: 3395–404

11 Stütz AM, Woisetschläger M. Functional synergism of STAT6 with either NF-κB or PU.1 to mediate IL-4-induced activation of IgE germline gene transcription. *J Immunol* 1999; **163**: 4383–91

12 Qui G, Stavnezer J. Overexpression of BSAP/Pax5 inhibits switching to IgA and enhances switching to IgE in the I.29µ B-cell line. *J Immunol* 1998; **161**: 2906–18

13 Coffman RL, Lebman DA, Rothman PB. Mechanism and regulation of immunoglobulin isotype switching. *Adv Immunol* 1993; **54**: 229–70

14 Stavnezer J. Antibody class switching. *Adv Immunol* 1996; **61**: 79–146

15 Siebenkotten G, Radbruch A. Switch transcripts and cytokine regulation of class switching. In: Vercelli D. (ed) *IgE regulation*. Chichester: Wiley, 1997; 143–54

16 Bottaro A, Alt FW. Class switch recombination: mechanism and specificity. In: Vercelli D. (ed) *IgE regulation*. Chichester: Wiley, 1997; 155–78

17 Stavnezer, J. Molecular processes that regulate class switching. *Curr Top Microbiol Immunol* 2000; **245**: 128–67

18 Lewis SM. The mechanism of V(D)J joining: lessons from molecular immunological, and comparative analyses. *Adv Immunol* 1994; **64**: 27–150

19 Gellert M. Recent advances in understanding V(D)J recombination. *Adv Immunol* 1997; **64**: 39–64

20 Oettinger MA. V(D)J recombination: on the cutting edge. *Curr Opin Cell Biol* 1999; **11**: 325–9

21 Tian M, Alt FW. Transcription-induced cleavage of immunoglobulin switch regions by nucleotide excision repair nucleases *in vitro*. *J Biol Chem* 2000; **275**: 24163–72

22 Bogue M, Roth DB. Mechanisms of V(D)J recombination. *Curr Opin in Immunol* 1996; **8**: 175–180

23 Hiom K, Gellert M. Assembly of a 12/23 paired signal complex: a critical control point in V(D)J recombination. *Mol Cell* 1998; **1**; 1011–9

24 Roth DB, Gellert M. Guardians of the genome. *Nature* 2000; **404**: 823–5

25 Roth DB, Roth SY. Unequal access: regulating V(D)J recombination through chromatin remodelling. *Cell* 2000; **103**: 699–702

26 Snapper CM, Marcu KB, Zelazowski P. The immunoglobulin class switch: beyond 'accessibility'. *Immunity* 1997; **6**: 217–23

27 Fujieda S, Lin YQ, Saxon A, Zhang K. Multiple types of chimeric germ-line Ig heavy chain transcripts in human B-cells: evidence for *trans*-splicing of human Ig RNA. *J Immunol* 1996; **157**: 3450–59

28 Kinoshita K, Honjo T. Unique and unprecedented recombination mechanism in class switching. *Curr Opin Immunol* 2000; **12**: 195–8

29 Hiom K, Melek M, Gellert M. DNA transposition by the RAG1 and RAG2 proteins: a possible source of oncogenic translocations. *Cell* 1998; **94**; 463–70

30 Weaver DT. What to do at an end: DNA double-strand-break repair. *Trends Genet* 1995; **11**: 388–92

31 Jackson SP, Jeggo PA. DNA double-strand break repair and V(D)J recombination: involvement of DNA-PK. *Trends Biochem* 1995; **20**: 412–5

32 Critchlow SE, Jackson SP. DNA end-joining: from yeast to man. *Trends Biochem* 1998; **23**; 394–8

33 Featherstone C, Jackson SP. DNA double-strand break repair. *Curr Biol* 1999; **9**: R759–61

34 Ramsden DA, Gellert M. Ku protein stimulates DNA end joining by mammalian ligases: a direct role for Ku in repair of DNA double-strand breaks. *EMBO J* 1998; **17**: 609–14

35 Paull TT, Rogakou EP, Yamazaki V *et al*. A critical role for histone H2AX in recruitment of repair factors to nuclear foci after DNA damage. *Curr Biol* 2000; **10**: 886–95

36 Paull TT, Gellert M. A mechanistic basis for Mre11-directed DNA joining at microhomologies. *Proc Natl Acad Sci USA* 2000; **97**: 6409–14

37 Paull TT, Gellert M. Nbs1 potentiates ATP-driven DNA unwinding and endonuclease cleavage by the Mre11/Rad50 complex *Genes Dev* 1999; **13**: 1276–88

38 Muramatsu M, Sankaranand VS, Anant S *et al*. Specific expression of activation-induced cytidine deaminase (AID), a novel member of the RNA-editing deaminase family in germinal center B-cells. *J Biol Chem* 1999; **274**: 18470–6

39 Muramatsu M, Kinoshita K, Fagarasan S *et al*. Class switch recombination and hypermutation require activation-induced cytidine deaminase (AID), a potential RNA editing enzyme. *Cell* 2000; **103**: 553–63

40 Revy P, Muto T, Levy Y *et al*. Activation-induced cytidine deaminase (AID) deficiency causes autosomal recessive form of the hyper-IgM syndrome. *Cell* 2000; **102**: 565–75

41 Muto, T, Muramatsu M, Taniwaki M, Kinoshita K, Honjo T. Isolation, tissue distribution, and chromosomal localization of the human activation-induced cytidine deaminase (AID) gene. *Genomics* 2000; **68**: 85–8

42 Gordon J, Pound JD. Fortifying B-cells with CD154: an engaging tale of many hues. *Immunology* 2000; **100**: 269–8l

43 Gould HJ, Beavil RL, Reljic R *et al*. IgE homeostasis: is CD23 the safety switch? In: Vercelli D. (ed) *IgE regulation*. Chichester: Wiley, 1997; 37–60

44 Liu YJ, Malisan F, Bouteiller O *et al*. Within germinal centers, isotype switching of immunoglobulin genes occurs after the onset of somatic mutation. *Immunity* 1996; **4**: 241–50

45 Cerutti A, Zan H, Schaffer A *et al*. CD40 ligand and appropriate cytokines induce switching to IgG, IgA, and IgE and coordinated germinal center and plasmacytoid phenotypic differentiation in a human monoclonal IgM+IgD+ B-cell line. *J Immunol* 1998; **160**: 2145–57

46 Hasbold J, Lyons AB, Kehry MR, Hodgkin PD. Cell division number regulates IgG1 and IgE switching of B-cells following stimulation by CD40 ligand and IL-4. *Eur J Immunol* 1998; **28**: 1040–51

47 Lundgren M, Strom L, Bergqvist LO *et al*. Cell cycle regulation of germline immunoglobulin transcription: potential role of ets family members. *Eur J Immunol* 1990; **25**: 2042–51

48 Davey EJ, Thyberg J, Conrad DH, Severinson E. Regulation of cell morphology in B lymphocytes by IL-4: evidence for induced cytoskeletal changes. *J Immunol* 1998; **160**: 5366–73

49 Malisan F, Brière F, Bridon J-M *et al*. Interleukin IL-10 induces immunoglobulin G isotype switch recombination in human CD40-activated naïve B lymphocytes. *J Exp Med* 1996; **183**: 937–47

50 Liu, Y-J, Cairns JA, Holder MJ *et al*. Recombinant 25 kDa CD23 and interleukin 1α promote the survival of germinal center B-cells: evidence for bifurcation in the development of centrocytes rescued from apoptosis. *Eur J Immunol* 1991; **21**: 1107–14

51 Aubry J-P, Pochon S, Graber P, Jansen KU, Bonnefoy J-Y. CD21 is a ligand for CD23 and regulates IgE production. *Nature* 1992; **358**: 505–7

52 Sutton BJ, Beavil RL, Beavil AJ. Inhibition of IgE receptor interactions. *Br Med Bull* 2000; **56**: 1004–1018

53 Reljic R, Cosentino G, Gould HJ. Function of CD23 in the response of human B-cells to antigen. *Eur J Immunol* 1997; **27**: 572–5

Food anaphylaxis

Hugh A Sampson

Professor of Pediatrics and Biomedical Sciences, The Mount Sinai School of Medicine, New York, New York, USA

Food anaphylaxis is now the leading single cause of anaphylactic reactions treated in emergency departments in Westernized countries. In the US, it is estimated that there are 29,000 anaphylactic reactions to foods treated in emergency departments and 125–150 deaths each year. Peanuts, tree nuts, fish and shellfish account for the vast majority of severe food anaphylactic reactions. Immunopathogenic mechanisms responsible for food anaphylaxis may differ somewhat from other forms of anaphylaxis, since elevation of serum tryptase is rarely seen following food anaphylactic reactions. Education regarding the strict avoidance of food allergens, the early recognition of anaphylactic symptoms, and the early use of self-injectable epinephrine remain the mainstays of therapy. However, clinical trials are now underway for the treatment of patients with peanut anaphylaxis utilizing anti-IgE antibody therapy and novel immunomodulatory therapies utilizing 'engineered' recombinant proteins, overlapping peptides, and immunostimulatory deoxyoligonucleotide sequences are being tested in animal models of anaphylaxis.

Three years after Portier and Richet first described anaphylaxis[1], Schlossman reported the first case of food anaphylaxis in the US[2], but it was not until 1969 that the first series of food anaphylaxis in man was published[3]. Now food anaphylaxis is the leading single cause of anaphylaxis treated in American emergency departments[4,5], a change some feel has come about in the last 10–20 years. Food anaphylaxis is an allergic syndrome manifested by an abrupt onset of symptoms within minutes to hours of ingesting a food and is associated with the classic features of IgE-mediated hypersensitivity. The syndrome results from the generation and release of a variety of potent biologically active mediators and their combined effects on various target organs. Anaphylaxis is recognized by cutaneous, respiratory, cardiovascular, and gastrointestinal signs and symptoms occurring singly or in combination. The majority of food anaphylactic reactions in the US and Europe are the result of allergic reactions to peanuts, tree nuts, fish and shellfish.

Correspondence to:
Prof. Hugh A Sampson,
Department of Pediatrics
Box 1198, The Mount
Sinai School of Medicine,
One Gustave L Levy Place,
New York,
NY 10029-6574, USA

Prevalence

The prevalence of food anaphylactic reactions appears to vary somewhat with the dietary habits of a region. In Denmark, Sorensen found a prevalence of 3.2 cases per 100,000 inhabitants per year with ~5% fatality rate[6]. In a more recent US survey, Yocum reported an annual incidence of food anaphylaxis of 7.6 cases per 100,000 person-years and a food anaphylaxis occurrence rate of 10.8 per 100,000 person-years[5]. The figures were based on a review of the medical records of Olmsted County inhabitants followed in the Rochester Epidemiology Study from 1983 to 1987. Based on this survey, one would predict about 29,000 food anaphylactic episodes in the US each year resulting in approximately 2000 hospitalizations and 150 deaths. Food anaphylactic reactions accounted for over one-third of anaphylactic reactions treated in emergency departments and were most often due to peanut, tree nuts, fish or shellfish. Pumphrey[7] in the UK and Moneret-Vautrin[8] in France reported similar findings. A survey of South Australian preschool and school-age children revealed a parent-reported food anaphylaxis rate of 0.43 per 100 school children, which accounted for over one-half of all cases of anaphylaxis in this age group[9]. Similarly, Novembre reported that food allergy was responsible for about one-half of severe anaphylactic episodes in Italian children treated in emergency departments[10]. While food anaphylaxis accounts for one-third to one-half of anaphylaxis cases treated in emergency departments in North America, Europe and Australia[5,7,9–13], it seems to be uncommon in non-Westernized countries.

In 1988, Yunginger reported 7 cases of fatal food anaphylaxis evaluated during a 16 month period[14], and, in 1992, we reported 6 fatal and 7 near-fatal food anaphylactic reactions in children (ages 2–17 years) that occurred in 3 metropolitan areas over a 14 month period[15]. Common risk factors for these severe reactions included the following: asthma (even if well controlled); inability to identify the responsible food allergen in the meal, previous allergic reactions to the incriminated food, although in most cases symptoms had been much milder; and all patients had immediate symptoms with about half experiencing a quiescent period prior to a major respiratory collapse. In both series, no patient who died received adrenaline immediately; however, in more recent reports, 7–10% of patients receiving injected epinephrine failed to reverse anaphylactic symptoms.[7,14] In a series of 48 fatal cases of food anaphylaxis reviewed by Pumphrey[7], 3 patients received epinephrine from a self-administration kit appropriately at the onset of their reaction, which failed to prevent a fatal outcome. Of 32 fatal food anaphylaxis cases reported by Bock and co-workers[14], 2 of 32 individuals experiencing fatal outcomes had received intramuscular epinephrine immediately but failed to respond. Interestingly, in most cases of fatal food anaphylaxis in which serum tryptase was measured, a significant increase in tryptase was not found, raising some question about the exact mechanism involved in food anaphylaxis[15].

Table 1 Foods most frequently implicated in food anaphylaxis

Peanuts	
Tree nuts	Walnuts, hazel nuts (filberts), cashews, pistachios, Brazil nuts, pine nuts, almonds
Fish	Less often tuna
Shellfish	Shrimp, crab, lobster, oyster, scallop]
Milk	Cow, goat
Chicken eggs	
Seeds	Cotton seed, sesame seed, mustard seed, psyllium
Fruit	Kiwi

Reports of food anaphylaxis associated with exercise (food-associated exercise-induced anaphylaxis) have been reported with increasing frequency, possibly due to the increased popularity of aerobic exercising over the past decade. Two forms of food anaphylaxis associated with exercise have been described: reactions following the ingestion of specific foods (e.g. celery, shellfish, wheat)[16–18], and, rarely, reactions following the ingestion of any food[19]. In most cases, anaphylaxis occurs when an afflicted individual exercises within 2–4 h of ingesting a specific food. Otherwise, the patient can ingest the food without any apparent reaction and can exercise without any apparent reaction as long as the specific food has not been ingested within the past several hours. This disorder appears to be twice as common in females and > 60% of cases occur in individuals less than 30 years of age. In a recent survey of 199 individuals experiencing exercise-induced anaphylaxis, ingestion of food within 2 h of exercise was felt to be a factor in the development of attacks in about one-half of the cases[19]. Symptoms often start with pruritus about the scalp that becomes more generalized. Urticaria and flushing are common followed by respiratory obstruction, and sometimes cardiovascular collapse. Patients with specific food anaphylaxis associated with exercise usually have positive skin tests to the food that provokes symptoms and occasionally have a history of reacting to the food when they were younger.

Foods implicated in anaphylaxis

The list of foods implicated in anaphylactic reactions is unlimited and, in theory, any food protein is capable of causing an anaphylactic reaction. As indicated in Table 1, certain foods appear more likely to provoke severe or fatal anaphylaxis, although any food may be the cause. In Westernized countries, peanuts and tree nuts[4,7,14,15] fish (*e.g.* cod, whitefish), and shellfish (shrimp, lobster, crab, scallops, oyster)[11] are most often implicated. Unfortunately, these foods tend to induce 'life-long sensitivities' in contrast to other foods frequently associated with allergy, such as milk, eggs, and soybeans.

Signs and symptoms of food anaphylaxis

Symptoms of food anaphylaxis may appear within seconds to a few hours after the food allergen is ingested, with the vast majority developing within the first hour. In general, the more prolonged the onset of anaphylactic symptoms, the less severe the overall reaction. About one-third of patients will experience a biphasic reaction[15]. In such cases, patients develop classical symptoms of anaphylaxis, appear to recover (and may become asymptomatic) and then experience a recurrence of symptoms. Bronchospasm often is severe and largely refractory to β-agonists leading to severe hypoxia. While severe initial symptoms more often precede the biphasic response, this is not always the case and premature discharges from emergency departments have resulted in fatal outcomes due to the second phase response. The intervening 'quiescent' period typically lasts for up to 1–3 h, so patients should be observed for about 4 h after initial symptoms abate. In a report of 7 cases of near-fatal food anaphylaxis, three experienced protracted anaphylaxis, with symptoms lasting from 1 day to 3 weeks[15]. Most reports suggest that the earlier epinephrine is administered in the course of anaphylaxis the better the chance of a favourable outcome. However, this does not necessarily prevent biphasic or protracted symptoms, and as noted above, does not always prevent fatal anaphylaxis.

Table 2 Clinical signs and symptoms of anaphylaxis

Oral	Pruritus of lips, tongue and palate, and oedema of lips and tongue	
Gastrointestinal	Nausea, abdominal pain (colic), vomiting (large amounts of 'stringy' mucus), and diarrhoea	
Skin	Flushing, pruritus, urticaria, angio-oedema, morbilliform rash, and pilor erecti	
Respiratory (major shock organ		
	Laryngeal	Pruritus and 'tightness' in the throat, dysphagia, dysphonia and hoarseness, dry 'staccato' cough, and sensation of itching in the external auditory canals
	Lung	Shortness of breath, dyspnoea, chest tightness, 'deep' cough, and wheezing
	Nose	Pruritus, congestion, rhinorrhoea, and sneezing
Cardiovascular	Feeling of faintness, syncope, chest pain, arrhythmia, hypotension	
Other	Peri-orbital pruritus, erythema and oedema, conjunctival erythema, and tearing; uterine contractions in women, and aura of 'doom'	

The symptoms of anaphylaxis are generally related to the skin, gastro-intestinal tract, respiratory tract, and cardiovascular systems (Table 2). The sequence, timing and severity of symptoms are highly variable among individuals, and may even vary in the same individual in response to different foods. Subsequent anaphylactic reactions to a food often provokes similar allergic symptoms, but reactions in patients with asthma and peanut, nut and/or seafood allergy appear to be somewhat less predictable. Peanut allergic toddlers, who reacted with minimal cutaneous and gastrointestinal symptoms before developing asthma, frequently experience severe anaphylactic reactions after ingesting peanut in later years.

The first symptoms experienced in food anaphylaxis often involve the oral cavity and throat. Symptoms may include tingling, pruritus and oedema of the lips, oral mucosa, palate, and pharynx. Young children may be seen scratching at their tongue, palate, anterior neck, or external auditory canals. These symptoms should not be confused with a similar symptom complex in patients with oral allergy syndrome due to cross-reactivity with birch, ragweed, grass or mugwort pollens. Evidence of laryngeal oedema includes a 'dry staccato' cough and/or dysphonia and dysphagia. In Pumphrey's series, severe upper airway oedema was considered the cause of death in ~10% of cases[20], but this has not been reported in other series. Gastrointestinal symptoms frequently follow including nausea, colicky abdominal pain, vomiting and diarrhoea. Emesis may contain large amounts of 'stringy' mucus. Skin symptoms during anaphylaxis may include flushing, urticaria, angio-oedema, and/or an erythematous macular rash, but may be absent in severe reactions[15]. Respiratory symptoms often consist of a deep repetitive cough, stridor, dyspnoea, and/or wheezing. The development of cardiovascular symptoms along with airway obstruction is of greatest concern in anaphylactic reactions. In the second phase of the biphasic response, it is often extremely difficult to ventilate patients due to extreme broncho-spasm, and tension pneumothoraces are a frequent complication of high ventilatory pressure. Cardiovascular symptoms may include syncope, a feeling of faintness, palpitations and/or chest pain. Hypotension or shock may be the result of vascular collapse, cardiac arrhythmia, or asphyxia. Anaphylaxis may be complicated by myocardial ischaemia.

Other signs and symptoms reported frequently in food-induced anaphylaxis include peri-ocular and nasal pruritus, sneezing, diaphoresis, disorientation, faecal or urinary urgency or incontinence, and uterine cramping in women (lower back pain). Patients often report a 'sense of doom'. In some instances the initial manifestation of anaphylaxis may be the loss of consciousness. Death may ensue in minutes but has been reported to occur days to weeks after anaphylaxis[21]. In 6 cases of fatal food-induced anaphylaxis[15], initial symptoms developed within 3–30 min and severe respiratory symptoms within 20–150 min. Symptoms involved the lower respiratory tract in all children, the gastrointestinal tract in 5 of 6, and the skin in only 1 of 6 children. The clinician must be aware that skin symptoms may be absent in food anaphylaxis.

Several factors appear to predispose individuals to more severe food anaphylaxis including a personal history of atopy, older age, the presence of asthma, and the particular food to which they are allergic[15,22,23]. In the reports of Yunginger[14] and Sampson[15], individuals were highly atopic and all had histories of asthma. Although atopy reportedly does not predispose individuals to an increased risk of anaphylaxis[24], it does tend to predispose to more severe reactions.

Diagnostic features

In light of its abrupt and dramatic nature, the diagnosis of food anaphylaxis is generally readily apparent (Table 2). Occasionally disorders such as scombroid poisoning, aspiration with upper airway obstruction, myocardial infarction, or a hysterical reaction may be mistaken for food anaphylaxis. In the majority of cases where a food is implicated, the responsible food is apparent from the temporal relationship between the ingestion and the onset of symptoms. When evaluating the cause of anaphylaxis, a very careful history is critical, especially when the cause of the episode is not straightforward. Specific questions should include whether any other precipitating factors appear to be involved, such as exercise. In cases where the aetiology of the anaphylactic reaction is not apparent, a dietary history should review all ingredients of the suspected meal including any possible concealed ingredients or food additives. The food provoking the reaction may often be a minor ingredient in the meal or a contaminant[25].

The laboratory evaluation of a food anaphylaxis is generally directed at testing a patient for specific IgE antibodies to the food in question. Limited prick skin testing or RAST determinations are necessary to demonstrate whether the patient possesses IgE antibodies to the suspected aetiological agent. In individuals with negative prick skin test to a suspected food, intradermal skin tests are sometimes performed. However, a positive intradermal test following a negative prick test is of questionable significance, unlikely to reflect clinical sensitivity[26], and probably should not be performed. In addition, anaphylactic reactions (including fatal reactions) following intradermal skin tests to foods have been documented[27]. In typical anaphylactic reactions, massive activation of mast cells during anaphylaxis results in a dramatic rise in plasma histamine and somewhat later a rise in plasma or serum tryptase[28–30]. Following the onset of symptoms in a food anaphylactic reaction, plasma histamine rises over the first several minutes of a reaction and generally remains elevated for only a few minutes[28]. Quantitation of plasma histamine requires special collection techniques not generally available in emergency departments and consequently is impractical except in research situations. Whether measurement of urinary methyl-histamine is useful for confirming anaphylaxis remains to be demonstrated. In bee sting and drug-induced anaphylaxis, serum tryptase has been shown to rise over the first hour and may remain elevated for up to 12 h.[29,30] It is stable at room temperature and can be obtained from post-mortem specimens. Strangely, serum tryptase is rarely elevated in food anaphylaxis[15]. The reason for this is not clear, but suggests that other cells, such as basophils or monocytes/macrophages may be more important in the pathogenesis of food anaphylaxis.

Food challenges are usually contra-indicated in patients with an clear-cut history of anaphylaxis following the isolated ingestion of a food to which they have IgE antibodies. However, in many cases patients have ingested several foods prior to their anaphylactic reaction and have positive skin tests to several foods. In such cases it is essential that the responsible food be identified and physician-supervised food challenges are warranted. Many young children who experience food anaphylaxis eventually outgrow their clinical reactivity (except to peanuts, tree nuts, fish and shellfish), so an oral challenge is appropriate following an extended period of food elimination with no history of adverse reactions. In these patients, quantitating their level of food-specific IgE antibodies may be useful in determining when they have 'outgrown' their sensitivity and it is safe to challenge them[31].

Treatment

Acute management of food anaphylaxis

Treatment of food anaphylaxis is similar to treatment of anaphylaxis of other causes. A review of fatal anaphylactic reactions due to bee stings indicated that the longer the initial therapy is delayed, the greater the incidence of complications and fatalities[21]. Reports of fatal food anaphylaxis have suggested similar findings[7,14,15]. Initial treatment must be preceded by a rapid assessment to determine the extent and severity of the reaction, the adequacy of oxygenation, cardiac output, and tissue perfusion, any potential confounding medications, and the suspected cause of the reaction[32]. Initial therapy should be directed at the maintenance of an effective airway and circulatory system. Intra-muscular epinephrine (adrenaline) is the drug of choice in the treatment of anaphylaxis (0.01 ml/kg of aqueous epinephrine 1:1000; maximal dose 0.3–0.5 ml, or 0.3–0.5 mg)[33,34]. Although there are reports suggesting that inhalation of racemic epinephrine may be used as an alternative form of therapy for anaphylaxis[35,36], a recent controlled trial failed to confirm the efficacy of this therapeutic approach in children[20]. In patients with pulmonary symptoms, supplemental oxygen should be administered.

Epinephrine for self-administration should be prescribed to individuals at high risk for food anaphylaxis, *i.e.* food allergic patients who have asthma (regardless of the severity) or who have experienced a previous reaction involving the airway or cardiovascular systems. In addition, their family members and other care-providers should be instructed in the administration of epinephrine. Preloaded syringes with epinephrine generally are recommended for use in emergency situations, since both the patient and care-givers are typically very distraught and the scene often chaotic. In the US, there are two forms of premeasured epinephrine: Epi-Pen® and Ana-Kit®. The Epi-Pen® is a disposable drug delivery system with a spring-activated, concealed needle used for a single intramuscular injection. It comes in two forms: the Epi-Pen® – 0.3 mg for adults and the Epi-Pen Jr® – 0.15 mg for children less than 22–5 kg. The Ana-Kit® contains a syringe with two doses of 0.3 mg of epinephrine. Sustained-release preparations of epinephrine are not appropriate treatment for acute anaphylaxis. Inhaled epinephrine may be beneficial to reverse laryngeal oedema or persistent bronchospasm, but should not be considered first-line therapy.

Studies suggest that the combination of H_1 antihistamines (*i.e.* diphenhydramine – 1 mg/kg up to 75 mg) and H_2 antihistamines (*e.g.* 4 mg/kg up to 300 mg of cimetidine) may be more effective than either administered alone[37]. Patients at risk for food anaphylaxis should be provided with liquid forms of these preparations for immediate use if an inadvertent ingestion is suspected. Many authorities recommend giving prednisone (1 mg/kg orally) for mild-to-moderate episodes of anaphylaxis and solumedrol (1–2 mg/kg intravenously) for severe anaphylaxis in an attempt to modulate the late-phase response. If wheezing is prominent, an aerosolized β-adrenergic agent (*i.e.* albuterol) is recommended intermittently or continuously, depending upon the patient's symptoms and the availability of cardiac monitoring. Hypotension may be severe and prove refractory to epinephrine and antihistamines. Depending upon the blood pressure, large volumes of crystalloid (*e.g.* lactated Ringer's solution or normal saline) infused rapidly are frequently required to reverse the hypotensive state.

Long-term management of food anaphylaxis

The life-threatening nature of anaphylaxis makes prevention the cornerstone of therapy. The central focus of prevention necessitates appropriate identification and complete dietary avoidance of the responsible food allergen. Certain factors place some individuals at increased risk for more severe anaphylactic reactions: (i) history of a previous anaphylactic reaction; (ii) history of asthma, especially if poorly controlled; (iii) allergy to peanuts, nuts, fish, and shellfish; and (iv) patients on β-blockers or ACE-inhibitors. Education is imperative to ensure the patient and the family understand how to avoid all forms of the food allergen and the potential severity of a reaction if the food is inadvertently ingested. In addition, patients at risk for food anaphylaxis should carry medical information concerning their condition, *e.g.* Medic Alert® bracelet, emergency medications, and a treatment plan with them at all times. This information may be life-saving, since it can expedite the diagnosis and appropriate treatment of a patient experiencing an anaphylactic reaction.

Future management of food anaphylaxis

An attempt to 'desensitize' patients with peanut anaphylaxis with standard immunotherapy was found to have an unacceptable risk:benefit ratio[38,39]. Consequently, new strategies are being investigated to 'desensitize' food-allergic patients. A trial of anti-IgE therapy for the treatment of patients with peanut anaphylaxis is underway in the US. In addition, new immunotherapeutic approaches utilizing 'engineered' recombinant peanut proteins, overlapping peptides of peanut allergens, and the addition of oligodeoxynucleotide immunostimulatory sequences to peanut proteins have all appeared promising for reversing peanut anaphylaxis in our murine model of peanut allergy (Li *et al.* in press). While the aetiology of the apparent increase in atopy and food allergy in Westernized countries remain unknown, it is hoped that safe, efficacious forms of immunotherapy will be available within the next decade to treat food anaphylaxis.

References

1   Portier P, Richet C. De l'action anaphylactique de certains venins. *C R Soc Biol (Paris)* 1902; **54**: 170–2

2   Anderson JA, Sogn DD. *Adverse Reactions to Foods*. NIH Public. #84-2442, 2. Bethesda, MD: National Institute of Allergy & Infectious Disease 1984

3   Goldbert TM, Pattereon R, Pruzansky JJ. Systemic allergic reactions to ingested antigens. *J Allergy* 1969; **44**: 96–107

3   Yocum MW, Khan DA. Assessment of patients who have experienced anaphylaxis: a 3-year survey. *Mayo Clin Proc* 1994; **69**: 16–23

5   Yocum MW, Butterfield JH, Klein JS, Volcheck GW, Schroeder DR, Silverstein MD. Epidemiology of anaphylaxis in Olmsted County: a population-based study. *J Allergy Clin Immunol* 1999; **104**: 452–6

6   Sorensen H, Nielsen B, Nielsen J. Anaphylactic shock occurring outside hospitals. *Allergy* 1989; **44**: 288–90

7   Pumphrey RSH, Stanworth SJ. The clinical spectrum of anaphylaxis in north-west England. *Clin Exp Allergy* 1996; **26**: 1364–70

8   Moneret-Vautrin DA, Kanny G. Food-induced anaphylaxis. A new French multicenter survey. *Ann Gastroenterol Hepatol* 1995; **31**: 256–63

9   Boros CA, Kay D, Gold MS. Parent reported allergy and anaphylaxis in 4173 south Australian children. *J Paediatr Child Health* 2000; **36**: 36–40

10 Novembre E, Cianferoni A, Bernardini R *et al*. Anaphylaxis in children: clinical and allergologic features. *Pediatrics* 1998; **101**: E8-1–E8/8

11 Kemp SF, Lockey RF, Wolf BL *et al*. Anaphylaxis: a review of 266 cases. *Arch Intern Med* 1995; **155**: 1749–54

12 Nissim A, Schwarzbaum S, Siraganian R, Eshhar Z. Fine specificity of the IgE interaction with the low and high affinity Fcε receptor. *J Immunol* 1993; **150**: 1365–74

13 Helm BA, Sayers I, Higginbotton A *et al*. Identification of the high affinity receptor binding region in human immunoglobulin E. *J Biol Chem* 1996; **271**: 7494–500

14 Yunginger JW, Sweeney KG, Sturner WQ *et al*. Fatal food-induced anaphylaxis. *JAMA* 1988; **260**: 1450–2

15 Sampson HA, Mendelson LM, Rosen JP. Fatal and near-fatal anaphylactic reactions to food in children and adolescents. *N Engl J Med* 1992; **327**: 380–4

16 Dohi M, Suko M, Sugiyama H *et al*. Food-dependent, exercise-induced anaphylaxis: a study on 11 Japanese cases. *J Allergy Clin Immunol* 1991; **87**: 34–40

17 Romano A, Fonso M, Giuffreda F *et al*. Diagnostic work-up for food-dependent, exercise-induced anaphylaxis. *Allergy* 1995; **50**: 817–24

18 Kushimito H, Aoki T. Masked type I wheat allergy – relation to exercise-induced anaphylaxis. *Arch Dermatol* 1985; **121**: 355–60

19 Horan RF, Sheffer AL. Food-dependent exercise-induced anaphylaxis. *Immunol Allergy Clin North Am* 1991; **11**: 757–66

20 Gu X, Simons KJ, Johnston L, Gillespie C, Simons EF. Can epinephrine inhalations be substituted for epinephrine injection in children at risk for systemic anaphylaxis? *J Allergy Clin Immunol* 2000; **105**: S276

21 Barnard J. Studies of 400 *Hymentoptera* sting deaths in the United States. *J Allergy Clin Immunol* 1973; **52**: 259–64

22 Atkins FM, Steinberg SS, Metcalfe DD. Evaluation of immediate adverse reactions to foods in adult patients. I. Correlation of demographic, laboratory, and prick skin test data with response to controlled oral food challenges. *J Allergy Clin Immunol* 1985; **75**: 348–55

23 DeMartino M, Novembre E, Gozza G, DeMarco A, Bonazza P, Verucci A. Sensitivity to tomato and peanut allergens in children monosensitized to grass pollen. *Allergy* 1988; **43**: 206–13

24 Settipane GA, Klein DE, Boyd GK. Relationship of atopy and anaphylactic sensitization: a bee sting allergy model. *Clin Allergy* 1978; **8**: 259–64

25 Gern J, Yang E, Evrard H, Sampson H. Allergic reactions to milk-contaminated 'non-dairy' products. *N Engl J Med* 1991; **324**: 976–9

26 Bock S, Buckley J, Holst A, May C. Proper use of skin tests with food extracts in diagnosis of food hypersensitivity. *Clin Allergy* 1978; **8**: 559–64

27 Lockey R, Benedict L, Turkeltaub P, Bukantz S. Fatalities form immunotherapy and skin testing. *J Allergy Clin Immunol* 1987; **79**: 660–7

28 Sampson HA, Jolie PL. Increased plasma histamine concentrations after food challenges in children with atopic dermatitis. *N Engl J Med* 1984; **311**: 372–6

29 Schwartz L, Yunginger J, Miller J *et al*. The time course of appearance and disappearance of human mast cell tryptase in the circulation after anaphylaxis. *J Clin Invest* 1989; **83**: 1551–5

30 Schwartz L, Metcalfe D, Miller J *et al*. Tryptase levels as an indicator of mast cell activation in systemic anaphylaxis and mastocytosis. *N Engl J Med* 1987; **316**: 1622–6

31 Sampson H, Ho D. Relationship between food-specific IgE concentration and the risk of positive food challenges in children and adolescents. *J Allergy Clin Immunol* 1997; **100**: 444–51

32 Bochner BS, Lichtenstein LM. Anaphylaxis. *N Engl J Med* 1991; **324**: 1785–90

33 Simons EF, Roberts JR, Gu X, Simons KJ. Epinephrine absorption in children with a history of anaphylaxis. *J Allergy Clin Immunol* 1998; **101**: 33–7

34 Muller U, Mosbech H, Aberer W *et al*. EAACI position statement: adrenaline for emergency kits. *Allergy* 1995; **50**: 783–7

35 Heilborn H, Hjemdahl P, Daleskog M, Adamsson U. Comparison of subcutaneous injection and high-dose inhalation of epinephrine – implication for self-treatment to prevent anaphylaxis. *J Allergy Clin Immunol* 1986; **78**: 1174–9

36 Warren J, Doble N, Dalton N, Ewan P. Systemic absorption of inhaled epinephrine. *Clin Pharmacol Ther* 1986; **40**: 673–8

37 Kambam J, Merrill W, Smith B. Histamine-2 receptor blocker in the treatment of protamine-related anaphylactoid reactions: two case reports. *Can J Anesth* 1989; **36**: 463–5

38 Oppenheimer JJ, Nelson HS, Bock SA, Christensen F, Leung DYM. Treatment of peanut allergy with rush immunotherapy. *J Allergy Clin Immunol* 1992; **90**: 256–62

39 Nelson HS, Lahr J, Rule R, Bock SA, Leung DYM. Treatment of anaphylactic sensitivity to peanuts by immunotherapy with injections of aqueous peanut extract. *J Allergy Clin Immunol* 1997; **99**: 744–51

Mast cells and basophils in acquired immunity

Jochen Wedemeyer* and **Stephen J Galli*,†**

Departments of *Pathology and †Microbiology and Immunology, Stanford University Medical Center, Stanford, California, USA

In this review we describe the basic biology of mast cells and basophils and discuss their proposed effector and immunoregulatory roles in acquired immunity, particularly the IgE-associated immune responses. While mast cells and basophils share a number of similarities, they also differ in many aspects of natural history and function. Both mast cells and basophils express the high affinity receptor for immunoglobulin E (FcεRI) on their surface and can be activated to secrete diverse preformed, lipid and cytokine mediators after crosslinking of FcεRI-bound IgE with bi- or multivalent antigen. Thus, both cell types can represent important effector cells, as well as potential immunoregulatory cells, in IgE-mediated acquired immunity. However, mature mast cells are long-term residents of vascularized tissues, whereas basophils are granulocytic leukocytes that circulate in mature form and must be recruited into tissues that are sites of inflammatory or immune responses. The similarities and differences in the natural history, mediator content and other features of mast cells and basophils not only strongly indicate that these cells represent distinct hematopoietic lineages that can express complementary or overlapping functions, but also offer insights into the specific roles of these cells in acute, 'late phase' and chronic aspects of adaptive or pathological IgE-associated acquired immune responses.

Correspondence to:
Dr Stephen J. Galli,
Department of Pathology
L-235, Stanford University
Medical Center, 300
Pasteur Drive, Palo Alto,
CA 94305-5324, USA

While mast cells and basophils are widely regarded as important effector cells in IgE-associated immune responses, such as those that contribute to asthma and other allergic diseases and to host resistance to certain parasites, these cells also may express immunoregulatory function in such settings[1-6]. Mast cells contribute importantly to the expression of many acute allergic reactions, such as anaphylaxis or the acute wheezing provoked by allergen challenge in subjects with atopic asthma[2,3,5,6]. Basophils probably also contribute to the expression of some acute IgE-associated responses, particularly anaphylaxis[5]. By contrast, there is less agreement about the importance of mast cells and basophils in late phase reactions or chronic allergic inflammation. Before discussing recent evidence, much of it derived from *in vivo* studies in mice, that indicates that mast cells can indeed contribute importantly to late phase reactions and chronic allergic inflammation, we will first review the basic biology of these two cell types.

Basic basophil biology

Basophilic granulocytes (basophils) derive their name from the affinity of their cytoplasmic granules for certain basic dyes. Like the other granulocytes (*i.e.* neutrophils and eosinophils) basophils are of hematopoietic origin and typically mature in the bone marrow and then circulate in the peripheral blood, from where they can then be recruited into the tissues[1,7]. They are the least frequent of the granulocytes, in humans ordinarily accounting for less than 0.5% of circulating leukocytes[1,7]. The basophil's prominent metachromatic cytoplasmic granules allow unmistakable identification in Wright Giemsa- or May-Grünwald Giemsa-stained films of blood or bone marrow. Under physiological conditions, basophils have a short life-span of several days. Interleukin-3 (IL-3) promotes the production and survival of human basophils *in vitro* and can induce basophilia *in vivo*[1,8]. Findings in wild type and IL-3[−/−] mice (that can not produce IL-3) indicate that IL-3 is not necessary for the development of normal numbers of bone marrow or blood basophils, but is mandatory for the striking bone marrow and blood basophilia associated with certain Th-2 cell-associated immunological responses[1,7,9].

Mediators stored preformed in the cytoplasmic granules of basophils include chondroitin sulphates, proteases and histamine[1,7]. Chondroitin sulphates probably contribute to the storage of histamine and neutral proteases, and basophils are the source of most of the histamine found in normal human blood. Upon antigen crosslinking of IgE, aggregation of FcεRI can induce 'degranulation' and the extracellular release of the preformed granule mediators. Furthermore, such FcεRI-dependent activation of basophils can induce the *de novo* production and secretion of leukotriene C_4. Although the ability of basophils to produce cytokines has been less extensively explored than has mast cell cytokine production, several reports have demonstrated that mature human basophils can release substantial amounts of IL-4 and IL-13 in response to FcεRI-dependent activation[10-12]. It is possible, although not yet proven, that the release of IL-4 and IL-13 by basophils may play a role in enhancing IgE production or driving Th-2 differentiation[1,7,10-12].

The extent of the biochemical and functional similarities between basophils and mast cells continue to be explored. Li *et al.*, in confirmation of earlier studies, found that the basophils in the peripheral blood of normal individuals expressed the basophil marker Bsp-1, but little or no surface kit or cell-associated tryptase, chymase, or carboxypeptidase A (CPA)[13]. However, the metachromatic cells in the peripheral blood of subjects with asthma, allergies, or drug reactions not only were increased in number, but many of them expressed surface kit, as well as tryptase, chymase, and CPA[13]. These findings indicate that the cytoplasmic granule content of human basophils and mast cells may exhibit even more overlap than had been previously supposed. As noted by Li *et al.*, their findings could reflect consequences of the cytokine-dependent regulation of basophil phenotype during allergic disorders.

Basic mast cell biology

Mast cells, like basophils, are derived from CD34[+] hematopoietic progenitor cells but, unlike basophils, mature mast cells ordinarily do not circulate in the blood. Mast cells typically complete their differentiation in vascularized tissues (and, especially in rodents, in serosal-lined cavities). However, unlike mature basophils, morphologically mature mast cells can be very long-lived and can retain their ability to proliferate under certain conditions[7,14]. Mast cells are found particularly around blood vessels, in close proximity to peripheral nerves, and beneath epithelial surfaces that are exposed to the external environment, such as those of the respiratory and gastrointestinal tract and skin[14-16].

Studies in murine rodents, non-human primates, and humans indicate that many aspects of mast cell development and survival are critically regulated by stem cell factor (SCF), the ligand for the c-kit tyrosine growth factor receptor, which is expressed on the mast cell surface[7,16,17]. For example, local treatment of mice with SCF can induce marked local increases in mast cell numbers, reflecting both enhanced recruitment/retention and/or maturation of mast cell precursors and proliferation of more mature mast cells[18]. By contrast, withdrawal of exogenous SCF induces apoptosis in mast cells *in vitro* as well as *in vivo*[16,19]. Besides its role in mast cell proliferation and differentiation, SCF can stimulate and/or enhance mast cell function. Not only can SCF augment IgE-dependent mast cell mediator release and directly induce secretion of mast cell products[1,3,7], but treatment with SCF in doses that do not increase the number of mast cells can result in higher survival rates in a mouse model of acute bacterial peritonitis[20]. Other cytokines and growth factors which regulate mast cell development and differentiation include IL-3, IL-4, IL-9, IL-10, and NGF[7,14].

Mast cells begin to express the high affinity receptor for Immunoglobulin E (FcεRI) early in their development, but apparently only after they undergo lineage-commitment[21]. Crosslinking of IgE bound to the FcεRI, with resulting aggregation of FcεRI, represents the best studied and most important trigger of mast cell activation in acquired immunological responses (see below).

Mast cell granules stain metachromatically with certain basic dyes, probably primarily reflecting the granules' content of proteoglycans such as chondroitin sulphates and heparin. Chondroitin sulphate and heparin proteoglycans are thought to bind histamine, neutral proteases, and carboxypeptidases primarily by ionic interactions and, therefore, contribute to the packaging and storage of these molecules in the cells' cytoplasmic granules. Mast cells are regarded as the only cells that store true heparin in their granules, a feature which distinguishes them from basophils[7,14]. Mice that lack the enzyme N-deacetylase/N-sulpho-transferase-2 (NDST-2) are unable to produce fully sulphated (i.e. 'true') heparin[22,23]. The phenotypic abnormalities of these 'heparin knock-out' mice so far appear to be confined to mast cells, which exhibit severe defects in their granules, with impaired storage of certain proteases and reduced content of histamine[22,23]. When mast cells' cytoplasmic granule matrices are exposed to physiological conditions of pH and ionic strength during degranulation, the various mediators associated with the proteoglycans dissociate at different rates – histamine very rapidly but tryptase and chymase much more slowly[14].

Studies in genetically mast cell-deficient and congenic normal mice indicate that mast cells account for nearly all of the histamine stored in normal tissues, with the exception of the glandular stomach and the central nervous system (CNS)[24]. Histamine mediates its action via the histamine receptors 1–3, which can transduce signals leading to a variety of responses including vasodilation, bronchoconstriction, and markedly enhanced permeability of post-capillary venules[25]. Accordingly, histamine (in humans) or histamine and serotonin (in mice and rats) are key mediators for some of the prominent signs and symptoms associated with acute allergic reactions[7,14].

Another important group of preformed, cytoplasmic granule-associated mediators is the neutral proteases. The two most important types of serine proteases found in mast cell granules are chymases and tryptases. In the mouse, at least 5 different cytoplasmic granule-associated chymases and 2 different granule-associated tryptases have been described at the protein level[4]. There appear to be multiple forms of human tryptase as well[26]. The specific protease content of individual mast cells can vary depending on the mast cells' micro-environment and, therefore can contribute significantly to the phenotypic (and therefore, functional) heterogeneity of mast cells[4,7,14]. For example, populations of mast cells found in mucosal tissue ('mucosal mast cells', MMCs) in mice express a different pattern of proteases than do populations of mast cells in the connective tissues or serosal cavities ('connective tissue mast cells', CTMC, or 'serosal mast cells')[4,7,14]. Several biochemical functions have been associated with the different proteases, e.g. cleavage of angiotensin I and procollagenase and degradation of neuropeptides such as vasoactive intestinal peptide (VIP) or calcitonin gene-related peptide (CGRP)[4,14]. A useful approach to reveal further information about the diverse potential biological roles of the many mouse mast cell proteases is to study gene-targeted mice that lack specific mast cell proteases. So far, only findings from mice that have been 'knocked out' for mouse mast cell protease-1 (mMCP-1) have been reported[27]. However, C57BL/6 mice have been found to lack mMCP-7 (a tryptase), mice with certain mutations at the *mi* locus have significantly decreased expression of mMCP-4, mMCP-5 and mMCP-6[28,29], and NDST-2[−/−] 'heparin knock-out' mice exhibit markedly reduced storage of mMCP-4, mMCP-5 and mMC carboxypeptidase A[22,23].

The most important mast cell-derived lipid mediators are certain cyclooxygenase and lipoxygenase metabolites of arachidonic acid, which can have potent inflammatory activities and which may also play a role in modulating the release process itself[1,7,14]. The major cyclooxygenase product of mast cells is prostaglandin D_2 (PGD_2), and the major lipoxygenase products derived from mast cells are the sulphiodopeptide leukotrienes (LTs): LTC_4 and its peptidolytic derivates LTD_4 and LTE_4[7,14]. Human mast cells can also produce LTB_4, although in much smaller quantities than PGD_2 or LTC_4, and some mast cell populations represent a potential source of PAF.

Studies with mouse and/or human mast cells indicate that mast cells represent a potential source of a vast array of cytokines and growth factors including IL-1, IL-2, IL-3, IL-4, IL-5, IL-6, IL-8, IL-13, IL-16, GM-CSF, TNF-α, TGF-β, bFGF, FGF-2, PDGF, NGF, VPF/VEGF and several C-C chemokines[1,3,7,14]. It appears that one of the more important cytokines produced and released by mast cells is TNF-α. In contrast to findings in other potential sources of TNF-α such as macrophages, T-cells and B-cells, several lines of evidence indicate that certain mature resting mouse or human mast cells contain pools of stored TNF-α that are available for immediate release[7,14,30,31]. Certain mast cell populations may also have preformed stores of VPF/VEGF[7,16,32]. Many other cytokines have been identified in various mast cell populations by immunohistochemical or immunocytochemical methods; these may represent additional cytokines which can be released in part from stored pools. Thus, in IgE-dependent reactions, mast cells are likely to represent an important initial source of TNF-α and perhaps other cytokines, while other cytokines whose production is induced from new mRNA transcripts as a result of FcεRI-dependent mast cell activation may contribute to late phase responses or even to certain aspects of chronic allergic inflammation.

Mast cell knock-in mice

A particularly useful approach to study mast cell function *in vivo* is to employ genetically mast cell-deficient WBB6F1-Kit^W/Kit^{W-v} mice (W/W^v mice), which lack expression of a functional c-kit receptor due to spontaneous mutations in both copies of c-kit[33,34]. This marked reduction in c-kit-dependent signalling produces a complex group of phenotypic abnormalities, including a moderate anaemia and a virtual absence of tissue mast cells, germ cells, melanocytes and interstitial cells of Cajal[7,33,34]. However the mast cell activity in W/W^v mice can be selectively reconstituted by the adoptive transfer of immature mast cells cultured from the bone marrow cells of the congenic wild type mice (bone marrow-derived cultured mast cells; BMCMCs). These BMCMCs can be administered systemically, by i.v. injection, or locally, by i.p or i.d. injection or by direct injection into the anterior wall of the stomach, thus producing 'mast cell knock-in mice'[7]. This approach enables investigators to assess whether the expression of acquired immune responses (and many other biological processes) differs in the presence or absence of mast cells. The selective local reconstitution of mast cells in the skin or stomach of W/W^v mice has the advantage of permitting the analysis of mast cell-deficient and mast cell-containing tissues simultaneously in the same animals.

In addition to using BMCMCs of congenic wild type origin to repair selectively the mast cell deficiency of W/W^v mice, one can substitute mast cells generated *in vitro* from various transgenic or knock out mice. An additional new approach, that uses embryonic stem cell derived mast cells (ESMCs) to reconstitute mast cell-deficient mice[35], has the great advantage of permitting the *in vivo* analysis of the effects of even 'embryonic lethal' mutations of genes that can be expressed in mast cells[35]. Unfortunately, there is no 'basophil knock-in' system available at this time. Even mice that are null for the major basophil growth factor IL-3 have normal baseline levels of bone marrow and circulating basophils and therefore can not be regarded as strictly 'basophil-deficient' mice[9].

Activation via FcεRI and other mechanisms

Mast cells and basophils share the ability to bind IgE antibodies to FcεRI, the high affinity receptor for IgE[36,37]. Indeed high 'constitutive' levels of FcεRI expression are restricted to mast cells and basophils, while low levels of expression can be detected in human peripheral blood dendritic cells and monocytes, Langerhans' cells, and eosinophils[37,38]. By contrast, in the absence of genetic manipulation, mice express FcεRI solely on mast cells and basophils[37,38]. In mast cells and basophils, FcεRI has a tetrameric structure composed of a single IgE binding α-chain, a single β-chain (which functions as a signal amplifier) and two identical disulphide-linked γ-chains[36,37]. All three subunits must be present for efficient cell surface expression in rodents, while human cells can express FcεRI function in the absence of the β-chain[37,38]. In humans, FcεRI+ cells other than mast cells and basophils (*e.g.* monocytes) express primarily the $\alpha\gamma_2$ form of the receptor[37,38].

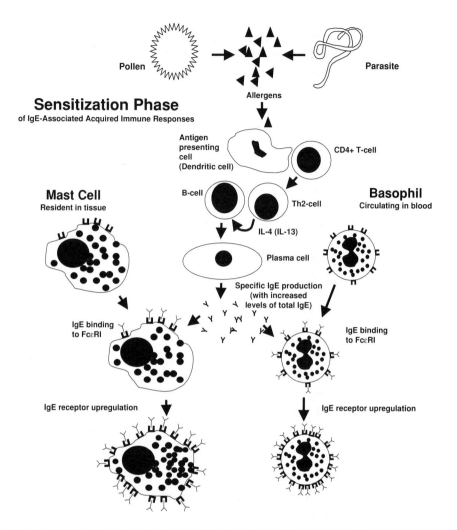

Fig. 1 Cellular interactions in the sensitization phase of IgE-associated immune responses. Antigen presenting cells (APC) (*e.g.* dendritic cells) acquire allergens at or close to epithelial surfaces (skin, airways, intestines); these cells then migrate to regional lymphoid tissue, where they can present peptide–MHC complexes to naive T-cells and induce T-cell activation and Th-2 development, with production of IL-4 and IL-13. This subsequently leads to B-cell activation and induces specific IgE production. IgE is bound to mast cells and basophils expressing FcεRI on their cell surface. IgE bound to FcεRI up-regulates FcεRI expression on both cell types. Mast cells and basophils are thereby primed to respond vigorously to a second exposure to specific allergen.

In mast cells and basophils, the aggregation of FcεRI that are occupied by IgE (*e.g.* by binding of IgE to multivalent antigens) is sufficient for initiating down-stream signal transduction events that activate the cells to degranulate and also induce the *de novo* synthesis and secretion of lipid mediators and cytokines[36-38]. It is of considerable interest, given that the FcεRI β-chain functions as an amplifier of signalling which can markedly up-regulate the magnitude of the mediator release response to FcεRI aggregation[38], that certain mutations that result in amino acid substitutions in the human β-chain may be linked to atopic diseases[38,39].

In vitro and *in vivo* studies in both mice and humans have revealed that levels of FcεRI surface expression on mast cells and basophils are regulated by levels of IgE (Fig. 1)[7,40,41]. For example, genetically IgE-deficient mice exhibit a greater than 80% reduction in mast cell and basophil FcεRI expression compared to the corresponding wild type mice, and this abnormality can be corrected by administration of exogenous monomeric IgE[7,40]. Up-regulation of FcεRI expression can permit mouse or human mast cells to secrete increased amounts of mediators after anti-IgE or antigen challenge and to exhibit IgE-dependent mediator release at lower concentrations of specific antigen[7,40,41]. Furthermore, mast cells that have undergone IgE-dependent up-regulation of surface FcεRI expression, upon subsequent FcεRI-dependent activation, may secrete cytokines and growth factors that are released in very low levels, or perhaps not at all, by mast cells with low levels of FcεRI expression[7,32,40]. Thus, basophils and mast cells in subjects with high levels of IgE (as typically characterizes patients with allergic disorders or parasite infections) can be significantly enhanced in their ability to express IgE-dependent effector functions or, via production of cytokines that can influence Th-2 polarization and IgE production, such as IL-4, IL-13, and MIP-1α, may also express potential immuno-regulatory functions. While the mechanism(s) by which monomeric IgE regulates FcεRI expression are not yet fully understood (at least in part, the phenomenon reflects the ability of IgE binding to stabilize the expression of FcεRI on the cell surface), research in this area may suggest novel therapeutic approaches for the management of allergic disease.

While we most commonly think of mast cells and basophils as effectors of IgE-associated acquired immunity, several recent studies have suggested that the roles of these cells in host defence may be considerably broader than previously supposed. The HIV glycoprotein 120, as well as protein Fv (pFv), which is released into the intestinal tract in patients with viral hepatitis, can interact with the V_H3 domain of IgE and thereby induce histamine, IL-4 and IL-13 release from human basophils and/or mast cells[42,43]. Human basophils also have been shown to respond to stimulation with immobilized secretory IgA (sIgA) by releasing both histamine and LTC_4, but only if the cells had first been primed by pretreatment with IL-3, IL-5, or GM-CSF[44]. Since IgA is the most abundant immunoglobulin isotype in mucosal secretions, this finding suggests that sIgA may contribute to basophil activation during immune responses at mucosal sites[44].

A growing body of evidence also indicates that mast cells can contribute significantly to several aspects of host defence during innate immune response to bacterial infection[16]. Mast cell knock-in mice were used to show that mast cells can represent a central component of host defence against bacterial infection, that the recruitment of circulating leukocytes with bactericidal properties is dependent on mast cells, and that TNF-α is one important element of this response[45,46]. While certain bacterial products – including lipopolysaccharide and at least one fimbrial adhesin[47] – can directly induce the release of some mast cell products, pathogens may also activate mast cells indirectly during innate immune responses via activation of the complement system[16,48].

IgE-associated allergic inflammation and related diseases

Allergen challenge of sensitized individuals can elicit three types of IgE-associated responses which occur in distinct temporal patterns: (i) acute allergic reactions, which develop within seconds or minutes of allergen exposure; (ii) late-phase reactions, which develop within hours of allergen exposure, often after at least some of the effects of the acute reaction have partially diminished; and (iii) chronic allergic inflammation, which can persist for days to years. While allergic disorders like anaphylaxis, hayfever or asthma can be thought of as exhibiting various proportions of these three reaction patterns, specific signs and symptoms may reflect composite responses that incorporate overlapping components of the three classical reaction patterns (Fig. 2).

Acute allergic reactions

The major features of acute allergic reactions primarily reflect the actions of preformed mediators released from mast cells, and in some responses such as anaphylaxis, perhaps also from basophils[3,7,14]. Passive cutaneous anaphylaxis represents one of the simplest experimental models used to study such acute IgE-associated allergic reactions. In this model, IgE antibodies of defined allergenic specificity are injected into the skin and, at 24 h thereafter, the specific allergen is administered intravenously. The ensuing FcϵRI aggregation in dermal mast cells results in the secretion of all classes of mast cell-derived mediators at the site where the IgE was injected. These products in turn produce multiple local effects, including enhanced local vascular permeability (leading to leakage of plasma proteins, including fibrinogen, resulting in local deposition of crosslinked fibrin and tissue swelling), increased cutaneous blood flow, with intravascular trapping of red cells due to arteriolar

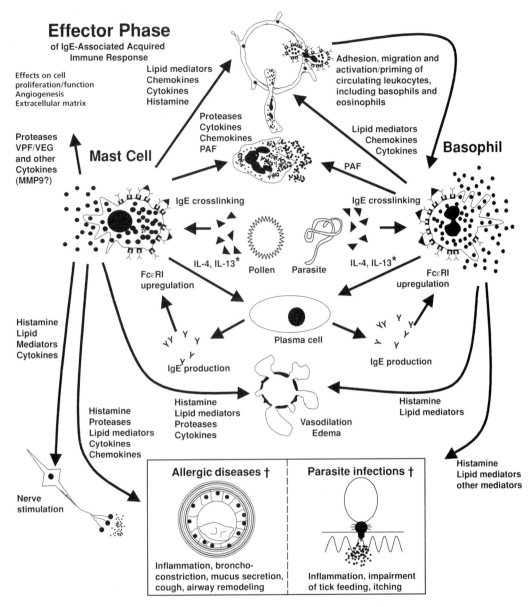

Fig. 2 Cellular interactions in the effector phase of IgE-associated immune responses. Binding of multivalent allergen to IgE bound to FcεRI on the mast cell surface initiates downstream signal transduction, events that activate the cells to degranulate and also induce the *de novo* synthesis and secretion of lipid mediators and cytokines. Besides a wide array of other effects on various target cells and tissues, this mast cell mediator/cytokine production can have effects that induce the recruitment of basophils and other leukocytes from the circulating blood into the tissues. Subsequently, binding of IgE to multivalent antigens can induce basophil activation and degranulation.

*Activated mast cells and basophils represent potential sources of IL-4 and IL-13, but both cytokines can also be secreted by other cells as well (*e.g.* T-cells).

†While only one example of an IgE-associated disease (asthma) or protective immune responses (to the feeding of larval ticks) is illustrated, similar mechanisms may also contribute to the expression of other IgE-associated allergic disorders or acquired immune responses to parasites.

dilation and increased loss of intravascular fluid from postcapillary venules producing erythema, and other effects such as itching, due to stimulation of cutaneous sensory nerves by histamine.

We have shown that mast cell-deficient W/W^v mice are not able to express detectable IgE-dependent PCA reactions[49]. By contrast, IgE-dependent PCA reactions can readily be expressed in W/W^v mice that have been selectively repaired of their mast cell deficiency[49]. Similar approaches have been used to show that essentially all of the assessed features of acute IgE-dependent reactions elicited in the respiratory tract or stomach of mice are also mast cell-dependent[7]. While humans contain cells distinct from mast cells and basophils that express FcεRI (*e.g.* Langerhans' cells) and these cells might, therefore, also represent effector cells in acute allergic reactions, there is little actual evidence for this. Moreover, many of the signs and symptoms associated with acute allergic disorders can be explained by mast cell degranulation; these include the swelling, itching and redness detected in positive allergen prick tests, as well as the rhinitis and itching associated with hayfever and allergic conjunctivitis. In contrast to the local elicitation of allergic reactions in diseases like hayfever and asthma, systemic anaphylaxis represents an acute hypersensitivity response to allergen that typically involves multiple organ systems and which, if untreated, can lead to death. Again, studies with mast cell-deficient W/W^v mice indicate that the expression of most models of IgE-dependent anaphylaxis requires mast cells[7]. By contrast, active anaphylaxis to penicillin V, which is thought to be mediated primarily by IgE, can be elicited in W/W^v mice, perhaps reflecting an important role of basophils in this response[50]. W/W^v mice can also express multiple pathophysiological features of IgG_1-dependent anaphylaxis, since the major receptor for IgG_1 (FcεRIII) occurs on mouse hematopoietic cells in addition to mast cells[7].

Late phase reactions (LPRs) and chronic allergic inflammation

In addition to their roles in classic acute IgE-associated immediate hypersensitivity responses, such as anaphylaxis, several lines of evidence indicate that mast cells and basophils can also contribute to late-phase reactions. Late-phase reactions occur when antigen challenge is followed, hours after initial IgE-dependent mast cell activation, by the recurrence of signs (*e.g.* cutaneous oedema) and symptoms (*e.g.* bronchoconstriction)[2,7]. Unlike acute allergic reactions, for which suitable animal models have been available for many years, models for LPRs in non-human subjects have been slower to develop and to gain widespread acceptance. Several points about human LPRs appear to be well-established: (i) the response can be elicited by appropriate allergen challenge in the skin and upper airways as well as in the lungs; (ii) the symptoms are usually (but not always) preceded by an acute allergic reaction, and at least some of the key pathological features of these acute responses usually resolve before the onset of the LPR; (iii) the signs and symptoms characteristic of LPRs are associated with the recruitment of circulating leukocytes to the sites of the reactions; and (iv) a variety of treatments which are associated with a reduction in the leukocyte recruitment that is elicited at sites of LPRs can also reduce the signs and symptoms that are characteristic of these responses. In humans, basophils are recruited to LPRs in the skin, nose and lower airways[51-53].

It is possible that the cellular infiltrates at sites of chronic allergic inflammation represent, at least in part, the result of multiple, overlapping LPRs elicited by persistent or repeated exposure to allergen. Indeed, the inflammatory infiltrates present at sites of human experimental LPRs and naturally occurring chronic allergic inflammation are similar in composition (prominent eosinophils and T-cells, with smaller numbers of monocytes, macrophages and basophils). Nevertheless, controversy persists regarding the mechanisms involved in the initiation of late phase responses or the development of chronic allergic inflammation. Several groups have shown that various features of late phase reactions or chronic allergic inflammation can be expressed in mice that lack IgE, B-cells or mast cells[7,54]. As a result, interest has focused increasingly on eosinophils and Th-2 lymphocytes as key effector cells of late phase reactions[55]. However, we feel that the key question is not whether IgE and mast cells, as opposed to eosinophils or T-cells, are mainly responsible for the pathology associated with chronic allergic diseases, since each cell type is likely to contribute, but to identify the extent to which particular clinically-significant characteristics of these disorders reflect the specific contributions of distinct potential effector cell types[3].

Our group has formulated the hypothesis that a mast cell–leukocyte cytokine cascade can critically contribute to the initiation, amplification, and perpetuation of IgE-associated allergic inflammation in the airways and other sites[7]. Specifically, we propose that the activation of mast cells through the FcεRI can initiate both the acute and late-phase components of the response, the latter orchestrated in part through the release of TNF-α and other cytokines that can influence the recruitment and function of additional effector cells. These recruited cells then promote the further progression of the inflammatory responses by providing additional sources of certain cytokines that may also be produced by mast cells stimulated by ongoing exposure to allergen, as well as new sources of cytokines and other mediators that may not be produced by mast cells. Certain mast cell cytokines, such as TNF-α, VPF/VEGF, and TGF-β, may also contribute to chronic allergic inflammation through effects on fibroblasts, vascular endothelial cells, and other cells resident at the sites of these reactions.

Certain aspects of this hypothetical model of allergic inflammation have already been confirmed by studies in mast cell knock-in mice and are also supported by more indirect lines of evidence, including data derived from studies in human subjects. Our studies in mast cell knock-in mice showed that mast cells were required for essentially all of the leukocyte infiltration observed in the skin after challenge with IgE and specific antigen and that ~50% of such IgE- and mast cell-dependent leukocyte recruitment was inhibitable with a neutralizing antibody to recombinant mouse TNF-α[56]. Furthermore, we showed that either dexamethasone or cyclosporine A (CsA) can substantially suppress: (i) the IgE-dependent secretion of TNF-α by mouse mast cells *in vitro*; (ii) the leukocyte recruitment induced by the injection of recombinant mouse TNF-α into mouse skin *in vivo*; and (iii) the mast cell-, IgE- and TNF-α-dependent leukocyte infiltration observed at cutaneous reaction sites in mice *in vivo*[57].

Are mast cells important in orchestrating eosinophil infiltration into the airways, a hallmark of human asthma? Many studies of asthma models in mice have suggested that the answer to this question is no. For example, at least four studies using mast cell-deficient W/W^v mice reported that mast cells were not essential for the development of antigen-induced infiltration of the airways with eosinophils[58–61]. However, in each of these studies, the investigators used strong procedures of sensitization and challenge, often in conjunction with an adjuvant such as alum; approaches that favour the production of strong non-specific antibody responses. In contrast, human subjects often express dramatic patho-physiological responses after sensitization and challenge with very low doses of specific antigen. Notably, Kung *et al.*, using a protocol in which aerosol challenge with OVA was performed only twice on a single day, found that eosinophil infiltration of the airways in W/W^v mice was < 50% of that in the wild-type mice[62]. Subsequently, using mast cell knock-in mice, we showed that mast cells can importantly contribute to the recruitment of eosinophils to the airways, especially in a model of asthma that does not employ alum as an adjuvant during sensitization[54]. Based on these findings, we hypothesize that mast cells can indeed be critical in regulating eosinophil infiltration during allergic inflammation in mice.

The specific mechanisms by which mast cells might regulate eosinophil recruitment and/or activation remain to be determined, but it seems reasonable to suggest that chemokines, and particularly eotaxin, may be involved. Persistent chronic allergic inflammation can result in remodelling of the affected tissues and these structural changes are often associated with functional alterations. For instance, some patients with asthma develop irreversible changes in lung function, despite apparently appropriate and aggressive anti-inflammatory therapy[63], and many subjects with asthma exhibit a decline in lung function over time[64,65]. Moreover, airway tissues from patients with asthma can exhibit structural abnormalities such as epithelial thickening, smooth muscle hypertrophy, mucus gland hyperplasia, blood vessel proliferation and collagen deposition beneath the epithelial basement membrane[66].

We feel that it is too soon to conclude whether and to what extent mast cells contribute to the tissue remodelling associated with chronic allergic inflammation. However, several lines of evidence suggest that mast cells may indeed participate in this process. Mast cell-derived proteases, cytokines, growth factors and other mediators have been shown to have a number of *in vitro* or *in vivo* effects that are consistent with the hypothesis that mast cells can promote tissue remodelling. For example, Kanbe *et al.* recently showed that human skin, lung and synovial mast cells are strongly positive for matrix metalloproteinase-9 (MMP-9) by immunohisto-chemistry[67]. Because they can promote the degradation of extracellular matrix, matrix metalloproteinases are believed to play a role in the pathogenesis of certain disorders associated with tissue remodelling. Various populations of mast cells also have been identified as sources of several growth-promoting peptide mediators, including TNF-α, VPF/VEGF, FGF-2, PDGF, TGF-β and NGF[7,9,14,32]; in aggregate, these products might contribute to the neovascularization, connective tissue remodelling and/or epithelial repair associated with chronic tissue remodelling, in the context of allergic disease and in other settings, such as IgE-associated responses to parasites and perhaps even carcinogenesis.

Mast cells and basophils in host defence and parasite immunity

It does not seem very likely that Th-2 and IgE-associated acquired immune responses evolved so that we can experience allergic disorders. What then is the adaptive advantage of these immune responses? Several lines of evidence now indicate that mast cells and basophils may represent important components of acquired immunity to at least some parasites. Infections with many parasites, particularly helminths, induce strong primary and secondary IgE responses, with some of the IgE being specific for parasite-derived antigens. Such responses also can be associated with increased levels of circulating basophils and eosinophils, increased numbers of mast cells at sites of parasite infection and infiltration of the affected tissues with basophils and, especially, eosinophils.

Nevertheless, it has been difficult to prove that individual components of IgE-associated responses to helminths, such as IgE, mast cells, eosinophils or basophils, are truly essential for the expression of protective host immunity. For example, IgE-deficient mice exhibit relatively modest abnormalities in their immune responses to *Schistosoma mansoni*[68]. Several studies demonstrated that W/W^v mice develop little or no mast cells at sites of parasite entry and, depending on the parasite, W/W^v mice may also exhibit a delay in parasite clearance; however, W/W^v mice, unlike T-cell-deficient nude mice, ultimately are able to clear these infections[7]. Moreover, perhaps because of difficulties in achieving selective reconstitution of intestinal mucosal mast cells populations in W/W^v mice, in many cases it is not clear to what extent the defects in parasite resistance in W/W^v mice reflect the mast cell deficiency of the mice, as opposed to c-kit related abnormalities in other hematopoietic cells and/or the lack of interstitial cells of Cajal. Notably, W/W^v mast cell-deficient mice which are also genetically devoid of IL-3 exhibit a striking impairment in their ability to expel a primary infection with the nematode *Strongyloides venezuelensis*[9]; this impairment is much greater than that exhibited by W/W^v mice that can produce IL-3 or by IL-3$^{-/-}$ mice with normal c-kit[9]. W/W^v, IL-3$^{-/-}$ mice also fail to develop increases in bone marrow and blood basophils in response to the infection, and they exhibit virtually no hyperplasia of mucosal mast cells in the intestines at sites of infection.

Taken together, these findings are consistent with the hypothesis that mast cells and basophils provide overlapping or complementary function during IgE-associated acquired immune responses to certain parasites. Indeed, in other settings, basophils may have a more important role in acquired immunity to parasites than do mast cells. For example, in the guinea pig, basophils (and eosinophils) appear to be required for the full expression of immune resistance to infestation of the skin by larval ixodid ticks of the species *Amblyomma americanum*[69], whereas expression of IgE-dependent immune resistance to the cutaneous infestation of larval *Haemaphysalis longicornis* ticks in mice is dependent on mast cells[70]. By contrast, W/W^v mice can express immune resistance to the feeding of larval ticks of the species *Dermacentor varibilis*, and the tick feeding sites exhibit prominent infiltration of basophils by electron microscopy[71]. Such studies support the notion that, in most cases, the maintenance of effective acquired immune resistance to helminths or ectoparasites may simply be too critical to permit the response to be ablated by the loss of a single effector component, such as IgE, mast cells, basophils or eosinophils. As noted previously, studies in mast cell knock-in mice have shown that mast cells can also contribute significantly to innate immunity in host defence against some bacterial infections[20,45,46].

Finally, mast cells and/or basophils represent potential sources of mediators and cytokines that can have potential down-regulating effects in inflammation; some of these cells also express cell surface receptors that can mediate down-regulation of FcεRI-dependent signalling[7,37,38,72]. Thus mast cells and basophils represent potential participants in the down-regulation or attenuation, as well as in the initiation and/or perpetuation, of acquired immune responses.

Conclusions

It seems very likely that mast cells and basophils express complex, and partially overlapping, roles in acquired immunity, and that these roles include both effector cell and immunoregulatory activities. Clearly, IgE-dependent mast cell activation importantly contributes to the expression of many acute allergic reactions, including acute allergen-induced bronchoconstriction in human atopic asthma, and both mast cells and basophils are activated during IgE-associated anaphylaxis. Studies in mice, and correlative analysis in humans, indicate that mast cells can contribute to the leukocyte infiltration associated with allergic inflammation as well. Moreover, in humans, basophils are prominent in the leukocytic infiltrates elicited at sites of late phase reactions in the skin, nose, and airways. Based on the known function of the wide spectrum of cytokines and growth factors that can be produced by mast cells, these cells may represent important contributors to many of the structural and functional changes observed in tissues at sites of chronic inflammation.

Notably, two newly recognized aspects of FcεRI function or expression (β-chain amplifier function, IgE-dependent up-regulation of FcεRI surface expression) provide strong support for the hypothesis that mast cells and basophils may have particularly important roles as effector cells in initiating and or amplifying IgE-dependent inflammatory reactions, especially in response to low dose antigen challenge. Mast cells and basophils may also express immunoregulatory functions in these settings, through the production of certain cytokines. For example, both mouse and human mast cells and basophils can produce IL-4 and/or IL-13, and other cytokines which can enhance IgE production. This fact, taken together with the findings about IgE-dependent regulation of FcεRI surface expression suggest a potential positive feedback mechanism ($\uparrow$IgE → $\uparrow$FcεRI surface expression → $\uparrow$antigen-, IgE-, and FcεRI-dependent release of IL-4 and/or IL-13 → $\uparrow$IgE) by which mast cells and possibly basophils may enhance the further evolution, and persistence, of Th-2 biased, IgE-associated immune responses. Finally, mast cells and basophils may enhance IgE production via expression of the CD40 ligand. The clinical significance of many of these new findings largely remains to be established. However, this work clearly supports a complex, but more unified, view of the pathogenesis of allergic disease and host defence mechanisms, which proposes that mast cells and basophils can have both effector cell and immunoregulatory roles in these contexts.

Acknowledgements

Some of the work reviewed in this chapter was supported by United States Public Health Service grants CA 72074, AI 23990, AI 31982, AI

41995 (project 1), by Deutsche Forschungsgemeinschaft grant WE 2300/1 and/or by AMGEN Inc.; Dr Galli consults for AMGEN Inc. under terms that accord with Stanford University conflict-of-interest guidelines.

References

1   Galli SJ. Mast cells and basophils. *Curr Opin Hematol* 2000; **7**: 32–9
2   Church MK, Okayama Y, Bradding P. The role of the mast cell in acute and chronic allergic inflammation. *Ann N Y Acad Sci* 1994; **725**: 13–21
3   Williams CMM, Galli SJ. The diverse potential effector and immunoregulatory roles of mast cells in allergic disease. *J Allergy Clin Immunol* 2000; **105**: 847–59
4   Huang C, Sali A, Stevens RL. Regulation and function of mast cell proteases in inflammation. *J Clin Immunol* 1998; **18**: 169–83
5   Bochner BS, Lichtenstein LM. Anaphylaxis. *N Engl J Med* 1991; **324**: 1785–90
6   Sutton BJ, Gould HJ. The human IgE network. *Nature* 1993; **366**: 421–8
7   Galli SJ, Lantz CS. Allergy. In: Paul WE. (ed) *Fundamental Immunology*. Philadelphia, PA: Lippincott-Raven, 1999; 1137–84
8   Valent P, Schmidt G, Besemer J *et al*. Interleukin-3 is a differentiation factor for human basophils. *Blood* 1989; **73**: 1763–9
9   Lantz CS, Boesiger J, Song CH *et al*. Role for interleukin-3 in mast-cell and basophil development and in immunity to parasites. *Nature* 1998; **392**: 90–3
10 Brunner T, Heusser CH, Dahinden CA. Human peripheral blood basophils primed by interleukin 3 (IL-3) produce IL-4 in response to immunoglobulin E receptor stimulation. *J Exp Med* 1993; **177**: 605–11
11 Li H, Sim TC, Alam R. IL-13 released by and localized in human basophils. *J Immunol* 1996; **156**: 4833–8
12 MacGlashan Jr D, White JM, Huang SK et al. Secretion of IL-4 from human basophils. The relationship between IL-4 mRNA and protein in resting and stimulated basophils. *J Immunol* 1994; **152**: 3006–16
13 Li L, Li Y, Reddel SW *et al*. Identification of basophilic cells that express mast cell granule proteases in the peripheral blood of asthma, allergy, and drug-reactive patients. *J Immunol* 1998; **161**: 5079–86
14 Schwartz LB, Huff TF. Biology of mast cells. In: Middleton EJ, Reed CE, Ellis EF, Yunginger JW, Adkinson NFJ, Busse WW. (eds) *Allergy: Principles and Practice*, vol. I. St Louis, MO: Mosby-Year Book, 1998; 261–76
15 McKay DM, Bienenstock J. The interaction between mast cells and nerves in the gastrointestinal tract. *Immunol Today* 1994; **15**: 533–8
16 Galli SJ, Maurer M, Lantz CS. Mast cells as sentinels of innate immunity. *Curr Opin Immunol* 1999; **11**: 53–9
17 Tsai M, Takeishi T, Thompson H *et al*. Induction of mast cell proliferation, maturation, and heparin synthesis by the rat c-kit ligand, stem cell factor. *Proc Natl Acad Sci USA* 1991; **88**: 6382–6
18 Tsai M, Shih LS, Newlands GF *et al*. The rat c-kit ligand, stem cell factor, induces the development of connective tissue-type and mucosal mast cells *in vivo*. Analysis by anatomical distribution, histochemistry, and protease phenotype. *J Exp Med* 1991; **174**: 125–31
19 Iemura A, Tsai M, Ando A, Wershil BK, Galli SJ. The c-kit ligand, stem cell factor, promotes mast cell survival by suppressing apoptosis. *Am J Pathol* 1994; **144**: 321–8
20 Maurer M, Echtenacher B, Hultner L *et al*. The c-kit ligand, stem cell factor, can enhance innate immunity through effects on mast cells. *J Exp Med* 1998; **188**: 2343–8
21 Rodewald HR, Dessing M, Dvorak AM, Galli SJ. Identification of a committed precursor for the mast cell lineage. *Science* 1996; **271**: 818–22
22 Humphries DE, Wong GW, Friend DS *et al*. Heparin is essential for the storage of specific granule proteases in mast cells. *Nature* 1999; **400**: 769–72

23 Forsberg E, Pejler G, Ringvall M *et al*. Abnormal mast cells in mice deficient in a heparin-synthesizing enzyme. *Nature* 1999; **400**: 773–6

24 Yamatodani A, Maeyama K, Watanabe T, Wada H, Kitamura Y. Tissue distribution of histamine in a mutant mouse deficient in mast cells: clear evidence for the presence of non-mast-cell histamine. *Biochem Pharmacol* 1982; **31**: 305–9

25 Arrang JM, Drutel G, Garbarg M *et al*. Molecular and functional diversity of histamine receptor subtypes. *Ann N Y Acad Sci* 1995; **757**: 314–23

26 Pallaoro M, Fejzo MS, Shayesteh L, Blount JL, Caughey GH. Characterization of genes encoding known and novel human mast cell tryptases on chromosome 16p13.3. *J Biol Chem* 1999; **274**: 3355–62

27 Wastling JM, Knight P, Ure J *et al*. Histochemical and ultrastructural modification of mucosal mast cell granules in parasitized mice lacking the beta-chymase, mouse mast cell protease-1. *Am J Pathol* 1998; **153**: 491–504

28 Hunt JE, Stevens RL, Austen KF *et al*. Natural disruption of the mouse mast cell protease 7 gene in the C57BL/6 mouse. *J Biol Chem* 1996; **271**: 2851–5

29 Kim DK, Morii E, Ogihara H *et al*. Different effect of various mutant MITF encoded by mi, Mior, or Miwh allele on phenotype of murine mast cells. *Blood* 1999; **93**: 4179–86

30 Gordon JR, Galli SJ. Mast cells as a source of both preformed and immunologically inducible TNF-α/cachectin. *Nature* 1990; **346**: 274–6

31 Gordon JR, Galli SJ. Release of both preformed and newly synthesized tumor necrosis factor alpha (TNF-α)/cachectin by mouse mast cells stimulated via the FcεRI. A mechanism for the sustained action of mast cell-derived TNF-α during IgE-dependent biological responses. *J Exp Med* 1991; **174**: 103–7

32 Boesiger J, Tsai M, Maurer M *et al*. Mast cells can secrete vascular permeability factor/vascular endothelial cell growth factor and exhibit enhanced release after immunoglobulin E-dependent upregulation of Fcε receptor I expression. *J Exp Med* 1998; **188**: 1135–45

33 Galli SJ, Tsai M, Gordon JR, Geissler EN, Wershil BK. Analyzing mast cell development and function using mice carrying mutations at W/c-kit or Sl/MGF (SCF) loci. *Ann N Y Acad Sci* 1992; **664**: 69–88

34 Nocka K, Tan JC, Chiu E *et al*. Molecular bases of dominant negative and loss of function mutations at the murine c-*kit*/white spotting locus: W^{37}, W^v, W^{41} and W. *EMBO J* 1990; **9**: 1805–13

35 Tsai M, Wedemeyer J, Ganiatsas S *et al*. *In vivo* immunological function of mast cells derived from embryonic stem cells: an approach for the rapid analysis of even embryonic lethal mutations in adult mice *in vivo*. *Proc Natl Acad Sci USA* 2000; **97**: 9186–90

36 Beaven MA, Metzger H. Signal transduction by Fc receptors: the FcεRI case. *Immunol Today* 1993; **14**: 222–6

37 Kinet J-P. The high-affinity IgE receptor (FcεRI): from physiology to pathology. *Annu Rev Immunol* 1999; **17**: 931–72

38 Turner H, Kinet J-P. Signalling through the high-affinity IgE receptor FcεRI. *Nature* 1999; **402**: B24–30

39 Hill MR, Cookson WO. A new variant of the β subunit of the high-affinity receptor for immunoglobulin E (FcεRI-β E237G): associations with measures of atopy and bronchial hyper-responsiveness. *Hum Mol Genet* 1996; **5**: 959–62

40 Yamaguchi M, Lantz CS, Oettgen HC *et al*. IgE enhances mouse mast cell FcεRI expression *in vitro* and *in vivo*: evidence for a novel amplification mechanism in IgE-dependent reactions. *J Exp Med* 1997; **185**: 663–72

41 Yamaguchi M, Sayama K, Yano K *et al*. IgE enhances Fc epsilon receptor I expression and IgE-dependent release of histamine and lipid mediators from human umbilical cord blood-derived mast cells: synergistic effect of IL-4 and IgE on human mast cell Fc epsilon receptor I expression and mediator release. *J Immunol* 1999; **162**: 5455–65

42 Patella V, Florio G, Petraroli A, Marone G. HIV-1 gp120 induces IL-4 and IL-13 release from human FcεRI⁺ cells through interaction with the V_H3 region of IgE. *J Immunol* 2000; **164**: 589–95

43 Patella V, Giuliano A, Bouvet JP, Marone G. Endogenous superallergen protein Fv induces IL-4 secretion from human FcεRI⁺ cells through interaction with the V_H3 region of IgE. *J Immunol* 1998; **161**: 5647–55

44   Iikura M, Yamaguchi M, Fujisawa T et al. Secretory IgA induces degranulation of IL-3-primed basophils. J Immunol 1998; **161**: 1510–5

45   Malaviya R, Ikeda T, Ross E, Abraham SN. Mast cell modulation of neutrophil influx and bacterial clearance at sites of infection through TNF-alpha. Nature 1996; **381**: 77–80

46   Echtenacher B, Mannel DN, Hultner L. Critical protective role of mast cells in a model of acute septic peritonitis. Nature 1996; **381**: 75–7

47   Malaviya R, Gao Z, Thankavel K, van der Merwe PA, Abraham SN. The mast cell tumor necrosis factor alpha response to FimH-expressing Escherichia coli is mediated by the glycosylphosphatidylinositol-anchored molecule CD48. Proc Natl Acad Sci USA 1999; **96**: 8110–5

48   Prodeus AP, Zhou X, Maurer M, Galli SJ, Carroll MC. Impaired mast cell-dependent natural immunity in complement C3-deficient mice. Nature 1997; **390**: 172–5

49   Wershil BK, Mekori YA, Murakami T, Galli SJ. ^{125}I-fibrin deposition in IgE-dependent immediate hypersensitivity reactions in mouse skin. Demonstration of the role of mast cells using genetically mast cell-deficient mice locally reconstituted with cultured mast cells. J Immunol 1987; **139**: 2605–14

50   Choi IH, Shin YM, Park JS et al. Immunoglobulin E-dependent active fatal anaphylaxis in mast cell-deficient mice. J Exp Med 1998; **188**: 1587–92

51   Charlesworth EN, Kagey-Sobotka A, Schleimer RP, Norman PS, Lichtenstein LM. Prednisone inhibits the appearance of inflammatory mediators and the influx of eosinophils and basophils associated with the cutaneous late-phase response to allergen. J Immunol 1991; **146**: 671–6

52   Bascom R, Wachs M, Naclerio RM et al. Basophil influx occurs after nasal antigen challenge: effects of topical corticosteroid pretreatment. J Allergy Clin Immunol 1988; **81**: 580–9

53   Liu MC, Hubbard WC, Proud D et al. Immediate and late inflammatory responses to ragweed antigen challenge of the peripheral airways in allergic asthmatics. Cellular, mediator, and permeability changes. Am Rev Respir Dis 1991; **144**: 51–8

54   Williams CMM, Galli SJ. Mast cells can amplify airway reactivity and features of chronic inflammation in an asthma model in mice. J Exp Med 2000; **192**:455–62

55   Kay AB. T cells in allergy and anergy. Allergy 1999; **54 (Suppl 56)**: 29–30

56   Wershil BK, Wang Z-S, Gordon JR, Galli SJ. Recruitment of neutrophils during IgE-dependent cutaneous late phase reactions in the mouse is mast cell-dependent. Partial inhibition of the reaction with antiserum against tumor necrosis factor-alpha. J Clin Invest 1991; **87**: 446–53

57   Wershil BK, Furuta GT, Lavigne JA et al. Dexamethasone or cyclosporin A suppress mast cell-leukocyte cytokine cascades. Multiple mechanisms of inhibition of IgE- and mast cell-dependent cutaneous inflammation in the mouse. J Immunol 1995; **154**: 1391–8

58   Nogami M, Suko M, Okudaira H et al. Experimental pulmonary eosinophilia in mice by Ascaris suum extract. Am Rev Respir Dis 1990; **141**: 1289–95

59   Brusselle GG, Kips JC, Tavernier JH et al. Attenuation of allergic airway inflammation in IL-4 deficient mice. Clin Exp Allergy 1994; **24**: 73–80

60   Nagai H, Yamaguchi S, Tanaka H. The role of interleukin-5 (IL-5) in allergic airway hyperresponsiveness in mice. Ann N Y Acad Sci 1996; **796**: 91–6

61   Takeda K, Hamelmann E, Joetham A et al. Development of eosinophilic airway inflammation and airway hyperresponsiveness in mast cell-deficient mice. J Exp Med 1997; **186**: 449–54

62   Kung TT, Stelts D, Zurcher JA et al. Mast cells modulate allergic pulmonary eosinophilia in mice. Am J Respir Cell Mol Biol 1995; **12**: 404–9

63   Jeffery PK, Godfrey RW, Adelroth E et al. Effects of treatment on airway inflammation and thickening of basement membrane reticular collagen in asthma. A quantitative light and electron microscopic study. Am Rev Respir Dis 1992; **145**: 890–9

64   Peat JK, Woodcock AJ, Cullen K et al. Rate of decline of lung function in subjects with asthma. Eur J Respir Dis 1987; **70**: 171–9

65   Brown PJ, Greville HW, Finucane KE. Asthma and irreversible airflow obstruction. Thorax 1984; **39**: 131–6

66   Pare PD, Bai TR, Roberts CR. The structural and functional consequences of chronic allergic inflammation of the airways. Ciba Found Symp 1997; **206**: 71–86

67   Kanbe N, Tanaka A, Kanbe M et al. Human mast cells produce matrix metalloproteinase 9. Eur J Immunol 1999; **29**: 2645–9

68 King CL, Xianli J, Malhotra I *et al*. Mice with a targeted deletion of the IgE gene have increased worm burdens and reduced granulomatous inflammation following primary infection with *Schistosoma mansoni*. *J Immunol* 1997; **158**: 294–300

69 Brown SJ, Galli SJ, Gleich GJ, Askenase PW. Ablation of immunity to *Amblyomma americanum* by anti-basophil serum: co-operation between basophils and eosinophils in expression of immunity to ectoparasites (ticks) in guinea pigs. *J Immunol* 1982; **129**: 790–6

70 Matsuda H, Watanabe N, Kiso Y *et al*. Necessity of IgE antibodies and mast cells for manifestation of resistance against larval *Haemaphysalis longicornis* ticks in mice. *J Immunol* 1990; **144**: 259–62

71 Steeves EB, Allen JR. Basophils in skin reactions of mast cell-deficient mice infested with *Dermacentor variabilis*. *Int J Parasitol* 1990; **20**: 655–67

72 Ujike A, Ishikawa Y, Ono M *et al*. Modulation of immunoglobulin (Ig) E-mediated systemic anaphylaxis by low-affinity Fc receptors for IgG. *J Exp Med* 1999; **189**: 1573–9

Th-2 cytokines in allergic disease

Douglas S Robinson

Allergy and Clinical Immunology, Imperial College School of Medicine at the National Heart and Lung Institute, London, UK

The Th-1/Th-2 paradigm

The description of two subtypes of T helper cells based on cytokine profiles by Mosman and Coffman in 1986 was a major step forward in thinking on control of immune responses[1]. Building on previous divisions of responses into predominantly humoral or predominantly cell-mediated[2], they described murine T cells clones that could be divided into either Th-1 producing IFN-γ and IL-2 but not IL-4 and IL-5 or Th-2 which produce IL-4 and IL-5 but not IFN-γ[1]. The functional consequences of this division follow from the observation that IFN-γ was required for activation of macrophage function and cytotoxic T-cell responses in cell mediated immunity[3], whereas IL-4 unopposed by IFN-γ was essential in switching B-cells to IgE synthesis[4] and IL-5 was involved in eosinophil development and survival[5]. This was seen most elegantly in the response of different mouse strains to *Leishmania* infection which was shown to largely determined by the genetic tendency to mount either a healing Th-1 response or an inappropriate Th-2 response leading to disseminated disease[6-8]. The potential relevance of Th-2 responses to atopic disease was rapidly apparent since IL-4 and IL-5 could explain both IgE and eosinophilic inflammation. These interactions are summarised in Figure 1.

Human Th-1 and Th-2 cells

Correspondence to:
Dr Douglas S Robinson,
Allergy and Clinical
Immunology, Imperial
College School of
Medicine, National Heart
and Lung Institute,
Dovehouse Street,
London SW3 6LY, UK

Although a variety of cytokine profiles were described from human T helper clones, the work of the groups of Romagnani and Kapsenberg firmly established that polarised Th-1 and Th-2 clones could indeed be derived from humans and, in particular that Th-2 responses were prominent in allergen specific CD4+ T-cell clones[9,10]. Although the principle of the Th-1/Th-2 concept applies in both mice and men, there are differences both in the cytokine profiles observed, the factors determining the response and the apparent stability of cytokine profile. Thus the work from study of murine T-cells and animal models needs to be confirmed in humans.

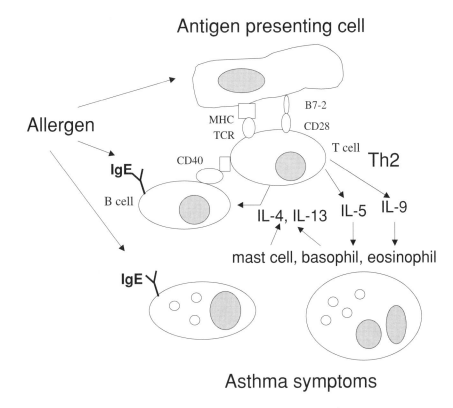

Fig. 1 Proposed interactions between allergen and Th-2 cells in asthma. Allergen is taken up by antigen presenting cells, cleaved into small peptides and complexed with MHC class II molecules. This complex is then recognised by Th-2 cells, which, with appropriate co-stimulation, proliferate and produce cytokines. IL-4 and IL-13 switch B-cells to IgE production, and IL-5 drives development, release and survival of eosinophils. IL-9 acts to increase IL-5 receptor expression. Mast cells, basophils and eosinophils themselves also produce type-2 cytokines and may thus amplify allergic inflammation. IgE cross linking on basophils and mast cells leads to histamine release and synthesis of lipid mediators and eosinophil degranulation and activation may contribute to airway hyper-responsiveness through lipid mediators and basic granule proteins.

Non-T-cell sources of type 2 cytokines

Fairly soon after the initial description of Th-1 and Th-2 cytokine patterns, it was shown that mast cells could produce type 2 cytokines[11]. It is now established that eosinophils, basophils and some structural cells such as epithelial and endothelial cells may also produce cytokines and chemokines that amplify the inflammatory cascade[12,13]. In addition, non-T-cell cytokines may influence the development of a Th-1 or Th-2 phenotype by responding T-cells: for example, IL-4 from basophils may help drive a Th-2 response, whereas NK cell-derived IFN-γ might favour a Th-1 phenotype. Basophils and mast can support IgE switching by B-cells[14]. How non-T-cell cytokine production is regulated and its role in the allergic response is at present uncertain.

The potential role of Th-2 cytokines in allergic disease

IgE regulation

The defining hallmark of atopic disease is production of specific IgE to allergens. The molecular regulation of IgE production from B-cells has been well defined[15,16]. In particular, IL-4 or IL-13 are essential for the first step in isotype switching: generation of the I_{eee} immature mRNA transcript. A second signal, such as that from CD40/CD40L interaction, is required for IgE production. Other cytokines including IL-5[17], IL-6[18], and IL-9[19] can enhance IgE production, whereas IFN-γ and IL-12 inhibit both isotype switch and IgE production. Thus, a Th-2 cytokine profile favours generation of specific IgE. It is of note that non-T-cells can also produce IL-4, and mast cells and basophils are capable of IgE switching[14]. However, without cognate MHC/TCR interaction such IgE will not be allergen specific. IL-13 can be produced by human Th-1 as well as Th-2 T-cells, although IFN-γ from Th-1 cells would inhibit IgE switching.

Interleukin-5 and eosinophils

Just before the description of Th-1 and Th-2 cells, IL-5 had been defined as a cytokine with specific action in the development, priming and survival of eosinophils[5]. Some activity is also seen on basophils and human B-cells[21,22]. Although IL-5 shares a common β receptor subunit with IL-3 and GM-CSF[23,24], and initial studies suggested that all three cytokines could act to cause eosinophil development from bone marrow progenitors[25], our recent studies suggest that IL-5 itself, but not IL-3 or GM-CSF up-regulates IL-5Rα expression and that human eosinophil development is largely IL-5 dependent[26].

Evidence for Th-2 cell involvement in atopic allergic disease

Baseline disease

Assessment of mRNA expression in broncho-alveolar lavage cells from atopic asthmatic subjects showed a predominant Th-2 pattern[27], and numbers of cells expressing both IL-4 and IL-5 mRNA were correlated with measures of disease severity, such as bronchial responsiveness or forced expiratory volume in 1 s[28]. In addition, IL-4 and IL-5, but not IFN-γ, protein levels were increased in BAL fluid from atopic asthmatics when compared to control subject[29], and allergen specific Th-2-type clones could be isolated from the respiratory mucosa of atopic subjects[30]. Similarly, allergen-specific Th-2 cells were isolated from lesional skin in atopic dermatitis, and a Th-2 cytokine mRNA profile was demonstrated in skin biopsies. More recently, allergen specific T-cell lines from BAL from atopic asthmatics were shown to produce IL-5: this was from both CD4 and CD8 cells[31]. In addition, by combining immunohistochemical staining to identify cell phenotype with *in situ* hybridization for cytokine mRNA, IL-4 and IL-5 mRNA were predominantly localised to CD4+ cells in the airway mucosa from asthmatic subjects, with lesser contributions from CD8+ cells, mast cells, and eosinophils[32]. Other Th-1 and Th-2 cytokines have been assessed in asthma: some reports find increased expression of IL-10[33], and increased IL-13 expression is also reported[34].

Non-atopic asthma

Non-atopic asthma is characterised by asthma, generally occurring later in life than atopic asthma, without clinical or laboratory evidence of IgE sensitization to aero-allergens. Bronchial biopsies from such asthmatics show eosinophil infiltration and activated T-cells in the bronchial mucosa, as in atopic asthma[35]. Although one study did not detect IL-4 in concentrated BAL fluid from non-atopic subjects, more recent biopsy studies have reported a Th-2 cytokine profile at both the mRNA and protein level[29,36]. In addition, increased numbers of cells bearing high affinity IgE receptors were detected in bronchial biopsies from non-atopic asthmatics when compared to control subjects[37]. What the role of IgE in this non-atopic variant of asthma is, and whether it is directed against specific antigens, remain to be established. It is of note that Valenta and colleagues have recently described a human IgE binding 'auto-allergen'[37].

Allergen challenge

The late phase response to allergen challenge has been used to model chronic allergic inflammation, and is characterised by T-cell activation and eosinophil and neutrophil infiltration[39,40]. Studies of cytokine mRNA expression also support activation of a Th-2-type response in skin, nose and lung biopsies obtained 24 h after allergen challenge[41–43].

Response to treatment

Numbers of cells expressing mRNA for IL-4 or IL-5 both fell after corticosteroid treatment of asthma in a double blind, placebo controlled study[44], and there was a small increase in IFN-γ mRNA expressing cells. That such changes might be relevant to clinical improvement was supported by the work of Leung *et al.* who showed a similar fall in IL-5 mRNA expressing cells in subjects responding to oral prednisone, but not in a group of subjects whose asthma did not improve with steroid therapy[45]. The role of T-cells in asthma was also supported by the demonstration of clinical efficacy and steroid-sparing activity of cyclosporin A in severe asthma, and by the inhibition of the late, but not early, asthmatic response to allergen challenge by this inhibitor of T-cell activation[46-48]. In addition, a non-depleting anti-CD4 monoclonal antibody was also shown to improve lung function in severe steroid-dependent asthmatics[49].

Allergen immunotherapy has been used to control atopic allergic disease for many years, and evidence also suggests that this too may target Th-2 T-cell activation, since reduced allergen induced IL-4 and IL-5 production with increased IFN-γ responses were seen after clinically successful treatment[50-52].

Animal models of allergic disease

Mouse models of allergic asthma yield varying data in different mouse strains and different sensitization and challenge regimens. Most models involve initial sensitization by intraperitoneal route with adjuvant and subsequent inhaled challenge. They are thus models of allergen challenge and some way from human asthma. Nonetheless, such models can elicit airway eosinophilia and hyper-responsiveness, and allow careful molecular dissection of the immunology of such responses. Although some caution must be applied in extrapolating to human disease, data from genetic studies and from gene manipulation in such models have elegantly identified themes for future research in human disease.

Gene knock-out studies and use of blocking antibodies established the importance of IL-4 and IL-5 in eosinophilic and IgE responses and AHR in animal models of allergen challenge, although the relative role of these cytokines varies according to the strain studied[53-55]. Targeting T-cells with anti-CD4 antibodies and experiments with adoptive transfer of antigen-specific Th-2 cells have shown that Th-2 cells can certainly induce airway eosinophilia and BHR[56,57]. Recent experiments suggest that IL-4 and IL-5 are not the only route to T-cell-dependent AHR. Hogan *et al.* showed that, in IL-4 gene targeted BALB/c mice, anti-IL-5 antibody treatment reduced airway eosinophila but did not block AHR, whereas depleting CD4[+] T-cells in mice lacking both IL-4 and IL-5 did abolish residual AHR[55]. More recently, an important role for IL-13 was suggested. Wills-Karp *et al.* showed that a soluble IL-13Rα–human IgG–Fc fusion protein, which blocks mouse IL-13 but not IL-4, could inhibit AHR in a mouse allergen challenge model, without reducing airway eosinophilia or serum antigen-specific IgE[58]. Grunig *et al.* showed similar data, although their experiments did suggest some reduction in eosinophilia, and went on to show that IL-4R deficient mice did not acquire the AHR upon Th-2 transfer that was seen in wild type controls[59]. These data suggest that IL-13 and IL-4 may act to produce AHR by mechanisms that do not involve IgE or eosinophils. Whether this is also so in humans remains to be established.

Transgenic expression of IL-5, IL-9, IL-11 or IL-13 under the control of a promoter directing lung specific over expression of these cytokines can induce AHR in mice without allergen challenge[60–63]. The airway pathology in such models varies, but variable mast cell and eosinophil expansion is seen. It is likely that such experiments induce a cascade of cytokines and chemokines in the lung, and definition of the patterns seen may pinpoint important contributors to the AHR seen in these models. Some such transgenic animals, in particular those overexpressing IL-11 and IL-13 also show some evidence of changes reminiscent of the airway remodelling that characterises chronic asthma, such as sub-epithelial collagen deposition, and may give information on these processes.

IL-9 may of particular interest in allergic disease. As mentioned above, transgenic overexpression of IL-9 alone is sufficient for eosinophilic airway inflammation and AHR in mice. Murine studies also show that IL-9 is genetically linked to BHR in different strains[64]. Human linkage studies have also implicated IL-9 in asthma. Receptor variants of IL-9 have been described which may explain differential sensitivity to the cytokine[65]. We have recently shown that IL-9 can up-regulate IL-5Rα on developing eosinophils and may act as an eosinophil survival factor[66].

Animal models have also defined the interaction of IL-5 with eotaxin and other chemokines in eosinophil mobilisation from the bone marrow. Collins *et al.* showed synergy between systemically delivered IL-5 with local eotaxin in recruitment of eosinophils, and both were shown to act in release of a bone marrow pool of eosinophils[67,68].

Factors regulating Th-2 development, recruitment and phenotype expression

Development of Th-1 and Th-2 cells

A variety of factors has been shown to act in driving developing naïve T-cell responses in either the Th-1 or Th-2 direction. The best defined is the cytokine environment, but the antigen dose, antigen presenting cell, local hormone and prostaglandin milieu can also influence the outcome[69]. As the molecular control of T-cell differentiation is defined, these data can be better understood. An important factor in Th-1/Th-2 development is the loss or retention of IL-12 responsiveness, determined at the level of expression of IL-12Rβ2. IL-4, unopposed by IFN-γ (or IFN-α in human cells) directs loss of IL-12Rβ2 expression and thus drives to Th-2 phenotype[70,71]. In contrast IFN-γ (IFN-α in humans) directs retention of IL-12Rβ2, and thus in the presence of IL-12, Th-1 development. More recently, the role of IL-1 family members induced in innate immune responses has been shown. In particular, IL-18 synergises with IL-12 in Th-1 phenotype expression, whereas Th-2 cells are responsive to IL-1α[72]. Indeed, IL-18R has been suggested as a phenotypic marker of Th-1 cells, whereas another IL-1R family member ST2/T1 appears restricted to Th-2 cells[73,74]. The ligand for ST2/T1 remains to defined.

Studies of transcriptional regulation of cytokine expression suggest a number of factors important in determining murine IL-4 production, including GATA3, c-maf, NIP-45 and NFAT[75]. Indeed overexpression of GATA3 was suggested to favour Th-2 development[76]. However, other investigators suggest that GATA3, together with NFκB, may be more important in control of IL-5 expression[77,78], and retroviral gene transfer to Th-1 cells down regulated IFN-γ production, suggesting that effects on IL-4 may be indirect[79]. It will be important to define whether similar mechanisms apply in regulating Th-2 phenotype expression in humans, although increased GATA3 expressing cells were seen in bronchial biopsies from asthmatic subjects[80]. Recent data suggest that IL-4, and IL-2, expression is regulated in a mono-allelic fashion[81]. Thus, only one of the two IL-4 alleles is expressed in developing Th-2 cells. In addition, further experiments are elucidating the epigenetic modification including histone de-acetylation and DNA methylation involved in directing gene expression, together with the role of cell cycling and passage of such epigenetic imprinting to determine, for example, IL-4 cells in progeny[82]. Understanding the molecular regulation of human Th-2 cytokine expression may help in understanding the complex genetics of asthma and atopy, and provide opportunities for regulating cytokine production in disease.

Although much work has been done on murine Th-1 and Th-2 development, and some of this has been extended to human T cells, there is still a need for information on the factors driving Th-2 responses during initiation of allergic disease and in maintaining the Th-2 phenotype in human allergen-specific memory T cells.

Recruitment of Th-1 and Th-2 cells

With the explosion of information on chemokines it has become clear that Th-1 and Th-2 cells can express different chemokine receptors and respond to different chemokines. It is also clear that chemokine receptor expression by T cells varies with activation status and cytokine environment, so that the picture *in vivo* may be different from that seen in isolated T cell clones. Current evidence suggests that human polarised Th-1 cells express CXCR3 and are more responsive to its ligand IP-10, whereas Th-2 lines express CCR3, CCR4 and CCR8 and respond to eotaxin, TARC and I-309[83,84]. Th-2 clones were reported to have reduced expression of CCR5. It will be interest to determine the chemokine receptor profile and responsiveness of allergen-specific T-cells *in vivo,* and to determine whether different chemokines are involved in recruitment, retention and activation of Th-2 cells at sites of allergic inflammation.

Differential responses of Th-1 and Th-2 cells to p- and e-selectin have been reported, and whether different adhesion pathways act in selection of Th-1 or Th-2 responses in humans remains to be established[85].

Conclusions and potential for regulating Th-2 responses

There is now considerable evidence that Th-2 type T-cell responses play a role in human atopic allergic disease. The factors that drive such a response in initiating the allergic diathesis will be important, and may act even *in utero*[86]. The relative role of continued 'new' Th-2 T-cells and memory responses in perpetuating human allergic disease and control of these processes will be important. The role of individual cytokines of the Th-2 'family' will become clearer with the use of blocking antibodies in human studies. Although initial understanding of the reciprocal regulation of Th-1 and Th-2 cells and data from immunotherapy studies were interpreted to suggest that inducing a Th-1 response might be beneficial in control of allergic inflammation, recent mouse studies suggest otherwise, and an allergen-specific Th-1 response might also induce pathology[87,88]. Of more interest is the possibility of inducing T-cell unresponsiveness, as had been described for both conventional allergen immunotherapy[89] and peptide therapy[90,91]. In particular, the description of regulatory T-cells, such as the murine Th-3, or murine and human Tr-1, that inhibit through cytokines such as IL-10 and TGF-β, is of interest[92,93]. Further understanding of normal immunological regulation of Th-1 and Th-2 responses may hold the key to targeted manipulation of pathological Th-2 responses in atopic allergic disease.

References

1   Mosmann TR, Cherwinski H, Bond MW, Gieldin MA, Coffman RL. Two types of murine helper T cell clone. I Definition according to profiles of lymphokine activities and secreted proteins. *J Immunol* 1986; **136**: 2348–57

2   Parish CR, Liew FY. Immune response to chemically modified flagellin. 3. Enhanced cell-mediated immunity during high and low zone antibody tolerance to flagellin. *J Exp Med* 1972; **135**: 298–311

3   Fong TA, Mosmann TR. The role of IFN-gamma in delayed-type hypersensitivity mediated by Th-1 clones. *J Immunol* 1989; **143**: 2887–93

4   Del Prete GF, Maggi E, Parronchi P *et al*. IL-4 is an essential factor for the IgE synthesis induced in vitro by human T cell clones and their supernatants. *J Immunol* 1988; **140**: 4193–8

5   Sanderson CJ. Interleukin 5, eosinophils and disease. *Blood* 1992; **79**: 3101–9

6   Heinzel FP, Sadick MD, Holaday BJ, Coffman RL, Locksley RM. Reciprocal expression of interferon gamma or interleukin 4 during the resolution or progression of murine leishmaniasis. Evidence for expansion of distinct helper T cell subsets. *J Exp Med* 1989; **169**: 59–72

7   Scott P, Natovitz P, Coffman RL, Pearce E, Sher A. Immunoregulation of cutaneous leishmaniasis. T cell lines that transfer protective immunity or exacerbation belong to different T helper subsets and respond to distinct parasite antigens. *J Exp Med* 1988; **168**: 1675–84

8   Guler ML, Gorham J, Hsieh CS *et al*. Genetic susceptibility to Leishmania: IL-12 responsiveness in TH1 cell development *Science* 1996; **271**: 984–7

9   Parronchi P, Macchia D, Piccinni MP *et al*. Allergen- and bacterial antigen-specific T-cell clones established from atopic donors show a different profile of cytokine production. *Proc Natl Acad Sci USA* 1991; **88**: 4538–42

10   Wierenga EA, Snoek M, de Groot C *et al*. Evidence compartmentalization of functional subsets of CD4$^+$ T lymphocytes in atopic patients. *J Immunol* 1990; **144**: 4651–6

11   Plaut M, Pierce JH, Watson CJ, Haney-Hyde J, Nordan RP, Paul WE. Mast cell lines produce lymphokines in response to cross-linkage of FcεRI or calcium ionophore. *Nature* 1989; **329**: 64–7

12   Moqbel R, Ying S, Barkans J *et al*. Identification of mRNA for interleukin-4 in human eosinophils with granule localization and release of the translated product. *J Immunol* 1995; **155**: 4939–47

13   Brunner T, Heusser CH, Dahinden CA. Human peripheral blood basophils primed by interleukin 3 (IL-3) produce IL-4 in response to immunoglobulin E receptor stimulation. *J Exp Med* 1993; **177**: 605–10

14   Gauchat J-F, Henchoz S, Mazzei G *et al*. Induction of human IgE synthesis in B cells by mast cells and basophils. *Nature* 1993; **365**: 340–3

15   Geha RS. Regulation of IgE synthesis in humans. *J Allergy Clin Immunol* 1992; **90**: 143–50

16   Sutton BJ, Gould HJ. The human IgE network. *Nature* 1993; **366**: 421–8

17   Pene J, Rousset F, Briere F *et al*. Interleukin 5 enhances interleukin 4-induced IgE production by normal human B cells. The role of soluble CD23 antigen. *Eur J Immunol* 1988; **18**: 929–35

18   Vercelli D, Jabara HH, Arai K, Yokota T, Geha RS. Endogenous IL-6 plays an obligatory role in IL-4-induced human IgE synthesis. *Eur J Immunol* 1989; **19**: 1419–22

19   Dugas B, Renauld JC, Pene J *et al*. Interleukin-9 potentiates the interleukin-4-induced immunoglobulin (IgG, IgM and IgE) production by normal human B lymphocytes. *Eur J Immunol* 1993l; **23**: 1687–92

20   Gauchat J-F, Henchoz S, Mazzei G *et al*. Induction of human IgE synthesis in B cells by mast cells and basophils. *Nature* 1993; **365**: 340–3

21   Denburg JA, Silver JE, Abrams JS. Interleukin-5 is a human basophilopoietin: induction of histamine content and basophilic differentiation of HL-60 cells and of peripheral blood basophil-eosinophil progenitors. *Blood* 1991; **77**: 1462–8

22   Huston MM, Moore JP, Mettes HJ, Tavana G, Huston DP. Human B cells express IL-5 receptor messenger ribonucleic acid and respond to IL-5 with enhanced IgM production after mitogenic stimulation with *Moraxella catarrhalis*. *J Immunol* 1996; **156**: 1392–401

23   Tavernier J, Devos R, Cornelis S *et al*. A human high affinity interleukin 5 receptor (IL-5R) is composed of an IL-5-specific alpha chain and a beta chain shared with the receptor for GM-CSF. *Cell* 1991; **66**: 1175–84

24   Kitamura T, Sato N, Arai K, Miyajima A. Expression cloning of the human interleukin 3 receptor cDNA reveals a shared beta subunit for the human IL-3 and GM-CSF receptors. *Cell* 1991; **66**: 1165–74

25 Clutterbuck EJ, Hirst EM, Sanderson CJ. Human interleukin 5 (IL-5) regulates the production of eosinophils in human bone marrow cultures: comparison and interaction with IL-1, IL-3, IL-6, and GM-CSF. *Blood* 1989; **73**: 1504–12

26 Tavernier J, Van der Heyden J, Verhee A *et al.* Interleukin 5 regulates the isoform expression of its own receptor α-subunit. Blood 2000; **96**: 1600–7

27 Robinson DS, Hamid Q, Sun Ying *et al.* Predominant Th-2-like bronchoalveolar T-lymphocyte population in atopic asthma. *N Engl J Med* 1992; **326**: 298–304

28 Robinson DS, Ying S, Bentley AM *et al.* Relationships among numbers of bronchoalveolar lavage cells expressing messenger ribonucleic acid for cytokines, asthma symptoms, and airway methacholine responsiveness in atopic asthma. *J Allergy Clin Immunol* 1993; **92**: 397–403

29 Walker C, Bode E, Boer L, Hansel TT, Blaser K, Virchow Jr J-C. Allergic and non-allergic asthmatics have distinct patterns of T-cell activation and cytokine production in peripheral blood and bronchoalveolar lavage. *Am Rev Respir Dis* 1992; **146**: 109–15

30 Del Prete GF, De Carli M, D'Elios MM *et al.* Allergen exposure induces the activation of allergen-specific Th-2 cells in the airway mucosa of patients with allergic respiratory disorders. *Eur J Immunol* 1993; **23**: 1445–9

31 Till S, Li B, Durham S *et al.* Secretion of the eosinophil-active cytokines interleukin-5, granulocyte/macrophage colony-stimulating factor and interleukin-3 by bronchoalveolar lavage CD4+ and CD8+ T cell lines in atopic asthmatics, and atopic and non-atopic controls. *Eur J Immunol* 1995; **25**: 2727–31

32 Ying S, Humbert M, Barkans J *et al.* Expression of IL-4 and IL-5 mRNA and protein product by CD4+ and CD8+ T cells, eosinophils, and mast cells in bronchial biopsies obtained from atopic and nonatopic (intrinsic) asthmatics. *J Immunol* 1997; **158**: 3539–44

33 Robinson DS, Tsicopoulos A, Meng Q, Durham S, Kay AB, Hamid Q. Increased interleukin-10 messenger RNA expression in atopic allergy and asthma. *Am J Respir Cell Mol Biol* 1996; **14**: 113–7

34 Humbert M, Durham SR, Kimmitt P *et al.* Elevated expression of messenger ribonucleic acid encoding IL-13 in the bronchial mucosa of atopic and nonatopic subjects with asthma. *J Allergy Clin Immunol* 1997; **99**: 657–65

35 Bentley AM, Menz G, Storz Chr *et al.* Identification of T-lymphocytes, macrophages and activated eosinophils in the bronchial mucosa in intrinsic asthma: relationship to symptoms and bronchial responsiveness. *Am Rev Respir Dis* 1992; **146**: 500–6

36 Humbert M, Durham M, Ying S *et al.* IL-4 and IL-5 mRNA and protein in bronchial biopsies from atopic and non-atopic asthmatics: evidence against 'intrinsic' asthma being a distinct immunopathological entity. *Am J Respir Crit Care Med* 1996; **154**: 1497–504

37 Humbert M, Grant JA, Taborda-Barata L *et al.* High affinity IgE receptor (FcεRI)-bearing cells in bronchial biopsies from atopic and nonatopic asthma. *Am J Respir Crit Care Med* 1996; **153**: 1931–7

38 Valenta R, Natter S, Seiberler S *et al.* Molecular characterization of an autoallergen, Hom s 1, identified by serum IgE from atopic dermatitis patients. *J Invest Dermatol* 1998; **111**: 1178–83

39 Frew AJ, Kay AB. The relationship between infiltrating CD4+ lymphocytes, activated eosinophils, and the magnitude of the allergen-induced late phase cutaneous reaction in man. *J Immunol* 1988; **141**: 4158–64

40 Robinson DS, Hamid Q, Bentley AM, Sun Ying, Kay AB, Durham SR. CD4+ T cell activation, eosinophil recruitment and interleukin 4 (IL-4), IL-5 and GM-CSF messenger RNA expression in bronchoalveolar lavage after allergen inhalation challenge of atopic asthmatics. *J Allergy Clin Immunol* 1993; **92**: 313–24

41 Kay AB, Ying S, Varney V *et al.* Messenger RNA expression of the cytokine gene cluster, interleukin 3 (IL-3), IL-4, IL-5, and granulocyte/macrophage colony-stimulating factor, in allergen-induced late-phase cutaneous reactions in atopic subjects. *J Exp Med* 1991; **173**: 775–8

42 Durham SR, Sun Ying, Varney VA *et al.* Cytokine messenger RNA expression for IL-3, IL-4, IL-5 and granulocyte macrophage colony-stimulating factor in the nasal mucosa after allergen provocation: relationship to tissue eosinophilia. *J Immunol* 1992; **148**: 2390–4

43 Bentley AM, Qiu Meng, Robinson DS, Hamid Q, Kay AB, Durham SR. Increases in activated T lymphocytes, eosinophils, and cytokine messenger RNA expression or IL-5 and GM-CSF in

bronchial biopsies after allergen inhalation challenge in atopic asthmatics. *Am J Respir Cell Mol Biol* 1993; **8**: 35–42

44   Robinson DS, Hamid Q, Sun Ying *et al*. Prednisolone treatment in asthma is associated with modulation of bronchoalveolar lavage cell interleukin-4, interleukin-5 and interferon-gamma cytokine gene expression. *Am Rev Respir Dis* 1993; **148**: 401–6

45   Leung DYM, Martin RJ, Szefler SJ *et al*. Dysregulation of interleukin 4, interleukin 5, and interferon γ gene expression in steroid-resistant asthma. *J Exp Med* 1995; **181**: 33–40

46   Alexander AG, Barnes NC, Kay AB. Trial of cyclosporin A in corticosteroid-dependent chronic severe asthma. *Lancet* 1992; **339**: 324–8

47   Lock SH, Kay AB, Barnes NC. Double-blind, placebo-controlled study of cyclosporin A as a corticosteroid-sparing agent in corticosteroid-dependent asthma. *Am J Respir Crit Care Med* 1996; **153**: 509–14

48   Sihra BS, Durham SR, Walker S, Kon OM, Barnes NC, Kay AB. Inhibition of the allergen-induced late asthmatic response by cyclosporin A. Effect of cyclosporin A on the allergen-induced late asthmatic reaction. *Thorax* 1997; **52**: 447–52

49   Kon OM, Sihra BS, Compton CH, Leonard TB, Kay AB, Barnes NC. Randomised, dose-ranging, placebo-controlled study of chimeric antibody to CD4 (keliximab) in chronic severe asthma. *Lancet* 1998; **352**: 1109–13

50   Jutel M, Pichler WJ, Skrbic D, Urwyler A, Dahinden C, Muller UR. Bee venom immunotherapy results in decrease of IL-4 and IL-5 and increase of IFN-gamma secretion in specific allergen-stimulated T cell cultures. *J Immunol* 1995; **154**: 4187–94

51   Secrist H, Chelen CJ, Wen Y, Marshall JD, Umetsu DT. Allergen immunotherapy decreases interleukin 4 production in CD4+ T cells from allergic individuals. *J Exp Med* 1993; **178**: 2123–30

52   Durham SR, Ying S, Varney VA *et al*. Grass pollen immunotherapy inhibits allergen-induced infiltration of CD4+ T lymphocytes and eosinophils in the nasal mucosa and increases the number of cells expressing messenger RNA for interferon-gamma. *J Allergy Clin Immunol* 1996; **97**: 1356–65

53   Corry DB, Folkesson HG, Warnock ML *et al*. Interleukin-4, but not interleukin-5 or eosinophils, is required in a murine model of acute airway hyperreactivity. *J Exp Med* 1996; **183**: 109–17

54   Foster PS, Hogan SP, Ramsay AJ, Matthaei KI, Young IG. IL-5 deficiency abolishes eosinophilia, airways hyperreactivity, and lung damage in a mouse asthma model. *J Exp Med* 1995; **183**: 195–201

55   Hogan SP, Matthaei KI, Young JM, Koskinen A, Young IG, Foster PS. A novel T cell-regulated mechanism modulating allergen-induced airways hyperreactivity in BALB/c mice independently of IL-4 and IL-5. *J Immunol* 1998; **161**: 1501–9

56   Gavett SH, Chen X, Finkelman F, Wills-Karp M. Depletion of murine CD4+ T lymphocytes prevents antigen-induced airway hyperreactivity and pulmonary eosinophilia. *Am J Respir Cell Mol Biol* 1994; **10**: 587–93

57   Li-XM, Schofield BH, Wang QF, Kim KH, Huang SK. Induction of pulmonary allergic responses by antigen-specific Th-2 cells. *J Immunol* 1998; **160**: 1378–84

58   Wills-Karp M, Luyimbazi J, Xu X *et al*. Interleukin-13: central mediator of allergic asthma. *Science* 1998; **282**: 2258–61

59   Grunig G, Warnock M, Wakil AE *et al*. Requirement for IL-13 independently of IL-4 in experimental asthma. *Science* 1998; **282**: 2261–3

60   Wang J, Palmer K, Lotval J *et al*. Circulating, but not local lung IL-5 is required for the development of antigen-induced airways eosinophilia. *J Clin Invest* 1998; **102**: 1132–41

61   Temann UA, Geba GP, Rankin JA, Flavell RA. Expression of interleukin 9 in the lungs of transgenic mice causes airway inflammation, mast cell hyperplasia and bronchial hyperresponsiveness. *J Exp Med* 1998; **188**: 1307–20

62   Tang W, Geba GP, Zheng T *et al*. Targeted expression of IL-11 in the murine airway causes lymphocytic inflammation, bronchial remodeling, and airways obstruction. *J Clin Invest* 1996; **98**: 2845–53

63   Zhu Z, Homer RJ, Wang Z *et al*. Pulmonary expression of interleukin 13 causes inflammation, mucus hypersecretion subepithelial fibrosis, physiologic abnormalities and eotaxin production. *J Clin Invest* 1999; **103**: 779–88

64 Wills-Karp M, Ewart SL. The genetics of allergen-induced airway hyperresponsiveness in mice. *Am J Respir Crit Care Med* 1997; **156**: S89–96

65 Grasso L, Huang M, Sullivan CD *et al.* Molecular analysis of human interleukin-9 receptor transcripts in peripheral blood mononuclear cells. *J Biol Chem* 1998; **273**: 24016–24

66 Soussi Gounni A, Gregory B, Nutku E *et al.* Interleukin-9 enhances interleukin-5 receptor expression, differentiation and survival of human eosinophils. Blood 2000; **96**: 2163–71

67 Collins PD, Marleau S, Griffiths-Johnson DA, Jose PJ, Williams TJ. Co-operation between interleukin-5 and the chemokine eotaxin to induce eosinophil accumulation *in vivo. J Exp Med* 1995; **182**: 1169–74

68 Palframan RT, Collins PD, Williams TJ, Rankin SM. Eotaxin induces a rapid release of eosinophils and their progenitors from the bone marrow. *Blood* 1998; **91**: 2240–8

69 O'Garra A. Cytokines induce the development of functionally heterogeneous T helper cell subsets. *Immunity* 1998; **8**: 275–83

70 Szabo SJ, Dighe AS, Gubler U, Murphy KM. Regulation of the interleukin (IL)-12R beta 2 subunit expression in developing T helper 1 (Th-1) and Th-2 cells. *J Exp Med* 1997; **185**: 817–24

71 Rogge L, Barberis-Maino L, Biffi M *et al.* Selective expression of an interleukin-12 receptor component by human T helper 1 cells. *J Exp Med* 1997; **185**: 825–31

72 Robinson D, Shibuya K, Mui A *et al.* IGIF does not drive Th-1 development but synergizes with IL-12 for interferon-gamma production and activates IRAK and NFkappaB. *Immunity* 1997; **7**: 571–81

73 Xu D, Chan WL, Leung BP *et al.* Selective expression of a stable cell surface molecule on type 2 but not type 1 helper T cells. *J Exp Med* 1998; **187**: 787–94

74 Xu D, Chan WL, Leung BP *et al.* Selective expression and functions of interleukin 18 receptor on T helper (Th) type 1 but not Th-2 cells. *J Exp Med* 1998; **188**: 1485–92

75 Szabo SJ, Glimcher LH, Ho IC. Genes that regulate interleukin-4 expression in T cells. *Curr Opin Immunol* 1997; **9**: 776–81

76 Zheng W, Flavell RA. The transcription factor GATA-3 is necessary and sufficient for Th-2 cytokine gene expression in CD4 T cells. *Cell* 1997; **89**: 587–96

77 Zhang DH, Yang L, Ray A. Differential responsiveness of the IL-5 and IL-4 genes to transcription factor GATA-3. *J Immunol* 1998; **161**: 3817–21

78 Yang L, Cohn L, Zhang DH, Homer R, Ray A, Ray P. Essential role of nuclear factor kappaB in the induction of eosinophilia in allergic airway inflammation. *J Exp Med* 1998; **188**: 1739–50

79 Ouyang W, Ranganath SH, Weindel K *et al.* Inhibition of Th-1 development mediated by GATA-3 through an IL-4-independent mechanism. *Immunity* 1998; **9**: 745–55

80 Nakamura Y, Ghaffar O, Olivenstein R *et al.* Gene expression of the GATA3 transcription factor is increased in atopic asthma. *J Allergy Clin Immunol* 1999; **103**: 215–22

81 Riviere I, Sunshine MJ, Littman DR. Regulation of IL-4 expression by activation of individual alleles. *Immunity* 1998; **9**: 217–28

82 Bird J, Brown DR, Mullen AC *et al.* Helper T cell differentiation is controlled by the cell cycle. *Immunity* 1998; **9**: 229–37

83 Sallusto F, Lenig D, Mackay CR, Lanzavecchia A. Flexible programs of chemokine receptor expression on human polarised T helper 1 and 2 lymphocytes. *J Exp Med* 1998; **187**: 875–83

84 Zingoni A, Soto H, Hedrick JA *et al.* The chemokine receptor CCR8 is preferentially expressed in Th-2 but not Th-1 cells. *J Immunol* 1998; **161**: 547–51

85 Austrup F, Vestweber D, Borges E *et al.* P- and E-selectin mediate recruitment of T-helper-1 but not T-helper-2 cells into inflamed tissues. *Nature* 1997; **385**: 81–3

86 Prescott SL, Macaubas C, Smallacombe T, Holt BJ, Sly PD, Holt PG. Development of allergen-specific T-cell memory in atopic and normal children. *Lancet* 1999; **353**: 196–200

87 Randolph DA, Carruthers CJ, Szabo SJ, Murphy KM, Chaplin DD. Modulation of airway inflammation by passive transfer of allergen-specific Th-1 and Th-2 cells in a mouse model of asthma. *J Immunol* 1999; **162**: 2375–83

88 Hansen G, Berry G, DeKruyff RH, Umetsu DT. Allergen-specific Th-1 cells fail to counterbalance Th-2 cell-induced hyperreactivity but cause severe airway inflammation. *J Clin Invest* 1999; **103**: 175–83

89 Akdis CA, Akdis M, Blesken T *et al*. Epitope-specific T cell tolerance to phospholipase A$_2$ in bee venom immunotherapy and recovery by IL-2 and IL-15 *in vitro*. *J Clin Invest* 1996; **98**: 1676–83

90 Norman PS, Ohman Jr JL, Long AA *et al*. Treatment of cat allergy with T-cell reactive peptides. *Am J Respir Crit Care Med* 1996; **154**: 1623–8

91 Haselden BM, Kay AB, Larche M. IgE-independent MHC-restricted T cell peptide epitope-induced late asthmatics reactions. *J Exp Med* 1999; **189**: 1885–94

92 Fukaura H, Kent SC, Pietrusewicz MJ, Khoury SJ, Weiner HL, Hafler DA. Induction of circulating myelin basic protein and proteolipid protein-specific transforming growth factor-beta1-secreting Th3 T cells by oral administration of myelin in multiple sclerosis patients. *J Clin Invest* 1996; **98**: 70–7

93 Groux H, O'Garra A, Bigler M *et al*. A CD4$^+$ T-cell subset inhibits antigen-specific T-cell responses and prevents colitis. *Nature* 1997; **389**: 737–42

Molecular aspects of T-cell differentiation

Anjana Rao and **Orly Avni**

The Center for Blood Research and the Department of Pathology, Harvard Medical School, Boston, Massachusetts, USA

Differentiated T helper 1 (Th1) and T helper 2 (Th2) T-cells show striking differences in their patterns of cytokine expression. This process is initiated by stimulation with antigen and the cytokines IL-12 and IL-4, respectively, and requires antigen-induced transcription factors such as NFAT and cytokine-induced transcription factors such as STAT4, induced by IL-12, and STAT6, induced by IL-4. This results in induction and maintained expression of subset-specific transcription factors including T-bet in Th1 cells and GATA3 in Th2 cells, which are involved in ensuring the commitment of T-cells to Th1 or Th2 lineages. Here we review the signalling pathways and transcription factors that mediate T-cell differentiation, and describe the epigenetic changes in chromatin structure, locus accessibility and DNA methylation that are known to accompany this process.

T-cells undergoing an immune response show varying patterns of cytokine production. The most discernible patterns are represented in both T helper and T cytolytic populations, and have been termed type 1 and type 2 (reviewed by Mossman & Coffman[1]). The patterns were originally identified by analysis of murine CD4+ T helper cell clones. T helper 1 (Th1) cells were defined as producing IFN-γ, TNF and lymphotoxin, but not IL-4, IL-5 or IL-13; while Th2 cells were defined as producing IL-4, IL-5, IL-9, IL-10 and IL-13 but not IFN-γ. While many established T-cell clones completely fit the Th1/Th2 paradigm in terms of non-overlapping patterns of IL-4 and IFN-γ expression, under physiological conditions the paradigm is more applicable to populations than to single cells (reviewed by Kelso[2]). The strongest *in vivo* levels of Th1/Th2 polarisation are elicited by chronic antigen stimulation; in particular, highly polarised Th1 and Th2 patterns of cytokine production are associated with states of chronic microbial and parasitic infections, respectively (reviewed by Abbas *et al*[3]). With less chronic exposure to antigen, Th1 and Th2 patterns of cytokine expression may still be apparent at the population level, but individual T-cells show varied and complex patterns of cytokine expression (reviewed by Fitzpatrick & Kelso[4]).

There are several features other than cytokine production that, at least at a population level, distinguish Th1 and Th2 cell populations (reviewed elsewhere[5–7]). Among these are several cytokine, chemokine

Correspondence to:
Dr Anjana Rao, The
Center for Blood
Research and the
Department of
Pathology, Harvard
Medical School, Warren
Alpert Building, 200
Longwood Avenue,
Boston, MA 02115, USA

and adhesion receptors, which presumably influence the migration and homing of differentiated T-cells and their responses to their immediate environment. Thus the IL-12 receptor β chain, the IFN-γ receptor β chain on Th1 cells, and the chemokine receptors CXCR3 and CCR5 are preferentially expressed on Th1 cells, while CCR3 (the eotaxin receptor), a novel IL-1-like molecule, T1/ST2, and the chemokine receptors CCR4 and CCR8 are preferentially expressed on Th2 cells. Th1 and Th2 cells are also distinguished by their differential expression of certain transcription factors (ERM and T-bet in Th1 cells, GATA-3 and cMaf in Th2 cells) that are important in maintaining the differential patterns of cytokine expression. The functional importance of some of these molecules will become apparent in the discussions below.

This review deals with the molecular basis for production of the signature cytokines of Th1 and Th2 cells, IFN-γ and IL-4/IL-5/IL-13. The latter three genes are grouped together since they are closely linked and reside within a ~200 kb genomic interval on a single chromosome in all mammalian species tested[8,9]. The IL-4, IL-5 and IL-13 genes are also co-expressed in mast cells, suggesting that their expression is coordinately regulated over a large chromosomal interval (although there is also evidence for non-coordinate regulation). The signalling pathways, the transcription factors, and the chromatin-based processes involved in IFN-γ and IL-4/IL-5/IL-13 gene transcription are briefly described.

The Th1/Th2 classification in disease

The Th1/Th2 classification has been most useful when relating overall patterns of cytokine production to clinical outcomes in a variety of pathological states (reviewed by Abbas *et al*[3]). Th1 patterns of cytokine production have protective functions in microbial infections. This is particularly apparent in leprosy, where the healing (tuberculoid) form of leprosy is associated with a predominant Th1 cytokine pattern and strong delayed-type hypersensitivity (DTH) responses, while uncontrolled lepromatous lesions are characterised by a Th2 cytokine pattern and weak DTH but high antibody titres. The clinical outcomes of microbial infections can be predicted based on the biological functions of the cytokines produced (reviewed by Abbas *et al*[3]). The principal Th1 effector cytokine, IFN-γ, activates effector macrophages, promoting their ability to ingest and destroy microbes. Together with IL-2, IFN-γ promotes the differentiation of CD8 T-cells into actively cytotoxic cells. Together with TNF-β, it recruits and activates inflammatory leukocytes. Thus Th1-dominated immune responses are associated with the presence of activated macrophages and cytolytic T-cells. In industrialised countries where there is less exposure to microbial infections, Th1-type cytokine patterns are observed clinically in cases of chronic inflammation, tissue injury, and autoimmune disease.

In contrast, Th2-type cytokine patterns are strongly apparent in parasitic infections, although whether they are truly protective is controversial (reviewed by Abbas et al[3]). Th2 cytokine responses are clearly associated with deleterious allergic reactions to environmental antigens and with the development of chronic bronchial inflammation and airways hyper-responsiveness in asthma (reviewed elsewhere[10,11]). The Th2 cytokine IL-4 is the principal agent that induces B cell switching to IgE production. IgE binds almost irreversibly to the IgE receptor on mast cells, and its crosslinking by multivalent antigens leads to the release of diverse inflammatory mediators[11]. The biological functions of IL-13 partially overlap with those of IL-4, possibly because the receptors for these two cytokines share a common subunit, the α-chain of the IL-4 receptor[12]. In mice, IL-13 induces many features of asthma, such as airway hyper-responsiveness and hypersecretion of mucus, without inducing eosinophilic inflammation[13]. The later stages of allergic asthma, which are characterised by eosinophilia and chronic tissue inflammation, appear to be mediated by IL-5, the principal cytokine responsible for eosinophil activation[14]. IL-5 is highly effective at releasing eosinophils and their precursors from the bone marrow. A single injection of anti-IL-5 diminishes the number of circulating eosinophils in an effect that lasts for several weeks, and 'knockout' mice lacking IL-5 or its receptor show marked defects in eosinophil responses to helminths (reviewed elsewhere[3,10,11]).

Signalling pathways and transcription factors underlying T-cell differentiation

The signalling pathways that contribute to Th differentiation are relatively well understood, with the best-characterised being those initiated by cytokines (reviewed elsewhere[5-7]). IL-12, IFN-α and IL-18 play a major role in promoting Th1 differentiation, while IL-4 (and to some extent IL-13) are the key cytokines that determine Th2 differentiation (Fig. 1). However, the nature of the antigen-presenting cell, the strength of stimulation with antigen, and the level and nature of co-stimulation also play important roles. This review will focus only on the most well-established pathways; for a discussion of other factors, the reader is referred to several excellent and recent reviews[3-7].

Th1 differentiation

Several signalling inputs that influence Th1 differentiation and IFN-γ production have been identified (reviewed elsewhere[5-7,15,16] and Fig.1). In

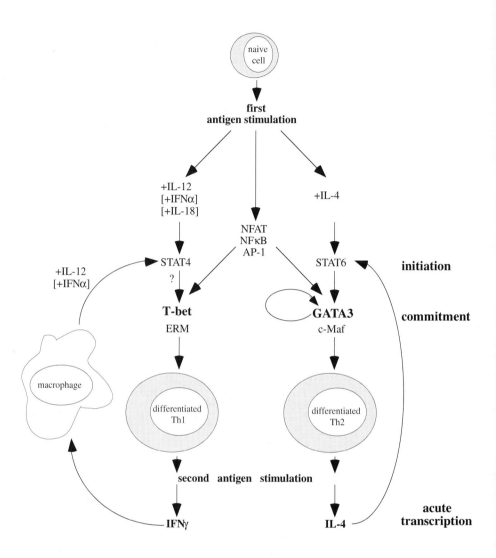

Fig. 1 Signalling pathways and transcription factors underlying T cell differentiation

the mouse, IL-12 induces Th1 differentiation while IFN-α has no effect; in contrast, Th1 differentiation of human T-cells can be induced by either IL-12 or IFN-α, although IFN-α may play the predominant role in controlling IFN-γ production *in vivo*. In humans, both IL-12 and IFN-α act through the STAT transcription factor STAT4, while only IL-12 induces STAT4 in the mouse. Mice deficient in IL-12 or STAT4 show a strong defect in IFN-γ production by CD4 T-cells, although IFN-γ production by CD8 T-cells is much less affected. Moreover, mice deficient in both STAT4 and STAT6 are capable of mounting Th1 responses, apparently because of the existence of an alternate STAT4-independent pathway of IFN-γ production that is suppressed by STAT6[17]. Indeed, STAT1, which is also induced by both IFN-α and IL-12, may substitute for STAT4 in human T-cells and in murine CD8 T-cells.

The cytokine IL-18 is related to IL-1 and, like IL-1, is coupled to activation of the transcription factor NFκB (reviewed by Akira[18]). IL-18 synergises powerfully with IL-12 to promote Th1 differentiation, in part by increasing the efficiency of Th1 differentiation and in part by acting on differentiated Th1 cells to enhance cytokine expression. Mice deficient in both IL-12 and IL-18 have a much more severe defect in IFN-γ production than mice lacking IL-12 or IL-18 alone.

The control of Th1 differentiation by IL-12 and IFN-α forms the basis for a powerful positive feedback loop that enhances IFN-γ production during microbial and viral infections (reviewed elsewhere[3-7] and Fig. 1). In the first arm of the positive feedback loop, microbial products such as endotoxin activate macrophages and induce IL-2 production. Likewise viral infections increase the production of type I interferons such as IFN-α by the infected cells. These cytokines, IL-12 and IFN-α, then act on naive T-cells to induce Th1 differentiation and IFN-γ production. The positive feedback loop is completed when IFN-γ produced by the differentiated Th1 cells further activates macrophages and potentiates their ability to produce IL-12. Thus the initial response of macrophages to microbial infections (IL-12 production) is exactly that needed to promote the development of the T-cell subset which, by producing IFN-γ, further activates them and enhances their microbicidal activity.

Two transcription factors, T-bet and ERM, have been described that are induced by STAT4 and T-cell receptor stimulation (reviewed elsewhere[5,6,16])[19,20]. As expected, both T-bet and ERM are preferentially expressed in Th1 cells relative to Th2 cells. However, ERM does not promote IFN-γ production when introduced into differentiating Th2 cells. In contrast, ectopic expression of T-bet in a variety of cell types leads to strong expression of IFN-γ and several Th1-specific cell surface receptors. Moreover, T-bet overexpression leads to down-regulation of the expression of IL-2 and several Th2-specific cytokines, suggesting that this transcription factor play a central role in promoting not only the development and maintenance of the Th1 phenotype but also suppression of the Th2 phenotype. The mechanistic basis for T-bet function is not yet well-understood; in particular, it is unclear whether expression of the IFN-γ gene and other Th1-specific genes requires direct binding of T-bet to one or more regulatory regions of these genes, or whether T-bet induces secondary transcription factors that contribute to gene expression.

Th2 differentiation

The cytokine IL-4, acting through the IL-4-induced transcription factor STAT6, exerts the single most powerful positive influence on T-cell differentiation towards the Th2 phenotype (reviewed elsewhere[3–7,15] and Fig.1). T-cells from STAT6-deficient mice are strongly suppressed for Th2 differentiation, although a small number of IL-4 producing cells can occasionally be observed[21]. T-cells from IL-4-deficient mice show a less striking phenotype on average; this is attributed to the fact that IL-13 also induces STAT6, since mice doubly deficient for IL-4 and IL-13 are as defective as STAT6$^{-/-}$ mice in their ability to produce Th2 cells. Ectopic expression of activated STAT6 in differentiating T-cells induces IL-4 production as shown by the use of a conditional STAT6-oestrogen receptor fusion protein that can be activated by tamoxifen without the need for IL-4[22]. These conditions also result in up-regulation of two transcription factors, GATA3 and cMaf (Maf), that are known to be preferentially expressed in Th2 cells relative to Th1 cells[23–25].

STAT6 may in large part exert its effects on Th2 differentiation by up-regulating the expression of GATA3[21–23,26]. While studies with cMaf-transgenic and knockout mice indicate that Maf controls transcription of only the IL-4 gene, and not the other cytokines and cell surface markers characteristic of the Th2 phenotype[27,28], it is becoming clear that GATA3 plays a major role in the expression of several Th2 cytokines and in the overall development of the Th2 phenotype itself. In fact, examination of the few IL-4-producing cells from STAT6-deficient mice indicates that these cells have stochastically up-regulated their level of GATA3 expression[21]; conversely, ectopic expression of GATA3 in differentiating Th1 cells results in IL-4 production[21,26]. Functional binding sites for GATA3 have been described in the IL-5 promoter[24] and a 3′ IL-4 enhancer[29]; and GATA3-transgenic mice show up-regulation of the Th2 cytokines IL-4, IL-5, and IL-10[23].

As described for Th1 cells above, Th2 differentiation is strongly potentiated by a powerful positive feedback loop involving autocrine activation of IL-4 gene transcription by extracellular IL-4 (reviewed elsewhere[3–7] and Fig. 1). The intracellular correlate of this positive feedback loop is the ability of ectopically-expressed GATA3 to up-regulate expression of the endogenous GATA3 gene, indicating the existence of an intracellular positive regulatory loop in which GATA3 autoactivates its own expression[21]. This property of GATA3 provides a very satisfactory explanation for how the Th2 phenotype (*i.e.* the characteristic expression of cell-surface receptors and the ability to produce IL-4, IL-5 and IL-13 upon subsequent stimulation) is maintained in resting Th2 cells in the absence of overt stimulation with IL-4 or intracellular activation of STAT6.

An alternate STAT6-independent pathway for Th2 differentiation has become apparent through studies of the transcriptional repressor BCL-6. Mice lacking BCL-6 display a profound Th2 bias[30], possibly because BCL-6 competes with STAT6 for binding sites in DNA and then is capable of recruiting transcriptional co-repressor complexes containing histone deacetylases to the relevant genes[30,31]. Interestingly, the Th2 bias observed in BCL-6-deficient T-cells is not dependent on STAT6, since a very similar degree of Th2 bias is observed in T-cells singly deficient for BCL-6 or doubly deficient for both BCL-6 and STAT6[32]; in contrast, T-cells lacking only STAT6 are only poorly capable of Th2 differentiation[3–7]. The possibilities are that BCL-6 inhibits a STAT6-independent pathway of Th2 differentiation, or that in the absence of the repressive influence exerted by BCL-6, the positive influence of STAT6 becomes less crucial for achieving the differentiated Th2 phenotype.

Negative feedback effects, mixed inputs and mixed phenotypes

In addition to the positive feedback pathways, there are strong negative feedback mechanisms by which IL-4, STAT6, GATA3 and Maf act to maintain the Th2 phenotype of differentiated T-cells and to down-regulate Th1 cytokine expression (Fig. 2). IL-4 has long been known to down-regulate IFN-γ production, and this effect appears to be mediated through the STAT6 target gene products GATA3 and Maf. Ectopic expression of GATA-3 or Maf, even in IL-4-deficient naive T-cells, results in marked inhibition of IFN-γ production by Th1 cells[21,26,28]. In contrast, forced expression of GATA-3 in established Th1 clones had little effect, indicating that the down-regulatory effects of GATA3 were not due to direct repression of IFN-γ gene transcription in stimulated Th1 cells, but rather were exerted at an earlier step of differentiation[21,26].

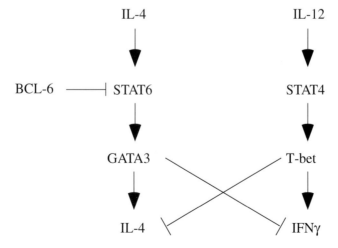

Fig. 2 Negative feedback effect of GATA3 and T-bet on production of the opposing cytokines

Conversely, ectopic expression of the Th1 transcription factor T-bet in differentiating T-cells led to down-regulation of IL-2 and several Th2-specific cytokines, suggesting that the role of this transcription factor in the Th1 lineage is analogous to that of GATA3 in the Th2 lineage[20].

In the mouse, differentiating Th2 cells lose expression of the β-2 subunit of the IL-12 receptor, thus dampening their ability to respond by IFN-γ production to stimulation with IL-12, and focusing their cytokine production towards IL-4 (reviewed elsewhere[5,6]). Ectopic expression of GATA3 in murine Th1 cells also resulted in down-regulation of IL-12Rβ2 chain expression, indicating that this down-regulation is also mediated by GATA3[33].

It is important to note, however, that cytokine production under conditions of mixed Th1/Th2 stimulation conditions reflects a balance between the different inputs prevailing in the culture environment (reviewed elsewhere[3–7]). When IL-4 and IL-12 are both present in cultures of naive murine T-cells at the time of antigen contact, the T-cells differentiate into IL-4-producing Th2 cells and lose IL-12Rβ2 chain expression, indicating that Th2 differentiation in the mouse is dominated by the positive autocrine effect of IL-4 and is less susceptible to negative feedback from IL-12. However, when high levels of IFN-γ are present in addition to IL-4, expression of the IL12Rβ2 chain is maintained, and cells producing both IL-4 and IFN-γ are obtained. Similarly human T-cells frequently co-express IL-4 and IFN-γ, possibly because the IFN-α receptor, unlike the IL12Rβ2 chain, is not lost during Th2 differentiation and continues to activate STAT1 and STAT4 which promote IFN-γ expression.

Regulation of cytokine gene expression at the level of chromatin accessibility

General considerations

The inference from all these studies is that the conditions prevailing during the first antigen stimulation of a naive T-cell play a major role in determining the pattern of cytokine production by the differentiated progeny of that T-cell. Furthermore, many studies have established that naive T-cells make very low levels of cytokines relative to a fully-differentiated Th1 or Th2 cell[34,35]. For instance, a naive T-cell produces in a 24–48 h period an amount of cytokine protein that is typically at least 1000-fold lower than that produced by a fully-differentiated T-cell within 2–4 h after stimulation[34,35]. Several days of antigen/cytokine exposure are typically needed to achieve the fully-differentiated state, and this has been traced to a requirement for cell division[36,37]. While the cytokine IL-2 is produced by antigen-stimulated naive T-cells even prior to S phase, production of other cytokines becomes detectable by intracellular cytokine staining only after a characteristic number of cell divisions. For instance, IFN-γ production becomes apparent after one cycle of cell division, while IL-4 production is observed after 3–4 cycles[36,37].

What is the basis for high-level cytokine production by differentiated, but not naive, Th1 and Th2 cells? Several studies support the notion that in naive T-cells, the IFN-γ gene and the linked IL-4/IL-5/IL-13 cytokine genes reside in a chromatin environment that is inaccessible to transcription factors, RNA polymerase, and the core transcriptional machinery (reviewed in elsewhere[40–43])[36,38,39]. As summarised below, the first exposure of the naive T-cell to antigen and cytokine results in specific changes in chromatin structure and DNA methylation of the relevant cytokine genes. These changes are termed **epigenetic** because they are determined not by the intrinsic nucleotide sequence information encoded in the DNA, but rather by modification of nucleosomal histones and of cytosine residues in DNA. So far the best-studied epigenetic modifications are histone acetylation and DNA methylation (reviewed elsewhere[44,45]); genes that are active ('open') in a particular tissue or cell type show increased histone acetylation and decreased methylation of cytosine–guanine (CpG) pairs, while genes that are inactive ('closed') are characterised by highly condensed chromatin, decreased histone acetylation, and dense CpG methylation. These modifications determine the level of cell type-specific gene transcription by modulating the accessibility of the relevant genes to the correct transcription factors, co-activator proteins, basal transcription apparatus, and RNA polymerase II. Epigenetic patterning is heritable, ensuring that once 'open', the cytokine loci remain accessible even in cells that have been rested for long periods in the absence of stimulation. This feature of effective irreversibility is characteristic of differentiative processes in general, and in the immune system may underlie T-cell memory.

Why are several cycles of cell division necessary for optimal differentiation? Data from other systems suggest that the process of locus 'opening' involves many sequential steps which may take several days to complete. The initial changes in chromatin structure often involve repositioning of nucleosomes away from transcription factor-binding regulatory regions of the gene, as well as long-range changes in the modification status of histones and in the methylation state of cytosine residues in DNA. These processes are likely to be initiated through the coordinate actions of antigen- and cytokine-induced transcription factors such as NFAT and STAT proteins, respectively, but be maintained by subset-specific transcription factors such as GATA3, Maf and T-bet (reviewed by Agarwal et al[42]). Together, the early and late-acting factors are thought to recruit chromatin remodeling complexes and histone-modifying enzymes to key regulatory regions of the cytokine genes. The subset-specific factors and the secondary proteins may not be present at sufficient levels or be able to gain sufficient access to DNA unless the cells have gone through one or more cycles of DNA replication when chromatin disassembly occurs, thus explaining the cell cycle requirement for optimal cytokine production.

Summary of experimental evidence

DNase I hypersensitivity

A useful technique for gauging gene 'accessibility' in the chromatin context is to monitor the sensitivity of the relevant DNA sequences to digestion with DNase I in intact nuclei (reviewed by Ng & Bird[46]). Many kilobases of DNA within and around the gene of interest can be monitored by this method. In general, genes located in active chromatin, that are actively transcribed or have the potential to be transcribed upon appropriate stimulation, are more sensitive to DNase I digestion than genes present in inactive or 'closed' chromatin, which are not expressed in the cell type or developmental stage under investigation. The technique is generally used, however, to identify regions of strong DNase I 'hyper' sensitivity, which often reflect perturbations introduced by protein binding to nucleosomal DNA and thus correlate with critical regulatory regions of the gene (*e.g.* inducible or tissue-specific enhancers, locus control regions, matrix attachment regions, insulators/boundary elements, or sites of relief from transcriptional attenuation (reviewed by Gross & Garrard[47]). Careful mapping of DNase I hypersensitive sites can reveal binding sites for key transcription factors within or immediately adjacent to the hypersensitive regions themselves[29].

Two recent studies showed that Th1 and Th2 differentiation are accompanied by long-range changes in DNase I hypersensitivity of the cytokine genes that are destined to be transcribed by the differentiated T-cells upon secondary stimulation (reviewed elsewhere[41,42])[38,39]. Naive T-cells have very simple patterns of DNase I hypersensitivity on the IFN-γ, IL-4 and IL-13 genes. During Th1 differentiation, a complex pattern of DNase I hypersensitivity, with appearance of three DNase I hypersensitive sites, develops specifically on the IFN-γ gene but not on the IL-4 and IL-13 genes[38]; conversely, Th2 differentiation is accompanied by development of at least 10 Th2-specific clusters of DNase I hypersensitive sites in the IL-4 and IL-13 genes but no change in the IFN-γ gene[38,39]. These changes in DNase I hypersensitivity are apparent within 48 h of initial stimulation of the naive T-cells, and require stimulation with both antigen and the appropriate cytokine[38].

The above experiments were performed on resting cells that were not actively transcribing the cytokine genes. Agarwal *et al*[29] showed that, upon stimulation, one of the DNase I hypersensitive sites in the IFN-γ gene was attenuated in its intensity, while a new, strongly inducible site developed in the 3′ region of the IL-4 gene. This region bound the Th2-specific transcription factor GATA3 *in vivo* and behaved as an inducible, Th2-specific enhancer in transient reporter assays. Moreover, this 3′ IL-4 enhancer bound selectively to the antigen-inducible transcription factor NFAT in Th2 cells but not Th1 cells, despite the equivalent activation of NFAT in both Th1 and Th2 cell types. This result indicated that the selective expression of the IL-4 gene in Th2 cells was, in part, due to its selective accessibility at the chromatin level.

Two constitutive and Th2-specific DNase I hypersensitive sites, HSS1 and HSS2, are present in the intergenic region between the IL-4 and IL-13 genes[39]. These sites are contained within a region, CNS-1 (conserved non-coding sequence-1) whose sequence is strongly conserved in all mammalian species[9]. Transgenic mice carrying yeast artificial chromosomes containing the human IL-4/IL-5/IL-13 locus showed appropriate expression of the human cytokines in Th1, Th2 and NK T-cells; when CNS-1 was deleted from the transgene by Cre-mediated recombination, there was a 50–70% decrease in the number of Th2 cells expressing human IL-4 and IL-13, without a significant effect on the level of cytokine expression per cell. CNS-1 also affected expression of the human IL-5 gene, located 120 kb away; but did not affect expression of the nearby RAD50 and KIF3 genes (ubiquitous and brain-specific, respectively). Thus CNS-1 appears to act selectively over long distances to increase the probability of IL-4/IL-5/IL-13 gene expression in the context of chromatin. This behaviour is reminiscent of locus control regions and certain enhancers, which can induce uniform expression and suppress silencing of transgenes that have been integrated into repressive locations such as centromeres (reviewed elsewhere[48,49]).

DNA demethylation

In general, silent genes are embedded in regions of hypermethylated DNA, while active genes are marked by hypomethylation. This is because methylated DNA recruits the methyl-CpG-binding protein MeCP2, that in turn recruits co-repressors such as the SIN3 histone deacetylase complex (reviewed by Strahl & Allis[45]). Most DNA methylation occurs symmetrically on CpG dinucleotides. During DNA replication, unmethylated cytosine becomes incorporated into the newly synthesised DNA strand, and thus the daughter strands contain hemi-methylated CpGs. This structure is recognised and rapidly remethylated by DNA methyltransferases, which, therefore, recreate fully-methylated CpG dinucleotides and stably maintain DNA methylation status through multiple cycles of cell division (reviewed elsewhere[41,42,45]).

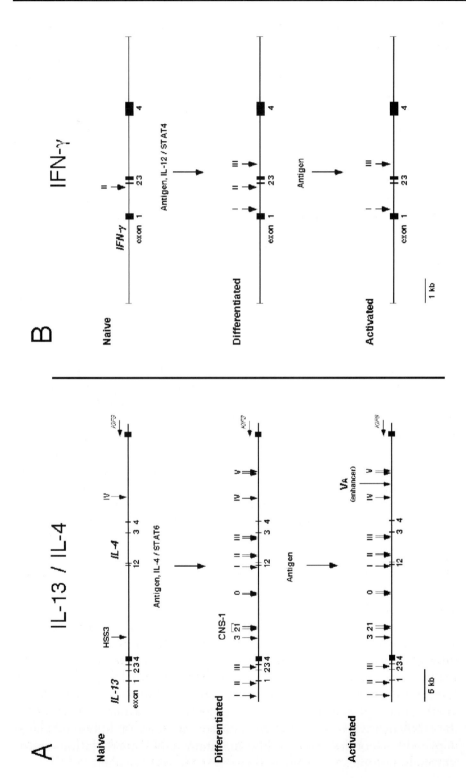

Fig. 3 Changes in DNase I hypersensitivity in the IL13/IL4 locus in Th2 cells and IFNγ in Th1 cells during T helper cell differentiation. Modified from Avni O. and Rao A. *Opin. Immunol* 2000; **12**: 654 with permission.

Bird *et al*[36] reported that IL-4 production by differentiating Th2 cells was accompanied by CpG demethylation of the IL-4 and IL-5 genes. Likewise, several groups have shown that hypomethylation of the IFN-γ gene correlates with increased IFN-γ gene expression in Th1 cells (reviewed elsewhere[41,42]). The mechanisms, which promote demethylation of cell type-specific genes, have not yet been elucidated. One possibility is that the nucleosome displacement that occurs during DNA replication allows cell-specific transcription factors to bind to DNA, and that the stable transcription complex established thereby interferes locally with maintenance methylation. This process would result in slow, cell-cycle-dependent demethylation. Alternatively, demethylation could occur in a cell-cycle-independent manner via an active demethylase.

An overall model for cytokine gene expression

We have proposed that cytokine gene expression may be envisioned as occurring in three distinct stages (reviewed elsewhere[41,42] see Fig.3).

Initiation phase

The initiation phase is highly dependent on antigen, antigen-induced transcription factors such as NFAT and NFκB, cytokines, and cytokine-induced STAT factors. Although these factors may initiate the process of locus remodelling, their activation is transient and is rapidly terminated in the absence of continued stimulation. As such, other factors and processes must be involved in **maintaining** the accessibility of cytokine loci in differentiated resting T-cells. We postulate that the transiently-activated transcription factors use a 'hit-and-run' mechanism to initiate locus remodelling and cytokine gene expression, by activating a differentiation-specific genetic programme following the initial stimulation with antigen and cytokines. This results in the stable expression of cell type-specific nuclear factors in the differentiated cells, including (but not necessarily limited to) GATA3 and Maf in Th2 cells and ERM and T-bet in Th1 cells.

Commitment phase

The commitment phase of T-cell differentiation is mediated by cell type-specific nuclear factors such as those listed above. During this phase, the differentiated phenotype is stabilised and maintained in the absence of further stimulation. A likely mechanism invokes the binding of these cell type-specific factors to dispersed regulatory elements in the cytokine genes, thereby recruiting histone acetyltransferases and chromatin remodelling enzymes to the appropriate genetic loci. The resulting chromatin configurations are stably inherited as described above, and persist in differentiated cells in the absence of active transcription.

Final phase

The final phase of acute gene transcription is elicited by secondary contact of the differentiated T-cells with antigen. This process involves binding of antigen-induced transcription factors such as NFAT to promoters and distal enhancer regions of cytokine genes. We have demonstrated[29] that, despite the fact that antigen-induced transcription factors are equivalently induced in both Th1 and Th2 cells, their access to these regulatory regions is limited by the prior process of cell type-specific chromatin remodelling that has occurred on the cytokine genes during the earlier differentiative phase. It has been shown in other systems that even the acute phase of gene transcription involves recruitment of ATP-dependent chromatin remodelling enzymes and histone acetyltransferases to promoter/enhancer regions of genes[50].

Conclusions

It should be apparent from this discussion that gene transcription is a truly dynamic process. The first steps of gene expression occur concomitantly with cell differentiation, and involve extensive changes in chromatin structure, sometimes occurring over hundreds of kilobases of DNA. These changes typically involve increased sensitivity to digestion by nucleases and restriction enzymes, increased histone acetylation of nucleosomal DNA, and decreased density of DNA methylation on CpG dinucleotides. The changes signal the acquisition of transcriptional competence, which precedes the overt transcription of lineage-specific genes. In the case of peripheral T-cells, the differentiation programme is initiated in response to first antigen contact, while overt gene transcription is delayed until later encounters with antigen. Full commitment to a specific lineage is established gradually and eventually becomes irreversible.

Acknowledgements

This work was supported by NIH grants CA42471 and AI44432. OA is supported by a postdoctoral fellowship from the Cancer Research Institute.

References

1   Mossman TR, Coffman RL. Th1 and Th2 cells: Different patterns of lymphokine secretion lead to different functional properties. *Annu Rev Immunol* 1989; **7**: 145–73
2   Kelso A. Th1 and Th2 subsets: paradigms lost? *Immunol Today* 1995; **16**: 374–9

3   Abbas AK, Murphy KM, Sher A. Functional diversity of helper T lymphocytes. *Nature* 1996; **383**: 787–93

4   Fitzpatrick DR, Kelso A. Nature versus nurture in T-cell cytokine production. *J Leukoc Biol* 1999; **66**: 869–75

5   Murphy KM, Ouyang W, Farrar JD *et al*. Signaling and transcription in T helper development. *Annu Rev Immunol* 2000; **18**: 451–549

6   Glimcher LH, Murphy KM. Lineage commitment in the immune system: the T helper lymphocyte grows up. *Genes Dev* 2000; **14**:1693-711

7   O'Garra A, Steinman L, Giijbels K. CD4⁺ T-cell subsets in autoimmunity. *Curr Opin Immunol* 1997; **9**: 872–3

8   Frazer KA, Ueda Y, Zhu Y, Gifford VR, Carofalo MR, Mohandas N. Computational and biological analysis of 680 kb of DNA sequence from the human 5q31 cytokine gene cluster region. *Genome Res* 1997; **7**: 495–512

9   Loots GG, Kocksley RM, Blankespoor CM *et al*. Identification of a coordinate regulator of interleukins 4, 13, and 5 by cross-species sequence comparisons. *Science* 2000; **288**: 136–40

10 Holgate ST. The epidemic of allergy and asthma. *Nature* 1999; **402**: B2–4

11 Corry DB, Kheradmand F. Induction and regulation of the IgE response. *Nature* 1999; **402**: B18–23

12 Zurawski SM, Vega Jr F, Huyghe B, Zurawski G. Receptors for interleukin-13 and interleukin-4 are complex and share a novel component that functions in signal transduction. *EMBO J* 1993; **12**: 2663–70

13 Chomarat P, Banchereau J. Interleukin-4 and interleukin-13: their similarities and discrepancies. *Int Rev Immunol* 1998; **17**: 1–52

14 Egan RW, Umland SP, Cuss FM, Chapman RW. Biology of interleukin-5 and its relevance to allergic disease. *Allergy* 1996; **51**: 71–81

15 Wurster AL, Tanaka T, Grusby MJ. The biology of STAT4 and STAT6. *Oncogene* 2000; **19**: 2577–84

16 Farrar JD, Murphy KM. Type I interferons and T helper development. *Immunol Today* 2000; **21**: 484–9

17 Kaplan MH, Wurster AL, Grusby MJ. A signal transducer and activator of transcription (STAT) 4-independent pathways for the development of T helper type 1 cells. *J Exp Med* 1998; **188**: 1191–6

18 Akira S. The role of IL-18 in innate in immunity. *Curr Opin Immunol* 2000; **12**: 59–63

19 Ouyang W, Jacobson NG, Bhattacharya D *et al*. The Ets transcription factor ERM is Th1-specific and induced by IL-12 through a STAT4-dependent pathway. *Proc Natl Acad Sci USA* 1999; **96**: 3888–93

20 Szabo SJ, Kim ST, Costa GL, Zhang X, Fathman CG, Glimcher LH. A novel transcription factor, T-bet, directs Th1 lineage commitment. *Cell* 2000; **100**: 655–69

21 Ouyang W, Lohning M, Gao Z *et al*. STAT6-independent GATA-3 autoactivation directs IL-4 independent Th2 development and commitment. *Immunity* 2000; **12**: 227–37

22 Kurata H, Lee H, O'Garra A, Arai N. Ectopic expression of activated Stat6 induces the expression of Th2-specific cytokine and transcription factors in developing Th1 cells. *Immunity* 1999; **11**: 677–88

23 Zhang W, Flavell RA. The transcription factor GATA-3 is necessary and sufficient for Th2 cytokine gene expression in CD4 T-cells. *Cell* 1997; **89**: 587–96

24 Zhang D, Cohn L, Ray P, Bottomly K, Ray A. Transcription factor GATA-3 is differentially expressed in murine Th1 and Th2 cells and controls Th2-specific expression of the interleukin-5 gene. *J Biol Chem* 1997; **272**: 21597–603

25 Ho I-C, Hodge MR, Rooney JW, Glimcher LH. The proto-oncogene *c-maf* is responsible for tissue-specific expression of interleukin-4. *Cell* 1996; **85**: 973–83

26 Lee HJ, Takemoto N, Kurata H *et al*. GATA-3 induces T helper cell type 2 (Th2) cytokine expression and chromatin remodelling in committed Th1 cells. *J Exp Med* 2000; **192**: 105–16

27 Ho I-C, Lo D, Glimcher L. C-maf promotes Th2 and attenuates Th1 differentiation by both IL-4 dependent and independent mechanisms. *J Exp Med* 1998; **188**: 1859–66

28 Kim J, Ho I-C, Grusby M, Glimcher L. The transcription factor c-Maf controls the production of interleukin-4 but not other Th2 cytokines. *Immunity* 1999; **10**: 745–51

29 Agarwal S, Avni O, Rao A. Cell-type-restricted binding of the transcription factor NFAT to a distal IL-4 enhancer *in vivo*. *Immunity* 2000; **12**: 643–52

30 Dent A, Shaffer AL, Yu X, Allman D, Staudt LM. T helper type 2 inflammatory disease in the absence of interleukin 4 and transcription factor STAT6. *Science* 1997; **276**: 589–92

31 Dhordian P, Lin RJ, Quief S *et al*. The LAZ3 (BCL-6) oncoprotein recruits a SMRT/mSIN3A/histone deacetylase containing complex to mediate transcriptional repression. *Nucleic Acids Res* 1998; **26**: 4645–51

32 Dent AL, Hu-Li, Paul WE, Staudt LM. T helper type 2 inflammatory disease in the absence of interleukin 4 and transcription factor STAT6. *Proc Natl Acad Sci* USA 1998; **95**: 13823–8

33 Ouyang W, Ranganath S, Weindel K *et al*. Inhibition of Th1 development mediated by GATA-3 through an IL-4 independent mechanism. *Immunity* 1998; **9**: 745–55

34 Lederer JA, Perez VL, DesRoches L, Kim SM, Abbas AK, Lichtman AH. Cytokine transcriptional events during helper T-cell subset differentiation. *J Exp Med* 1996; **184**: 397–406

35 Croft M, Swain SL. Recently activated naïve CD4 T-cells can help resting B cells, and can produce sufficient autocrine IL-4 to drive differentiation to secretion of T helper 2-type cytokines. *J Immunol* 1995; **154**: 4269–82

36 Bird JJ, Brown DR, Mullen AC *et al*. Helper T-cell differentiation is controlled by the cell cycle. *Immunity* 1998; **9**: 229–37

37 Gett A, Hodgkin P. Cell division regulates the T-cell cytokine repertoire, revealing a mechanism underlying immune class regulation. *Proc Natl Acad Sci* USA 1998; **95**: 9488–93

38 Agarwal S, Rao A. Modulation of chromatin structure regulates cytokine gene expression during T-cell differentiation. *Immunity* 1998; **9**: 765–75

39 Takemoto N, Koyano-Nakagawa N, Yokota T *et al*. Th2-specific DNase I-hypersensitive sites in the murine IL-13 and IL-4 intergenic region. *Int Immunol* 1998; **10**: 1981–5

40 Agarwal S, Rao A. Long-range transcriptional regulation of cytokine gene expression. *Curr Opin Immunol* 1998; **10**: 345–52

41 Agarwal S, Viola JPB, Rao A. Chromatin-based regulatory mechanisms governing cytokine gene transcription. *J Allergy Clin Immunol* 1999; **103**: 990–9

42 Avni O, Rao A. T-cell differentiation: a mechanistic view. *Curr Opin Immunol* 2000; **12**: 654–9

43 Reiner S, Sader R. Dealing from the evolutionary pawnshop: how lymphocytes makes decisions. *Immunity* 1999; **11**: 1–10

44 Strahl BD, Allis CD. The language of covalent histone modifications. *Nature* 2000; **403**: 41–5

45 Ng H-N, Bird A. DNA methylation and chromatin modification. *Curr Opin Genet Dev* 1999; **9**: 158–63

46 Gross DS, Garrard WT. Nuclease hypersensitive sites in chromatin. *Annu Rev Biochem* 1988; **57**: 159–97

47 Ernst P, Smale ST. Combinatorial regulation of transcription I: general aspects of transcriptional control. *Immunity* 1995; **2**: 311–9

48 Blackwood E, Kadonaga J. Going the distance: a current view of enhancer action. *Science* 1998; **281**: 60–3

49 Festenstein R, Kioussis D. Locus control regions and epigenetic chromatin modifiers. *Curr Opin Genet Dev* 2000; **10**: 199–203

50 Agalioti T, Lomvardas S, Parekh B, Yie J, Maniatis T, Thanos D. Ordered recruitment of chromatin modifying and general transcription factors to the IFN-beta promoter. *Cell* 2000; **103**: 667–78

Eosinophils in asthma and other allergic diseases

A J Wardlaw, C Brightling, R Green, G Woltmann and **I Pavord**

Division of Respiratory Medicine, Institute for Lung Health, University of Leicester School of Medical, Glenfield Hospital, Leicester, UK

A hallmark of allergic disease is infiltration of the tissues with increased numbers of eosinophils. This is the result of the co-ordinated action of cytokines, particularly IL-5, CCR3 binding chemokines and the adhesion molecules P-selectin and VCAM-1, acting in concert to cause selective trafficking of eosinophils into allergic tissue. This process is orchestrated by the Th-2 allergen specific lymphocyte. While there is little data to support the view that eosinophils ameliorate the allergic process, although they could have an important role in the disordered repair that leads to permanently impaired function in some allergic diseases, the evidence that they cause many of the pathophysiological features of allergic disease, while strong, remains circumstantial. Much of the data could be interpreted just as easily to suggest that eosinophils are bystander cells; markers of a certain type of pathological process, but not impinging upon it. The most direct evidence for a pathological role rests on the toxicity of the eosinophil granule proteins for bronchial epithelium and the bronchoconstrictor actions of the sulphidopeptide leukotrienes. The actions of LT antagonists in asthma which are certainly beneficial, but in most cases are not as effective as glucocorticoids, could be interpreted both for and against the eosinophil. In this paper we have focused on the studies that ask most directly the question of whether eosinophils are important effector cells in the pathogenesis of allergic disease. We conclude with a qualified affirmative. Even if they are only bystander cells they remain clinically important as diagnostic markers and a guide to the management of allergic disease.

Correspondence to:
Prof. A J Wardlaw,
Department of
Respiratory Medicine,
Glenfield Hospital,
Groby Road,
Leicester LE3 9QP, UK

Eosinophils are a characteristic feature of the pathology of asthma and related diseases such as atopic dermatitis and rhinitis. Ideas about their role in these diseases have fluctuated with a view in the 1970s that they were an ameliorating influence, followed by a consensus since the 1980s that they are important pro-inflammatory cells. This view evolved from evidence that eosinophils were potentially cytotoxic. In the 1970s it was shown that eosinophils could effectively kill the larval stage of helminthic parasites[1]. This was followed by evidence demonstrating a toxic effect on mammalian cells, particularly bronchial epithelium, mediated by the eosinophil specific basic proteins[2]. Eosinophils were shown to produce large amounts of the sulphidopeptide leukotrienes (LTC4/D4 and E4) and platelet activating factor (PAF) which were thought to be involved in causing bronchospasm in asthma. Furthermore, it had long been known that one of the most noticeable effects of glucocorticoids in asthma was their ability to reduce the blood and airway eosinophilia. Further impetus for the hypothesis that eosinophils were inextricably involved in the asthma process (and by extension other allergic diseases) was provided by the development of the hypothesis in the 1990s that allergic disease is due to inappropriate activation of allergen specific Th-2 lymphocytes[3]. Th-2 cells through elaboration of IL-4 and IL-5 are inextricably linked with the development of blood and tissue eosinophilia with IL-5 being the major eosinophil specific growth factor[4] and IL-4 causing selective up-regulation of eosinophil specific endothelial adhesion and chemo-attractant pathways[5]. The view of asthma as a disease caused by an airway eosinophilia leading to bronchial hyper-responsiveness (BHR) has become firmly embedded in the literature to the extent that the widely used mouse model of asthma has been defined in terms of generation of an airway eosinophilia and BHR after antigen challenge.

The relevance of eosinophils to allergic disease has generated considerable interest in their biology which has been regularly reviewed in recent years[6-10]. Here we will give only a brief overview. Similarly the literature on eosinophils and allergic disease is extensive with over 3500 papers on *Medline* for asthma and eosinophils alone, most of which have been published in the last decade. It is not possible to do justice to all these papers, many of which deal with animal models of allergic disease. This review focuses on the key issue as to whether eosinophils really can be regarded as key effector cells in allergic disease. Attention is concentrated on studies of clinical disease rather than animal models which, while useful in dissecting out the possible role of individual molecules, particularly in trafficking, are of limited relevance to the disease process itself. Similarly the allergen challenge models in humans are of questionable value in understanding the pathogenesis of chronic allergic disease and these will be mentioned only in passing.

The biology of eosinophils

Eosinophils are end stage cells derived from the bone marrow under the influence of GM-CSF, IL-3 and the late differentiation factor IL-5, which in humans is only active on eosinophils and basophils[11]. In terms of their ontogeny, they are more closely related to the basophil than the neutrophil or monocyte. After leaving the bone marrow, eosinophils circulate briefly in tissue before migrating to the gastrointestinal mucosa under the direction of the eosinophil specific chemokine eotaxin and the gut homing adhesion receptor $\alpha4\beta7$ which binds to the gut expressed MAdCAM-1[12,13]. Once in the tissues, eosinophils survive for up to 2 weeks through autocrine production of GM-CSF as a result of $\alpha4$ mediated interactions with fibronectin[14]. Teleologically, it has been presumed that this is a surveillance mechanism related to the gut orientated life cycle of helminthic parasites, which are thought to be the major host defence target of eosinophils. In allergic disease, eosinophils migrate to extra-intestinal sites in a relatively selective fashion, with up to 100-fold enrichment of eosinophils over neutrophils in tissue. This is mediated by a multi-step process directed by Th-2 cytokine producing T-cells[5]. The first step is increased production and release of eosinophils from the bone marrow under the influence of the IL-5 and specific chemo-attractants such as eotaxin. Secondly, the target organ vasculature has increased adhesiveness for eosinophils through the specific effects of locally generated IL-4 and IL-13. These cytokines induce expression of VCAM-1 which binds eosinophils through VLA-4, a receptor not expressed by neutrophils, and P-selectin to which eosinophils bind with greater avidity than neutrophils[15–17]. CC chemokines such as eotaxin which bind CCR3, a receptor almost exclusively expressed by eosinophils and basophils, attract eosinophils into tissue where they survive for prolonged periods as a result of locally generated IL-5. The mechanisms by which IL-5 cause prolonged eosinophil survival (or delayed eosinophil apoptosis), are still imperfectly understood. IL-5 survival associated signalling is dependent on phosphorylation of Lyn and Jak2 kinases which bind to the common β chain of the IL-5 receptor, as well as Raf-1[18]. However survival is not dependent on activation on P-13 kinase, a pathway that mediates many IL-5 (and other agonist) mediated effects on eosinophils including increased adhesiveness and superoxide generation (personal observation). IL-5 prevents translocation of the pro-apoptotic Bcl-2 family member BAX, which is well expressed by eosinophils to the mitochondrial outer membrane. BAX translocation results in increased mitochondrial permeability, cytochrome c release and subsequent activation of downstream caspases, particularly caspase 3[19].

The relatively eosinophil specific basic proteins which are stored in the distinctive secondary granules are major basic protein (MBP) eosinophil cationic protein (ECP), eosinophil peroxidase (EPO) and eosinophil derived neurotoxin (EDN). All of these proteins are toxic to the larval stages of many helminthic parasites as well as bronchial epithelial cells. Inhaled MBP can also induce BHR in primates[20], and inhibit the actions of down-regulatory M2 muscarinic receptors[21]. Eosinophils, with mast cells and basophils, are the most prominent source of sulphidopeptide leukotrienes produced mainly by enzymes present in lipid bodies[22]. They also produce significant amounts of PAF although this is not specific to the eosinophil. Many of the diverse range of cytokines produced by eosinophils are released only in small amounts which may, nonetheless, have important autocrine effects[23]. For example, the small amounts of GM-CSF produced by the eosinophil is sufficient to prolong its own survival. The production of cytokines such as TGF-α and TGF-β by eosinophils has broadened the range of eosinophil functions emphasising their potential importance in, for example, wound healing.

The physiological triggers which lead to eosinophil mediator release in allergic disease remain uncertain. Engagement of Fcγ and Fcα receptors are the most reliable physiological triggers for degranulation of eosinophil basic proteins, especially when presented on the surface of a large particle, or in the context of co-engagement of the adhesion receptor Mac-1[24]. However, there is little evidence that immunoglobulin-mediated release is involved in allergic disease. Priming with eosinophil active growth factors such as IL-5 greatly enhances degranulation via Fc receptors and also causes degranulation directly[25]. PMA is an effective, albeit non-physiological, stimulus for superoxide production but not for degranulation or cytokine release. Calcium ionophore is a good stimulus for lipid mediator production. Chemo-attractants binding via G protein linked serpentine receptors stimulate superoxide production, but are not a good stimulus for other mediators. Cytochalasin B which inhibits cytoskeletal assembly has been used in many studies to enhance release and the relevance of this to a physiological setting is unclear. Eosinophils undergo piecemeal degranulation in most *in vivo* settings[26]. This involves the eosinophil releasing its granule products through pores in the plasma membrane without leading to cell death. With more vigorous stimuli, for example after allergen challenge, cytolysis is often prominent[27].

The immunopathology of asthma and other allergic diseases

Although there is a significant body of work detailing the presence of eosinophils in the tissue in all allergic diseases, most work has been undertaken in the context of asthma, particularly those studies relating disease severity to the degree of tissue eosinophilia. For this reason, most of the papers reviewed below relate to asthma. The pathology of asthma comprises infiltration of the bronchial submucosa and epithelium with eosinophils, monocytes and lymphocytes although the latter two cell types are relatively abundant in the normal airway. Epithelial des-quamation, or at least fragility, has been considered a hallmark of the disease, although detailed studies of the pathology of asthma deaths has called this dogma into question[28], and it is striking that induced sputum from asthmatics does not contain an increased number of bronchial epithelial cells. Thickening of the basement membrane beneath the epithelium is a constant feature as is increased smooth muscle hypertrophy leading to thickening of the bronchial wall, as well as increased vascularity. Mucus hypertrophy and mast cell degranulation have also been reported. In this review, attention will focus on the eosinophil, although it is important to note that this cell type is just one part of a distinctive mucosal inflammatory response which is the underlying cause of asthma and rhinoconjunctivitis.

Bronchoscopy studies

The observation that increased numbers of eosinophils were a feature of asthma has been known for many decades. Eosinophils and their granule products, including Charcot Leyden crystals were a hallmark of spontaneously induced sputum and were plentiful in the airways in *post-mortem* specimens[29]. Subsequent studies have confirmed this association[30], at the same time pointing out that a small proportion of patients dying of asthma, particularly those with sudden death, do not have an airway eosinophilia[31]. The inflammatory response in asthma deaths has been noted to effect both the large and small airways[32]. *Post-mortem* studies inevitably suffer from small numbers, lack of appropriate controls, a paucity of clinical details and the difficulty in controlling for the effects of treatment. It also represents an extreme end of the asthma severity spectrum. In the early 1980s, it was appreciated that bronchoscopy in asthma could be carried out safely as long as appropriate precautions were taken[33]. It then became apparent that even in very mild asthma there was evidence of airway inflammation and that the most obvious feature of the inflammatory response was the increased number of eosinophils in BAL fluid without an increase in neutrophils[34], as reviewed by Djukanovic and colleagues[35]. These studies demonstrated a considerable variability in the degree of BAL eosinophilia ranging from 1% to up to 30% (the normal being less than 1%). There was evidence that the eosinophils were actively secreting mediators with increased amounts of the eosinophil granule proteins and leukotrienes in BAL fluid[36,37] (and subsequently sputum[38]), although data regarding mediators in BAL fluid should always be treated with caution because of the lack of a good denominator to control for recovery of airway lining fluid. BAL eosinophils express the putative activation receptor CD69, have reduced expression of L-selectin, and increased expression of Mac-1 and ICAM-1 when compared to peripheral blood eosinophils. These changes in phenotype can be mimicked *in vitro* by treatment with IL-5 (for 24 h)[39], and suggest an activated phenotype.

Studies of BAL were followed by biopsy studies which allowed a more detailed immunopathological analysis of the inflammatory response in the bronchial tree[40–42]. One advantage of biopsy studies is that they allow accurate quantification of bronchial lymphocytes and mast cells which are anchored within the epithelium and do not migrate into the lumen so do not appear in BAL fluid (or sputum) in representative numbers. These studies confirmed the consistent increase in the number of eosinophils in the airway submucosa without an increase, in most cases, in neutrophils. Eosinophils which are very infrequent in the normal airway, are enriched by up to 100-fold in the airways of asthmatic subjects compared to neutrophils. All these studies involve a cross-sectional analysis and say little to nothing about the kinetics of migration of these cells into the airways. Endobronchial biopsy studies also demonstrated increased numbers of CD4 T-cells in asthmatic airways. Although most bronchoscopy studies have been undertaken in young adults with mild atopic asthma, increased numbers of eosinophils have also been reported in intrinsic asthma[43], and occupational asthma due to Western Red Cedar and toluene di-isocyanate[44,45], as well as aspirin sensitive asthma where more eosinophils were seen than in non-aspirin sensitive asthmatics[46]. In severe corticosteroid dependent asthma two patterns were observed. Out of 34 severe oral glucocorticoid dependent asthmatics, in 14 patients eosinophils were absent in endobronchial biopsies whereas in 20 subjects eosinophils were increased. Neutrophils were increased in both groups. The eosinophilic group had been intubated more often[47]. Few bronchoscopy studies have been undertaken in children with asthma, although increases in both eosinophils and neutrophils have been reported[48,49]. As well as asthma, eosinophils are also a characteristic feature of seasonal and perennial rhinitis[50]. Nasal polyposis is usually associated with an intense eosino-philia[51] as is non-atopic rhinitis with eosinophils (NARES). Atopic dermatitis is characterised by increased numbers of eosinophils and deposition of eosinophil basic proteins in the affected skin[52,53]. Eosinophils in bronchial biopsies often have a partially degranulated appearance[54] and after nasal allergen challenge were shown to have undergone degranulation through a combination of cytolysis and piecemeal degranulation[27]. Tissue eosinophils express a range of cytokines as shown by both *in situ* hybridization and immunohisto-chemistry[55]. The anti-ECP antibody EG2 has been widely used as a marker of eosinophil activation, although the validity of this has recently been called into question[56]. An airway eosinophilia is a consistent feature of the late response to allergen challenge in the bronchial and nasal mucosa as well as the skin[57–59]. This is often more marked than the often modest number seen in chronic disease. However, the extent to which allergen challenge is a model for clinical disease remains controversial.

Induced sputum

Bronchoscopy is invasive, potentially hazardous and expensive. Small numbers of individuals with generally mild disease are usually studied and repeat measurements are difficult. Measurement of the eosinophil count in induced sputum has overcome some of these problems. Although analysis of sputum in asthma has a long pedigree, it was hampered as an investigative tool by lack of standardization and the ability to obtain a sample in only a minority of cases. This problem was overcome by inducing sputum using hypertonic saline, a technique which is safe and reproducible. The sputum plugs are generally selected to reduce contamination with upper respiratory tract material (although not all groups do this), and the cells dissociated from mucus using a reducing agent such as dithiothreitol (DTT). Good quality cytospins can be routinely obtained and a reliable cell differential generated[60-62]. Eosinophil counts in sputum correlate reasonably well with bronchial biopsies, washings and BAL with the eosinophilia being often more marked in sputum[63,64]. The normal value for non-smokers has been reported as 0.4% with a 90th percentile of up to 1.1% with atopics higher than non-atopics[65]. We have found similar values. The range of eosinophil counts in asthma is wide from 1–50% or more. We have found that most, though not all, asthmatics have a raised eosinophil count (Fig. 1). Taking a cut off of 1% as indicating a raised sputum eosinophil count when compared with normal airways, a sputum eosinophilia as a test for asthma (defined by a Pc20 of < 8.0 mg/ml or a significant improvement in FEV1 after β2 agonists) gives a sensitivity of over 80% and a specificity of 95%. These values fall to 70% and 80%, respectively, when compared with subjects with respiratory symptoms which have led to a diagnosis of asthma but who subsequently turn out to have other conditions. In both cases this is considerably better than peak flow variability and much more sensitive than improvements in FEV1. Interestingly, in our experience, while the majority of patients with acute severe asthma have a very high eosinophil count, a small proportion had no eosinophils. Raised numbers of neutrophils in acute severe asthma have been reported by others[66,67], although in the Fahy study about a third had been on oral glucocorticoids which may have influenced the findings. Up to 64% of neutrophils are found in the normal airway which makes interpretation of a raised neutrophil count in asthma more difficult. A sputum eosinophilia is a feature of occupational asthma and may be useful in diagnosis[68]. As discussed below, the use of induced sputum has allowed a much more detailed assessment of the relationship between asthma and airway inflammation in terms of specificity, severity, asthma phenotype, bronchial hyper-responsiveness and response to treatment. For example, bronchoscopy

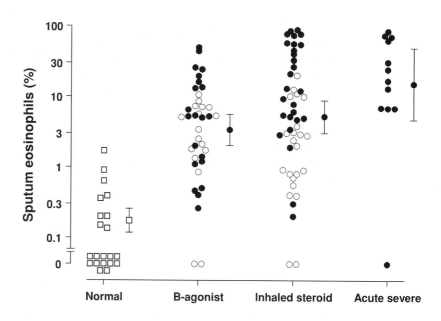

Fig. 1 Percentage of eosinophils in induced sputum from patients with asthma attending an out-patient clinic or admitted to hospital with acute severe asthma compared with normal non-smoking controls. The normal sputum eosinophil count was less than 1%. Closed symbols represent patients requiring a step-up in treatment. Most asthmatics had increased numbers of sputum eosinophils with numbers being greatest in the patients with acute severe asthma.

studies have suggested that, whereas asthma is characterised by an airway eosinophilia, COPD is associated with a neutrophilia[69], although eosinophils were noted to be present during exacerbations[70]. However, it is clear from sputum studies in which larger numbers of more severe patients can be studied that up to a third of patients with stable irreversible smoking associated COPD have a significant airway eosinophilia[71,72]. In addition, an airway eosinophilia is commonly associated with chronic cough (a condition labelled eosinophilic bronchitis) which occurs in the absence of variable airflow obstruction and BHR[73,74]. Increased numbers of eosinophils compared to controls are seen in the airways of atopics without asthma although the increase is less marked than in asthmatics[54,65,75].

Eosinophils and relationship to disease severity

Symptoms and lung function

If eosinophils were important in causing the pathophysiology of asthma and related diseases, then a correlation between the degree of tissue eosinophilia and disease severity might be expected. Early studies of peripheral blood eosinophil counts had suggested a correlation with lung function both in clinical disease[76] and after allergen challenge[77]. However, blood eosinophils are an insensitive and imprecise marker of tissue inflammatory responses[78]. In asthma deaths, the eosinophilic inflammation, particularly in the proximal bronchial tree, is more intense than in mild-to-moderate asthma[79]. In the early bronchoscopy studies, the presence of eosinophils in BAL fluid was associated with symptomatic asthma and was not seen in asthmatics in remission[34]. There was also a broad correlation between clinical severity and degree of airway eosinophilia[80]. In 17 patients with mild asthma, Walker *et al.* reported a correlation between the degree of BAL eosinophilia, lung function and BHR. This study also found a correlation between the numbers of eosinophils and activated T cells as did a bronchial biopsy study by Bradley *et al.* emphasising the relationship between T-cells and eosinophils in allergic disease[81]. Lim *et al.* found that there was a weak correlation between mucosal eosinophils and lung function in 16 asthmatics half of whom were taking inhaled glucocorticoids[82]. Most bronchoscopy studies have investigated mild asthma so it is difficult to get a spectrum of asthma severity in terms of symptoms and lung function. Induced sputum can be obtained safely even in moderately severe asthmatics and has allowed a more detailed analysis of the relationship between eosinophilic airways inflammation and asthma[83].

In a relatively early sputum study, Pin *et al.* found an inverse correlation between FEV1 and sputum eosinophil counts[84]. In contrast, another study of 20 asthmatics after an 8 week course of high dose inhaled steroids, no correlation between sputum eosinophils and clinical markers of severity was observed although there was a weak correlation with BHR[85]. In 20 atopic asthmatic children on inhaled steroids with moderate to severe chronic asthma, a weak correlation was observed between sputum eosinophil numbers and asthma severity in terms of lung function and an asthma severity index[86]. In a study which compared the degree of airways inflammation in mild and moderate asthma, the number of eosinophils, as well we other markers of inflammation, were more marked in the more severe disease group[87]. In a study of induced sputum in 74 asthmatics ranging from mild to severe persistent disease, asthma severity as assessed by lung function, symptoms scores and BHR, correlated with the degree of airway eosinophilia. A weak correlation was also seen between sputum neutrophilia and symptom scores[88]. In a study of 43 mild-to-severe asthmatics, the sputum eosinophil count was greater in the severe compared to the mild and moderate asthmatics as defined by the clinical Aas score, but only weak correlations with FEV1 and BHR were observed[89]. In an interesting study by Jatakanon *et al.*, asthma exacerbations were induced by withdrawing inhaled steroids. Baseline sputum eosinophilia was a predictor of subsequent exacerbations and the degree of sputum eosinophilia correlated with falls in PEF and FEV1[90]. Probably more important than numbers of eosinophils is the amount of mediators they are generating. In a study of 36 patients with asthma ranging in severity from mild to severe there was a higher concentration of ECP in the severe asthmatics compared to the mild-to-moderate patients. Taking all the subjects ECP levels correlated with symptom scores and inversely with PEF[91]). Similarly Virchow *et al.* found that, in 14 patients with asthma not taking corticosteroids, sputum ECP was a better marker of severity in terms of lung function than sputum eosinophil counts[92].

Studying the relationship between various markers of asthma severity and airway inflammation is difficult. Symptoms are not objective and peak flow measurements are unreliable. Cross-sectional studies involving a single measurement of FEV1 and eosinophil count (the usual study design) in a disease like asthma which is defined in terms of its variable severity are crude, particularly when the sampling errors involved in measuring the degree of airway eosinophilia are taken into account. There is a paucity of longitudinal studies correlating asthma severity with airway inflammation on an individual basis. Most of the reported studies are relatively under-powered and treatment with anti-inflammatory drugs adds another important variable.

Eosinophils and bronchial hyper-responsiveness (BHR)

BHR refers to the increased sensitivity of asthmatics to irritant inhaled stimuli. This is non-specific in the sense that it not antigen dependent and can be caused by a number of diverse agents ranging from smoke and dust through to cold air, exercise and perfumes. It can, therefore, be caused by agents such as methacholine and histamine that act directly on smooth muscle to cause bronchoconstriction or agents such as cold air that are thought to act indirectly possibly through a neural reflex. BHR is a hallmark of asthma and measurement of BHR, for example by constructing a histamine or methacholine dose response curve, is the most sensitive and specific test for asthma. BHR is regarded as a necessary ingredient for the integrity of asthma models either in humans or animals. However, the extent to which the increased bronchial reactivity seen after allergen challenge and in animal models is related to the BHR seen in clinical disease is debatable. Despite intensive research over the last 20 years the cause of BHR is still unknown. In particular, the extent to which BHR is caused by, or interacts with, airway inflammation and especially eosinophilic inflammation remains contentious. BHR and eosinophilic inflammation generally occur together. In the early bronchoscopy studies, although there was a clear association between BHR and an airway eosinophilia, there was little evidence of a correlation between the severity of the BHR and the number of BAL eosinophils[34]. Similarly, in the study by Foresi et al. quoted above of 15 asthmatics and 30 patients with seasonal allergic rhinitis, a good correlation ($P<0.005$) was seen between sputum eosinophils and BHR, but this was skewed by the inclusion of patients with seasonal rhinitis without asthma[75]. In a much larger study of 71 asthmatics, no relationship was seen between sputum eosinophilia and BHR although the eosinophil count did inversely correlate with lung function[93]. Some studies have seen a correlation. For example, Jatakanon et al. found a weak negative correlation (r −0.4) between the sputum eosinophil count and Pc20 in 35 stable asthmatics taking only β2 agonists. A stronger inverse correlation was seen with NO concentrations in exhaled air[94]. In our own experience of over 200 stable asthmatics attending our routine out-patient clinics (46% atopic and 44% taking inhaled steroids), there was no relationship between log sputum eosinophil count and log Pc20 in the non-atopic group but there was a significant inverse correlation in the atopic group ($P < 0.002$) in both patients taking inhaled steroids and those on β2 agonists alone, although the correlation was weak (r −0.365). A dissociation between BHR and airway eosinophilia has been observed in animal studies. For example, Henderson et al. found that an antibody against the α4 integrin when given intraperitoneally was able to inhibit eosinophil migration into the airways after ovalbumin challenge, but had no effect on BHR, whereas both BHR and the airway eosinophilia were inhibited by nasal delivery of the antibody[95]. One issue is that the Pc20 threshold may not be the best marker of BHR to use. Moller et al. found a good correlation between the plateau of the methacholine dose response curve (which in the majority of patients had to be modelled from a calculated sigmoid curve) and the airway eosinophil count in 20 asthmatics, but no correlation with Pc20[96].

Current evidence supports the idea that BHR and eosinophilic airway inflammation are independently regulated but closely interrelated, a view supported by a factor analysis undertaken by Rosi et al. in 99 mild asthmatics[97]. This would predict that in a cross-section of patients, for a given degree of inflammation, marked differences in BHR can result. This is consistent with the observation that eosinophilic inflammation can occur without BHR as in eosinophilic bronchitis and marked BHR can occur in the context of minimal airway eosinophilia. It would also suggest, however, that within an individual, changes in BHR may mirror changes in eosinophilic airway inflammation to the extent that airway inflammation could be used longitudinally to guide asthma management.

Eosinophils and anti-inflammatory drugs in asthma

If eosinophils are to be plausibly implicated in causing allergic disease, drugs which are effective in their treatment should also reduce eosinophil numbers and mediator release. With the exception of β2 agonists and anti-cholinergic bronchodilators, this appears to be the case as is most clearly seen with glucocorticoids (GCs), the most effective anti-inflammatory treatment for asthma. GCs cause a marked eosinopenia when given orally and both oral and topical GCs reduce the tissue eosinophilia in a wide range of eosinophilic conditions in a dose-dependent manner. In contrast, they have little effect on neutrophils, actually increasing the peripheral blood neutrophil count, and are ineffective in most diseases characterised by neutrophilic inflammation. GCs increase the rate of eosinophil apoptosis, although this effect is modest in degree and only seen at relatively high concentrations of steroids with an IC_{50} of about 10^{-6} M whereas they prolong neutrophil life-span[98]. The molecular basis for this difference is unknown. It is likely that the principle action of steroids in asthma is to inhibit cytokine and chemokine production by both leukocytes and resident airway cells, such as epithelial cells, fibroblasts and bronchial smooth muscle[99]. The evidence that GCs reduce eosinophil counts in asthma is consistent. For example, 6 days of treatment with oral glucocorticoids reduced the sputum eosinophil count (and ECP level) in 24 asthmatics from 14% to 1%, whereas no change was observed in the placebo group. Moreover, the increase in peak flow associated with steroid treatment correlated with the fall in the eosinophil count[100]. Oral prednisolone caused a fall in the sputum eosinophil count and ECP level in patients with severe exacerbations of their disease. The improvement in sputum eosinophils and ECP levels correlated with improvement in lung function[101]. In a bronchial biopsy study of 10 asthmatics, treatment with 2 mg of beclomethasone diproprionate for 6 weeks resulted in an improvement in lung function, symptoms, Pc20 and a reduction in markers of inflammation including the eosinophil count[102]. Inhaled budesonide resulted in a fall in eosinophil counts which correlated with the improvement in Pc20 in 14 asthmatics[103]. Oral prednisolone given for 2 weeks caused a significant fall in eosinophil counts which was not seen in the placebo limb of the study[99]. In all these studies, comparable effects were also seen on mast cell and T-cell counts emphasising the broad spectrum of anti-inflammatory actions of GCs, although neutrophil numbers were unaffected. However, the eosinophil count does appear to be a useful marker of steroid responsiveness in both asthma, COPD and rhinitis[71,104–108]. In all these studies, the airway eosinophilia was not abolished and in some patients only a modest fall was seen. It was striking that in our clinic population many patients still had a significant sputum eosinophilia despite being on inhaled GCs, although whether this was due to poor compliance, insufficient dose or GC resistance is not clear. As well as GCs, leukotriene antagonists modestly reduce the eosinophil count in asthma. Interestingly, they also promote eosinophil apoptosis[109,110]. Cyclosporin and a thomboxane A_2 antagonist have been shown to reduce eosinophil counts in asthmatic airways although whether this is related to their benefit in asthma is not clear as they have a wide range of other actions[111,112].

Novel anti-eosinophil therapies

The evidence supporting an important role for the eosinophil in causing allergic disease has led to a number of pharmaceutical companies developing specific anti-eosinophil therapies. The most advanced of these, and the only one where clinical studies have been reported, involved the use of two different anti-IL-5 antibodies. One was an allergen challenge study in mild asthma[113] and one was a study in severe asthma (not yet published). Both were designed primarily as dosing and safety studies and were not really powered for their clinical effects. Nonetheless, some interesting data have emerged. In both cases, the antibodies were well tolerated and effective in reducing the peripheral blood and, to a lesser extent, sputum eosinophilia. In the allergen challenge study, no affect was seen on either the early or late response or on the severity of BHR in these very mild subjects. Caveats to this study are the extent to which allergen challenge is a good model for asthma and the reliance on sputum so that we can not be sure that the eosinophil count in the bronchial submucosa was also inhibited. In the severe asthma study, there was a trend towards an improvement in the active group but this was not clear cut and the numbers of patients were too small to draw any firm conclusions.

Conclusions

The hypothesis that eosinophils are important effector cells in asthma and allergic disease rests on three main pillars of evidence. Firstly, that eosinophils are found in asthmatic airways (and relevant tissues in other allergic diseases); secondly, that their mediators are relevant to the disease process; and thirdly, that removal of eosinophils is associated with an improvement in the disease. Examining each of these in turn, there is a considerable body of literature documenting in detail the close relationship between the presence of eosinophils in the airway submucosa and asthma to the extent that it is a useful diagnostic marker.

Broadly speaking, the degree of eosinophilia correlates with disease severity, and in atopics at least BHR, although the correlation with BHR is weak suggesting an indirect relationship. Eosinophil specific mediators certainly appear relevant to asthma and to a lesser extent other allergic diseases, but their importance has been challenged by recent studies showing lack of evidence for epithelial damage in asthma and by the ineffectiveness of PAF antagonists and the modest benefits of LT antagonists. GCs undoubtedly have a profound effect on eosinophils and their beneficial effects in allergic disease appear to go hand-in-hand with their inhibition of tissue eosinophilia, but they are of course broad spectrum anti-inflammatory drugs.

Taking the evidence together, there is no doubt that eosinophils are intimately associated with asthma and the other atopic diseases. As there is virtually no evidence that eosinophils can ameliorate disease, we presume they must either be bystander cells or actively involved in pathogenesis. The current evidence is consistent with a role for eosinophils simply as markers of the inflammatory process, but not impinging upon it. Even if they are just markers, eosinophils are so closely related to at least asthma that they remain extremely useful as indicators of diagnosis and response to treatment in allergic diseases. The evidence would also be entirely consistent with eosinophils being important effector cells. Perhaps the most likely answer is that eosinophils are part of a complex inflammatory process in which they favour one aspect of the pathophysiology, cough for example or airway wall remodelling. If this is the case, using anti-eosinophilic drugs to assess their role may be more difficult than simply measuring FEV1 or BHR in short-term studies.

There is clearly a great deal more work that can be done to determine the extent to which the airway eosinophilia might guide management. In particular, in diagnosis and in longitudinal studies of individual patients to assess the value of the sputum eosinophil in guiding treatment with GCs. In contrast, getting closer to the question as to whether eosinophils cause asthma requires detailed studies with specific anti-eosinophilic therapies. We await these with interest.

References

1   Butterworth AE, Sturrock RF, Houba V, Mahmoud AA, Sher A, Rees PH. Eosinophils as mediators of antibody-dependent damage to schistosomula. *Nature* 1975; **256**: 727–9

2   Frigas E, Motojima S, Gleich GJ. The eosinophilic injury to the mucosa of the airways in the pathogenesis of bronchial asthma. *Eur Respir J* 1991; **Suppl 13**: S123–35

3   Corrigan CJ, Kay AB. T cells and eosinophils in the pathogenesis of asthma. *Immunol Today* 1992; **13**: 501–7

4   Sanderson CJ. Interleukin-5, eosinophils, and disease. *Blood* 1992; **79**: 3101–9

5   Wardlaw AJ. Molecular regulation of eosinophil trafficking: a multi-step paradigm. *J Allergy Clin Immunol* 1999; **104**: 917–26

6   Wardlaw AJ, Moqbel R, Kay AB. Eosinophils: biology and role in disease. *Adv Immunol* 1995; **60**: 151–266

7   Weller PF. Human eosinophils. *J Allergy Clin Immunol* 1997; **100**: 283–7

8   Gleich GJ, Adolphson CR, Leiferman KM. The biology of the eosinophilic leukocyte. *Annu Rev Med* 1993; **44**: 85–101

9   Walsh GM. Advances in the immunobiology of eosinophils and their role in disease. *Crit Rev Clin Lab Sci* 1999; **36**: 453–96

10   Rothenberg ME. Eosinophilia. *N Engl J Med* 1998; **338**: 1592–600

11   Denburg JA. Bone marrow in atopy and asthma: hematopoietic mechanisms in allergic inflammation. *Immunol Today* 1999; **20**: 111–3

12   Walsh GM, Symon FA, Lazarovils AL, Wardlaw AJ. Integrin alpha 4 beta 7 mediates human eosinophil interaction with MAdCAM-1, VCAM-1 and fibronectin. *Immunology* 1996; **89**: 112–9

13   Mishra A, Hogan SP, Lee JJ, Foster PS, Rothenberg ME. Fundamental signals that regulate eosinophil homing to the gastrointestinal tract. *J Clin Invest* 1999; **103**: 1719–27

14   Anwar AR, Moqbel R, Walsh GM, Kay AB, Wardlaw AJ. Adhesion to fibronectin prolongs eosinophil survival. *J Exp Med* 1993; **177**: 839–43.

15   Woltmann G, McNulty CA, Dewson G, Symon FA, Wardlaw AJ. Interleukin-13 induces PSGL-1/P-selectin-dependent adhesion of eosinophils, but not neutrophils, to human umbilical vein endothelial cells under flow. *Blood* 2000; **95**: 3146–52

16   Edwards BS, Curry MS, Tsuji H, Brown D, Larson RS, Sklar LA. Expression of P-selectin at low site density promotes selective attachment of eosinophils over neutrophils. *J Immunol* 2000; **165**: 404–10

17   Symon FA, Lawrence MB, Williamson ML, Walsh GM, Watson SR, Wardlaw AJ. Functional and structural characterization of the eosinophil P-selectin ligand. *J Immunol* 1996; **157**: 1711–9

18   Pazdrak K, Olszewska-Pazdrak B, Stafford S, Garofalo RP, Alam R. Lyn, Jak2, and Raf-1 kinases are critical for the anti-apoptotic effect of interleukin 5, whereas only Raf-1 kinase is essential for eosinophil activation and degranulation. *J Exp Med* 1998; **188**: 421–9

19   Dewson G, Cohen G, Wardlaw AJ. IL-5 inhibits eosinophil apoptosis by preventing BAX translocation to the mitochondria with resultant increased mitochondrial permeability, cytochrome c release, and caspase activation. 2001; Submitted

20   Gundel RH, Letts LG, Gleich GJ. Human eosinophil major basic protein induces airway constriction and airway hyperresponsiveness in primates. *J Clin Invest* 1991; **87**: 1470–3

21   Costello RW, Schofield BH, Kephart GM, Gleich GJ, Jacoby DB, Fryer AD. Localization of eosinophils to airway nerves and effect on neuronal M2 muscarinic receptor function. *Am J Physiol* 1997; **273**: L93–103

22   Bozza PT, Yu W, Penrose JF, Morgan ES, Dvorak AM, Weller PF. Eosinophil lipid bodies: specific, inducible intracellular sites for enhanced eicosanoid formation. *J Exp Med* 1997; **186**: 909–20

23   Lacy P, Moqbel R. Eosinophil cytokines. *Chem Immunol* 2000; **76**: 134–55

24   Kaneko M, Horie S, Kato M, Gleich GJ, Kita H. A crucial role for beta 2 integrin in the activation of eosinophils stimulated by IgG. J Immunol 1995; **155**: 2631–41

25   Kita H, Weiler DA, Abu-Ghazaleh R, Sanderson CJ, Gleich GJ. Release of granule proteins from eosinophils cultured with IL-5. *J Immunol* 1992; **149**: 629–35

26   Dvorak AM, Weller PF. Ultrastructural analysis of human eosinophils. *Chem Immunol* 2000; **76**: 1–28

27   Erjefalt JS, Greiff L, Andersson M *et al*. Allergen-induced eosinophil cytolysis is a primary mechanism for granule protein release in human upper airways. *Am J Respir Crit Care Med* 1999; **160**:304–12

28   Carroll N, Elliot J, Morton A, James A. The structure of large and small airways in nonfatal and fatal asthma. *Am Rev Respir Dis* 1993; **147**: 405–10

29   Filley WV, Holley KE, Kephart GM, Gleich GJ. Identification by immunofluorescence of eosinophil granule major basic protein in lung tissues of patients with bronchial asthma. *Lancet* 1982; **ii**: 11–6

30   Azzawi M, Johnston PW, Majumdar S, Kay AB, Jeffery PK. T lymphocytes and activated eosinophils in airway mucosa in fatal asthma and cystic fibrosis. *Am Rev Respir Dis* 1992; **145**: 1477–82

31 Sur S, Crotty TB, Kephart GM *et al*. Sudden-onset fatal asthma. A distinct entity with few eosinophils and relatively more neutrophils in the airway submucosa? *Am Rev Respir Dis* 1993; **148**: 713–9

32 Carroll N, Cooke C, James A. The distribution of eosinophils and lymphocytes in the large and small airways of asthmatics. *Eur Respir J* 1997; **10**: 292–300

33 Djukanovic R, Wilson JW, Lai CK, Holgate ST, Howarth PH. The safety aspects of fiberoptic bronchoscopy, bronchoalveolar lavage, and endobronchial biopsy in asthma. *Am Rev Respir Dis* 1991; **143**: 772–7

34 Wardlaw AJ, Dunnette S, Gleich GJ, Collins JV, Kay AB. Eosinophils and mast cells in bronchoalveolar lavage in subjects with mild asthma. Relationship to bronchial hyperreactivity. *Am Rev Respir Dis* 1988; **137**: 62–9

35 Djukanovic R, Roche WR, Wilson JW *et al*. Mucosal inflammation in asthma. *Am Rev Respir Dis* 1990; **142**: 434–57

36 Wardlaw AJ, Hay H, Cromwell O, Collins JV, Kay AB. Leukotrienes, LTC4 and LTB4, in bronchoalveolar lavage in bronchial asthma and other respiratory diseases. *J Allergy Clin Immunol* 1989; **84**: 19–26

37 Broide DH, Gleich GJ, Cuomo AJ *et al*. Evidence of ongoing mast cell and eosinophil degranulation in symptomatic asthma airway. *J Allergy Clin Immunol* 1991; **88**: 637–48

38 Pavord ID, Ward R, Woltmann G, Wardlaw AJ, Sheller JR, R Dworski JR. Induced sputum eicosanoid concentrations in asthma. *Am J Respir Crit Care Med* 1999; **160**: 1905–9

39 Hartnell A, Robinson DS, Kay AB, Wardlaw AJ. CD69 is expressed by human eosinophils activated *in vivo* in asthma and *in vitro* by cytokines. *Immunology* 1993; **80**: 281–6

40 Djukanovic R, Wilson JW, Britten KM *et al*. Quantitation of mast cells and eosinophils in the bronchial mucosa of symptomatic atopic asthmatics and healthy control subjects using immunohistochemistry. *Am Rev Respir Dis* 1990; **142**: 863–71

41 Azzawi M, Bradley B, Jeffery PK *et al*. Identification of activated T lymphocytes and eosinophils in bronchial biopsies in stable atopic asthma. *Am Rev Respir Dis* 1990; **142**: 1407–13

42 Poston RN, Chanez P, Lacoste JY, Litchfield T, Lee TH, Bousquet J. Immunohistochemical characterization of the cellular infiltration in asthmatic bronchi. *Am Rev Respir Dis* 1992; **145**: 918–21

43 Bentley AM, Menz G, Storz C *et al*. Identification of T lymphocytes, macrophages, and activated eosinophils in the bronchial mucosa in intrinsic asthma. Relationship to symptoms and bronchial responsiveness. *Am Rev Respir Dis* 1992; **146**: 500–6

44 Frew AJ, Chan H, Lam S, Chan-Yeung M. Bronchial inflammation in occupational asthma due to western red cedar. *Am J Respir Crit Care Med* 1995; **151**: 340–4

45 Saetta M, Di Stefano A, Maestrelli P *et al*. Airway mucosal inflammation in occupational asthma induced by toluene diisocyanate. *Am Rev Respir Dis* 1992; **145**: 160–8

46 Nasser SM, Pfister R, Christie PE *et al*. Inflammatory cell populations in bronchial biopsies from aspirin-sensitive asthmatic subjects. *Am J Respir Crit Care Med* 1996; **153**: 90–6

47 Wenzel SE, Schwartz LB, Langmack EL *et al*. Evidence that severe asthma can be divided pathologically into two inflammatory subtypes with distinct physiologic and clinical characteristics. *Am J Respir Crit Care Med* 1999; **160**: 1001–8

48 Kim CK, Chung CY, Choi SJ, Kim DK, Park Y, Koh YY. Bronchoalveolar lavage cellular composition in acute asthma and acute bronchiolitis. *J Pediatr* 2000; **137**: 517–22

49 Marguet C, Jouen-Boedes F, Dean TP, Warner JO. Bronchoalveolar cell profiles in children with asthma, infantile wheeze, chronic cough, or cystic fibrosis. *Am J Respir Crit Care Med* 1999; **159**: 1533–40

50 Christodoulopoulos P, Cameron L, Durham S, Hamid Q. Molecular pathology of allergic disease. II. Upper airway disease. *J Allergy Clin Immunol* 2000; **105**: 211–23

51 Lamblin C, Gosset P, Salez F *et al*. Eosinophilic airway inflammation in nasal polyposis. *J Allergy Clin Immunol* 1999; **104**: 85–92

52 Leiferman KM. Eosinophils in atopic dermatitis. *Allergy* 1989; **44 (Suppl 9)**: 20–6

53 Leiferman KM, Ackerman SJ, Sampson HA, Haugen HS, Venencie PY, Gleich GJ. Dermal deposition of eosinophil-granule major basic protein in atopic dermatitis. Comparison with onchocerciasis. *N Engl J Med* 1985; **313**: 282–5

54 Djukanovic R, Lai CK, Wilson JW *et al*. Bronchial mucosal manifestations of atopy: a comparison of markers of inflammation between atopic asthmatics, atopic non-asthmatics and healthy controls. *Eur Respir J* 1992; **5**: 538–44

55 Broide DH, Paine MM, Firestein GS. Eosinophils express interleukin 5 and granulocyte macrophage-colony- stimulating factor mRNA at sites of allergic inflammation in asthmatics. *J Clin Invest* 1992; **90**: 1414–24

56 Nakajima H, Loegering DA, Kita H, Kephart GM, Gleich GJ. Reactivity of monoclonal antibodies EG1 and EG2 with eosinophils and their granule proteins. *J Leukoc Biol* 1999; **66**: 447–54

57 Aalbers R, Kauffman HF, Vrugt B *et al*. Bronchial lavage and bronchoalveolar lavage in allergen-induced single early and dual asthmatic responders. *Am Rev Respir Dis* 1993; **147**: 76–81

58 Varney VA, Jacobson MR, Sudderick RM *et al*. Immunohistology of the nasal mucosa following allergen-induced rhinitis. Identification of activated T lymphocytes, eosinophils, and neutrophils. *Am Rev Respir Dis* 1992; **146**: 170–6

59 Tsicopoulos A, Hamid Q, Haczku A *et al*. Kinetics of cell infiltration and cytokine messenger RNA expression after intradermal challenge with allergen and tuberculin in the same atopic individuals. *J Allergy Clin Immunol* 1994; **94**: 764–72

60 Fahy JV, Liu J, Wong H, Boushey HA. Cellular and biochemical analysis of induced sputum from asthmatic and from healthy subjects. *Am Rev Respir Dis* 1993; **147**: 1126–31

61 Gibson PG, Girgis-Gabardo A, Morris MM *et al*. Cellular characteristics of sputum from patients with asthma and chronic bronchitis. *Thorax* 1989; **44**: 693–9

62 Pavord ID, Pizzichini MM, Pizzichini E, Hargreave FE. The use of induced sputum to investigate airway inflammation. *Thorax* 1997; **52**: 498–501

63 Maestrelli P, Saetta M, Di Stefano A *et al*. Comparison of leukocyte counts in sputum, bronchial biopsies, and bronchoalveolar lavage. *Am J Respir Crit Care Med* 1995; **152**: 1926–31

64 Fahy JV, Wong H, Liu J, Boushey HA. Comparison of samples collected by sputum induction and bronchoscopy from asthmatic and healthy subjects. *Am J Respir Crit Care Med* 1995; **152**: 53–8

65 Belda J, Leigh R, Parameswaran K, O'Byrne PM, Sears MR, Hargreave FE. Induced sputum cell counts in healthy adults. *Am J Respir Crit Care Med* 2000; **161**: 475–8

66 Fahy JV, Kim KW, Liu J, Boushey HA. Prominent neutrophilic inflammation in sputum from subjects with asthma exacerbation. *J Allergy Clin Immunol* 1995; **95**: 843–52

67 Norzila MZ, Fakes K, Henry RL, Simpson J, Gibson PG. Interleukin-8 secretion and neutrophil recruitment accompanies induced sputum eosinophil activation in children with acute asthma. *Am J Respir Crit Care Med* 2000; **161**: 769–74

68 Lemiere C, Pizzichini MM, Balkissoon R *et al*. Diagnosing occupational asthma: use of induced sputum. Eur Respir J 1999; **13**: 482–8

69 Jeffery PK. Differences and similarities between chronic obstructive pulmonary disease and asthma. *Clin Exp Allergy* 1999; **29 (Suppl 2)**: 14–26

70 Saetta M, Di Stefano A, Maestrelli P *et al*. Airway eosinophilia in chronic bronchitis during exacerbations. *Am J Respir Crit Care Med* 1994; **150**: 1646–52

71 Brightling CE, Monteiro W, Ward R *et al*. Sputum eosinophilia and short-term response to prednisolone in chronic obstructive pulmonary disease: a randomised controlled trial. *Lancet* 2000; **356**: 1480–5

72 Balzano G, Stefanelli F, Iorio C *et al*. Eosinophilic inflammation in stable chronic obstructive pulmonary disease. Relationship with neutrophils and airway function. *Am J Respir Crit Care Med* 1999; **160**: 1486–92

73 Gibson PG, Dolovich J, Denburg J, Ramsdale EH, Hargreave FE. Chronic cough: eosinophilic bronchitis without asthma. *Lancet* 1989; **i**: 1346–8

74 Brightling CE, Pavord ID. Eosinophilic bronchitis – what is it and why is it important? *Clin Exp Allergy* 2000; **30**: 4–6

75 Foresi A, Leone C, Pelucchi A *et al*. Eosinophils, mast cells, and basophils in induced sputum from patients with seasonal allergic rhinitis and perennial asthma: relationship to methacholine responsiveness [published erratum appears in *J Allergy Clin Immunol* 1997; **100**: 720]. *J Allergy Clin Immunol* 1997; **100**: 58–64

76 Horn BR, Robin ED, Theodore J, Van-Kessel A. Total eosinophil counts in the management of bronchial asthma. *N Engl J Med* 1975; **292**: 1152–5

77 Durham SR, Kay AB. Eosinophils, bronchial hyperreactivity and late-phase asthmatic reactions. *Clin Allergy* 1985; **15**: 411–8

78 Pizzichini E, Pizzichini MM, Efthimiadis A, Dolovich J, Hargreave FE. Measuring airway inflammation in asthma: eosinophils and eosinophilic cationic protein in induced sputum compared with peripheral blood. *J Allergy Clin Immunol* 1997; **99**: 539–44

79 Synek M, Beasley R, Frew AJ *et al*. Cellular infiltration of the airways in asthma of varying severity. *Am J Respir Crit Care Med* 1996; **154**: 224–30

80 Bousquet J, Chanez P, Lacoste JY *et al*. Eosinophilic inflammation in asthma. *N Engl J Med* 1990; **323**: 1033–9

81 Bradley BL, Azzawi M, Jacobson M *et al*. Eosinophils, T-lymphocytes, mast cells, neutrophils, and macrophages in bronchial biopsy specimens from atopic subjects with asthma: comparison with biopsy specimens from atopic subjects without asthma and normal control subjects and relationship to bronchial hyperresponsiveness. *J Allergy Clin Immunol* 1991; **88**: 661–74

82 Lim S, Jatakanon A, Meah S, Oates T, Chung KF, Barnes PJ. Relationship between exhaled nitric oxide and mucosal eosinophilic inflammation in mild to moderately severe asthma. *Thorax* 2000; **55**: 184–8

83 Rosi E, Scano G. Association of sputum parameters with clinical and functional measurements in asthma. *Thorax* 2000; **55**: 235–8

84 Pin I, Gibson PG, Kolendowicz R *et al*. Use of induced sputum cell counts to investigate airway inflammation in asthma. *Thorax* 1992; **47**: 25–9

85 Gibson PG, Saltos N, Borgas T. Airway mast cells and eosinophils correlate with clinical severity and airway hyperresponsiveness in corticosteroid-treated asthma. *J Allergy Clin Immunol* 2000; **105**: 752–9

86 Grootendorst DC, van den Bos JW, Romeijn JJ *et al*. Induced sputum in adolescents with severe stable asthma. Safety and the relationship of cell counts and eosinophil cationic protein to clinical severity. *Eur Respir J* 1999; **13**: 647–53

87 Vignola AM, Chanez P, Campbell AM *et al*. Airway inflammation in mild intermittent and in persistent asthma. *Am J Respir Crit Care Med* 1998; **157**: 403–9

88 Louis R, Lau LC, Bron AO, Roldaan AC, Radermecker M, Djukanovic R. The relationship between airways inflammation and asthma severity. *Am J Respir Crit Care Med* 2000; **161**: 9–16

89 Ronchi MC, Piragino C, Rosi E *et al*. Do sputum eosinophils and ECP relate to the severity of asthma? *Eur Respir J* 1997; **10**: 1809–13

90 Jatakanon A, Lim S, Barnes PJ. Changes in sputum eosinophils predict loss of asthma control. *Am J Respir Crit Care Med* 2000; **161**: 64–72

91 Fujimoto K, Kubo K, Matsuzawa Y, Sekiguchi M. Eosinophil cationic protein levels in induced sputum correlate with the severity of bronchial asthma. *Chest* 1997; **112**: 1241–7

92 Virchow Jr JC, Holscher U, Virchow Sr C. Sputum ECP levels correlate with parameters of airflow obstruction. *Am Rev Respir Dis* 1992; **146**: 604–6

93 Crimi E, Spanevello A, Neri M, Ind PW, Rossi GA, Brusasco V. Dissociation between airway inflammation and airway hyperresponsiveness in allergic asthma. *Am J Respir Crit Care Med* 1998; **157**: 4–9

94 Jatakanon A, Lim S, Kharitonov SA, Chung KF, Barnes PJ. Correlation between exhaled nitric oxide, sputum eosinophils, and methacholine responsiveness in patients with mild asthma. *Thorax* 1998; **53**: 91–5

95 Henderson Jr WR, Chi EY, Albert RK *et al*. Blockade of CD49d (alpha4 integrin) on intrapulmonary but not circulating leukocytes inhibits airway inflammation and hyperresponsiveness in a mouse model of asthma. *J Clin Invest* 1997; **100**: 3083–92

96 Moller GM, Overbeek SE, van Helden-Meeuwsen CG, Hoogsteden HC, Bogaard JM. Eosinophils in the bronchial mucosa in relation to methacholine dose-response curves in atopic asthma. *J Appl Physiol* 1999; **86**: 1352–6

97 Rosi E, Ronchi MC, Grazzini M, Duranti R, Scano G. Sputum analysis, bronchial hyperresponsiveness, and airway function in asthma: results of a factor analysis. *J Allergy Clin Immunol* 1999; **103**: 232–7

98 Meagher LC, Cousin JM, Seckl JR, Haslett C. Opposing effects of glucocorticoids on the rate of apoptosis in neutrophilic and eosinophilic granulocytes. *J Immunol* 1996; **156**: 4422–8

99 Bentley AM, Hamid Q, Robinson DS *et al*. Prednisolone treatment in asthma. Reduction in the numbers of eosinophils, T cells, tryptase-only positive mast cells, and modulation of IL-4, IL-5, and interferon-gamma cytokine gene expression within the bronchial mucosa. *Am J Respir Crit Care Med* 1996; **153**: 551–6

100 Claman DM, Boushey HA, Liu J, Wong H, Fahy JV. Analysis of induced sputum to examine the effects of prednisone on airway inflammation in asthmatic subjects. *J Allergy Clin Immunol* 1994; **94**: 861–9

101 Pizzichini MM, Pizzichini E, Clelland L *et al*. Sputum in severe exacerbations of asthma: kinetics of inflammatory indices after prednisone treatment. *Am J Respir Crit Care Med* 1997; **155**: 1501–8

102 Djukanovic R, Wilson JW, Britten KM *et al*. Effect of an inhaled corticosteroid on airway inflammation and symptoms in asthma. *Am Rev Respir Dis* 1992; **145**: 669–74

103 Lim S, Jatakanon A, John M *et al*. Effect of inhaled budesonide on lung function and airway inflammation. Assessment by various inflammatory markers in mild asthma. *Am J Respir Crit Care Med* 1999; **159**: 22–30

104 Little SA, Chalmers GW, MacLeod KJ, McSharry C, Thomson NC. Non-invasive markers of airway inflammation as predictors of oral steroid responsiveness in asthma. *Thorax* 2000; **55**: 232–4

105 Pizzichini E, Pizzichini MM, Gibson P *et al*. Sputum eosinophilia predicts benefit from prednisone in smokers with chronic obstructive bronchitis. *Am J Respir Crit Care Med* 1998; **158**: 1511–7

106 Fujimoto K, Kubo K, Yamamoto H, Yamaguchi S, Matsuzawa Y. Eosinophilic inflammation in the airway is related to glucocorticoid reversibility in patients with pulmonary emphysema. *Chest* 1999; **115**: 697–702

107 Kita H, Jorgensen RK, Reed CE *et al*. Mechanism of topical glucocorticoid treatment of hay fever: IL-5 and eosinophil activation during natural allergen exposure are suppressed, but IL-4, IL-6, and IgE antibody production are unaffected. *J Allergy Clin Immunol* 2000; **106**: 521–9

108 Pavord ID, Brightling CE, Woltmann G, Wardlaw AJ. Non-eosinophilic corticosteroid unresponsive asthma. *Lancet* 1999; **353**: 2213–4

109 Pizzichini E, Leff JA, Reiss TF *et al*. Montelukast reduces airway eosinophilic inflammation in asthma: a randomized, controlled trial. *Eur Respir J* 1999; **14**: 12–8

110 Lee E, Robertson T, Smith J, Kilfeather S. Leukotriene receptor antagonists and synthesis inhibitors reverse survival in eosinophils of asthmatic individuals. *Am J Respir Crit Care Med* 2000; **161**: 1881–6

111 Hoshino M, Sim J, Shimizu K, Nakayama, Koya A. Effect of AA-2414, a thromboxane A$_2$ receptor antagonist, on airway inflammation in subjects with asthma. *J Allergy Clin Immunol* 1999; **103**: 1054–61

112 Khan LN, Kon OM, Macfarlane AJ *et al*. Attenuation of the allergen-induced late asthmatic reaction by cyclosporin A is associated with inhibition of bronchial eosinophils, interleukin-5, granulocyte macrophage colony-stimulating factor, and eotaxin. *Am J Respir Crit Care Med* 2000; **162**: 1377–1382

113 Leckie MJ, ten Brinke A, Khan J *et al*. Effects of an interleukin-5 blocking monoclonal antibody on eosinophils, airway hyper-responsiveness, and the late asthmatic response. *Lancet* 2000; **356**: 2144–8

Inhibition of IgE-receptor interactions

Brian J Sutton, **Rebecca L Beavil** and **Andrew J Beavil**

The Randall Centre for Molecular Mechanisms of Cell Function, King's College London, London, UK

Immunoglobulin E plays a central role in allergic disease and, as our understanding of the network of interactions between IgE and its receptors improves, new opportunities for therapeutic intervention emerge. IgE binding to its 'high-affinity' receptor, FcεRI, first identified on mast cells and now known to be expressed on a variety of other cell types, is the best characterised interaction, and has attracted most attention. The 'low affinity' receptor, FcεRII/CD23, first found on B-cells, appears to be part of a more complex network that has yet to be fully elucidated. Two recent advances concerning the IgE-FcεRI interaction are noteworthy. The first is the development of a monoclonal anti-IgE antibody, now in advanced clinical trials, which inhibits this interaction and certainly proves the viability of this approach. The second is the publication of the crystal structure of the complex between IgE and FcεRI, which opens the way for the first structure-based design of small molecule inhibitors.

Correspondence to:
Dr Brian J Sutton,
The Randall Centre for
Molecular Mechanisms of
Cell Function, King's
College London, New
Hunt's House, Guy's
Hospital Campus,
London Bridge,
London SE1 1UL, UK

The interactions between immunoglobulin E (IgE) and its cellular receptors have been studied over many years with the aim not only of understanding the molecular mechanisms underlying the allergic response, but also of identifying molecular targets for therapeutic intervention. The first receptor to be identified, termed FcεRI by virtue of the fact that it binds to the Fc region of IgE, was found on mast cells and basophils. IgE binds to cells bearing this receptor with such a high affinity ($K_a \sim 10^{10}$ M^{-1}), that they are permanently coated with IgE, and thus sensitised for rapid activation when challenged with allergen. This activation, triggered by aggregation of as few as two receptor molecules by multivalent allergen, leads to release of molecules that promote an immediate inflammatory response. A second receptor was later discovered on B-cells, termed FcεRII and also identified as CD23 (the name that will be used in this review), to which IgE binds with lower affinity ($K_a \sim 10^7$ M^{-1}). This interaction is involved in both IgE regulation and allergen presentation by B-cells, but understanding the functional roles of CD23 is further complicated by the fact that it exists both as a cell surface molecule and in a soluble form generated by cleavage from the cell surface; furthermore, it exists in both monomeric and oligomeric states, as will be discussed in more detail below (see Sutton & Gould[1] for a review).

These two receptors, FcεRI and CD23 are very different in their molecular structure. FcεRI belongs to the immunoglobulin superfamily and is highly homologous in sequence and structure to the IgG Fc receptors, while CD23 is a member of the C-type lectin superfamily (which includes clearance proteins such as the asialoglycoprotein receptor). Despite the fact that CD23 is a lectin-like molecule and IgE is a glycoprotein, binding does not occur through the carbohydrate component of IgE, and the search for another ligand for CD23 led to the discovery of the interaction with another B-cell surface molecule, CD21 or CR2 (complement receptor 2)[2]. This extended the network of IgE interactions to the complement system. The more recent discovery of interactions between CD23 and the complement receptors CR3 (CD11b/CD18) and CR4 (CD11c/CD18), which are members of the integrin superfamily and also implicated in inflammatory mechanisms[3], extends the IgE network yet further. The early characterisation of these interactions, and the appreciation of this extended network have been

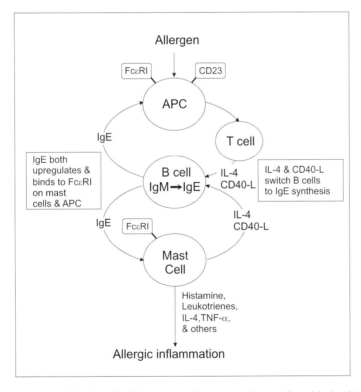

Fig. 1 Positive feedback between allergen uptake, mediated by both FcεRI and CD23 on antigen presenting cells (APC), and activation of effector cells such as mast cells and basophils, bearing FcεRI. Both activated effector cells and T-cells can provide necessary signals (IL-4 and CD40L) for induction of heavy-chain switching to IgE in B-cells. CD23 on B-cells (see Fig. 3) further contributes to the differentiation of committed B-cells into IgE-secreting B-cells.

reviewed elsewhere[1,4]. Here, we shall concentrate solely on the receptors FcεRI and CD23 and their interactions with IgE, since only these are understood in sufficient detail at present to allow consideration of intervention at the molecular level.

Functional diversity of FcεRI and CD23

FcεRI is now known to be expressed on a variety of cells in addition to mast cells and basophils. It has been found on Langerhans cells and dendritic cells where it is involved in antigen presentation, on eosinophils where it plays a role in defence against parasitic infection, and also monocytes (see Kinet[5] for a review). CD23 is also expressed on a variety of cells that include antigen-presenting cells[6]. Thus blocking of IgE-receptor interactions may have functional consequences at different stages of the allergic response, and inhibition of IgE-dependent uptake of allergen, for example, would clearly be desirable. Figure 1 schematically indicates the involvement of both receptors in allergen uptake and presentation to T-cells by antigen-presenting cells (APC), and the involvement of FcεRI in allergen-induced activation of mast cells. Both activated T-cells and effector cells can then provide the necessary signals (IL-4 and CD40-L) for switching B-cells to IgE synthesis, which in turn promotes sensitisation of both effector cells and APC in positive feedback, perpetuating the allergic state[7].

The binding of IgE to FcεRI, and to CD23 on the cell surface is depicted schematically in Figure 2. The IgE molecule has a bent structure (as discussed in the following section) and interacts with the second Ig-like extracellular domain of the FcεRI α-chain through its Cε3 domains, as revealed in a crystal structure of the complex[8]. In contrast, the IgE-binding lectin domains of CD23 are connected to the membrane by a triple-stranded α-helical 'stalk' region, and the interaction, again with the Cε3 domains of IgE, involves two 'heads'[7]. However, the structure of the CD23 head has yet to be determined (although it has been modelled on the structures of other C-type lectins), and the details of its binding to Cε3 are not known. The interactions shown in Figure 2 represent those involved in the presentation of allergen-IgE complexes by these two receptors, and also in the case of FcεRI, the sensitisation of mast cells and basophils by IgE for allergen-induced activation. Membrane-bound CD23 (mCD23) also delivers a down-regulatory signal for IgE synthesis by B-cells when engaged by IgE-allergen complexes (see Gould et al[7] for a review), and anti-CD23 antibodies have been investigated for their therapeutic potential[9-11]. Their mechanism of action is still debated, but one of these anti-CD23 antibodies, now in clinical trials, is thought to function by co-ligating mCD23 with the IgG receptor FcγRII/CD32 on the same cell through its Fc region[11].

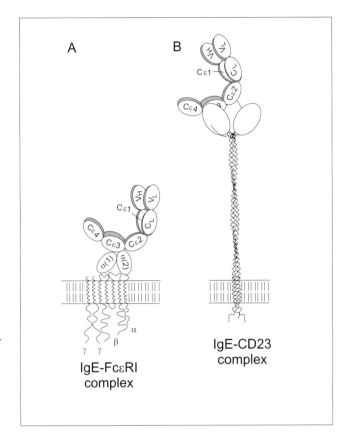

Fig. 2 Schematic representation of the binding of IgE to its receptors: (A) FcεRI α-chain and (B) CD23. FcεRI consists of four polypeptide chains, αβγ$_2$; mCD23 is a trimer of identical polypeptide chains.

CD23 also exists in a soluble form (sCD23), cleaved in the stalk region by an endogenous, membrane-bound metalloprotease[12]. It is this sCD23 that acts as a B-cell growth factor up-regulating the production of IgE, though only when it is trimeric, not when monomeric[13]. Since sCD23 binds to both IgE, including membrane-bound IgE (mIgE), and CD21[2], it has been proposed that trimeric sCD23 may promote IgE synthesis by cross-linking mIgE and CD21 on B-cells committed to IgE synthesis[1,7]. This is shown schematically in Figure 3, which also identifies potential points for intervention. Soluble fragments of these molecules such as monomeric CD23 heads[13], sCD21 domains[14] or antibodies to these molecules[9–11], are potential inhibitors of such events at the B-cell surface, as are inhibitors of the endogenous metalloprotease(s) that cleave CD23 from the cell surface[15]. *Der p1*, the major house dust mite allergen and a cysteine protease, also cleaves mCD23 (and CD25, the IL-2 receptor), and in this way may promote IgE synthesis by simultaneously removing the down-regulatory signal (*via* mCD23) and promoting the up-regulatory signal (*via* sCD23)[16]. Inhibitors of *Der p1* are being developed as a means to combat house dust mite allergy.

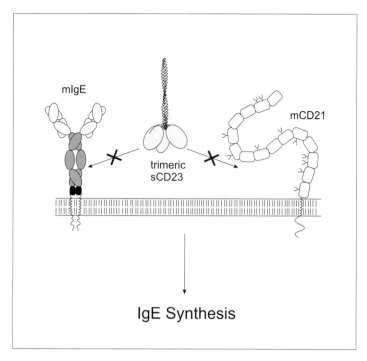

Fig. 3 Schematic representation of the cross-linking of mIgE and mCD21 by trimeric sCD23 at the surface of a B cell committed to IgE synthesis. Inhibition of either interaction, (indicated by X) may suppress IgE production. In mIgE, the additional domains linking the Cε4 domains to the membrane are shown; in mCD21, glycosylation sites on the domains of CD21 are indicated.

While all of these lines of research are actively being pursued in the quest for a means to down-regulate IgE production *via* CD23, they are at a relatively early stage and will not be considered further here. We now turn to the IgE molecule itself and its interaction with FcεRI, for it is here that the most promising developments have occurred recently.

The IgE molecule as a target

The Fc region of the IgE molecule, which contains binding sites for both FcεRI and CD23, consists of a disulphide-linked dimer of two polypeptide chains each folded into the Cε2, Cε3 and Cε4 domains – a total of six domains. The Cε2 domains have no counterpart in IgG, which instead has a flexible 'hinge' region linking the antigen-binding Fab regions to the (four-domain) receptor-binding Fc region. This replacement of a flexible hinge with a pair of disulphide-linked folded domains leads to a very different structure for IgE, compared with the flexible Y-shaped IgG molecule. Spectroscopic studies have shown that IgE adopts a compact, bent structure both in solution and when bound to FcεRI[17], as shown schematically in Figure 2A. Furthermore, X-ray scattering studies have shown that IgE Fc is bent, between the Cε2 and Cε3 domains[18]. Thus although IgE Fc consists of two identical chains, it has an asymmetric structure, with a 'concave' face and a 'convex' face. This asymmetry, and the topology of its binding to FcεRI α-chain domains, clearly shows why a single IgE molecule cannot simultaneously bind to two receptors – a necessity since such an event could lead to receptor aggregation and mast cell activation in the absence of allergen. In fact we now know that receptor binding also causes a conformational change in the Fc that precludes binding to a second receptor molecule[8]. With regard to the design and development of inhibitors of receptor binding, both the asymmetry and the conformational change turn out to be critical aspects of the IgE structure.

The first attempts to inhibit IgE binding to FcεRI involved synthesising short peptides from the IgE Fc region, and the earliest of these was a pentapeptide from the linker region between Cε2 and Cε3 identified by sequence comparison of IgE with IgG, IgA and IgM[19]. Although doubt was subsequently cast upon the inhibitory properties of this peptide[20], larger peptides including this segment were found to be inhibitory[21,22], and mutagenesis studies confirmed the importance of this region of the Fc[23]. The crystal structure of the complex[8] finally confirmed the key role of this N-terminal region of the Cε3 domains. However, competition of such a high affinity interaction with short peptides is clearly always going to be difficult, and the alternative of blocking with antibodies to IgE has long been considered a promising strategy.

Therapeutically useful antibodies to IgE must have the property of blocking IgE binding to the receptor, but clearly must not bind to receptor-bound IgE since this could lead to cross-linking of IgE/receptor complexes and cell activation. The asymmetric structure of receptor-bound IgE (Fig. 2A), and the conformational change in the Fc upon receptor binding, explains why a subset of anti-IgE antibodies directed to the receptor binding site may indeed have this property. However, soluble IgE is not the only target. mIgE is expressed on the surface of B-cells committed to IgE synthesis, and targeting mIgE could lead to the elimination of these B-cells and the suppression of IgE levels. Indeed, early studies with an anti-IgE established that the molecule must be bivalent in order to be effective[24], implying that cross-linking of mIgE was occurring, and even earlier studies in mice with anti-IgE demonstrated long-term inhibition of IgE synthesis[25,26]. Since mIgE has an additional region of polypeptide chain linking the Cε4 domains to the membrane that is not present in secreted IgE (see Fig. 3), this unique structural feature can be used to target antibodies specifically to mIgE[27].

An anti-IgE therapeutic antibody

Two distinct strategies have been employed to generate anti-IgE antibodies. One is to use a vaccine approach, raising the antibodies in a natural response to a short peptide[28,29] or larger fragments of IgE Fc (*e.g.* Cε2–Cε3)[30], but this will not be discussed further here. The other approach is to engineer a humanised monoclonal anti-IgE molecule for therapeutic application and, while a number of groups have pursued this route (*e.g.* Corne *et al*[31]), by far the most advanced is the humanised monoclonal IgG antibody rhuMab-E25 from Genentech Inc.[32,33]. This antibody has specificity for the receptor-binding region of IgE Fc, but cannot bind to receptor-bound IgE and thus cannot trigger mast cell or basophil degranulation. Its half-life in serum is approximately 14 days, much longer than that of free IgE, which is approximately 2 days, and its affinity for IgE is extremely high, 1.5×10^{10} M^{-1}. However, even this affinity is only just high enough to enable it to compete and block soluble IgE binding to FcεRI. Since the rate of dissociation of IgE from cell surface FcεRI is extremely slow ($k_d \sim 10^{-5}$ s^{-1}; *i.e.* 20 h for half of the IgE molecules to dissociate from the surface), and perhaps only 1% of receptors on a mast cell need to be occupied by IgE for allergen-induced triggering to occur, this mechanism alone is unlikely to account for the dramatic efficacy reported for this antibody. In human trials, with a single dose administered every one or two weeks (monthly in later trials), circulating IgE levels fell to less than 1% of their original value[34], strongly indicative of a direct effect upon the IgE-secreting B-cells. The precise molecular mechanism for this phenomenon has not been elucidated, but direct binding to B-cells has been demonstrated[35]. It may involve cross-linking of mIgE on the B cell, but inhibition of other B cell surface interactions required for proliferation, such as those depicted in Figure 3, or disruption of interactions between mIgE and the Ig-α and Ig-β chains of the B cell receptor that are required for signalling, could certainly also be effected by rhuMab-E25. As discussed in the following section, however, suppression of IgE synthesis by a soluble receptor fragment, sFcεRIα, has been shown to be due to a direct interaction with mIgE[36]; as this molecule is monovalent, cross-linking of mIgE is clearly not the only possibility.

A further beneficial effect of lowering the concentration of free IgE is that the cell-surface expression of FcεRI is down-regulated. This has been observed on a range of FcεRI-expressing cells, and shown directly for basophils following rhuMab-E25 administration[34]. The fact that this is a direct result of interaction between IgE and the receptor has also been demonstrated[37]. The reduction in circulating IgE, and consequent lowering of FcεRI expression, constitute a most effective negative feedback effect.

Figure 4 summarises the activities of rhuMab-E25 discussed so far, and also illustrates a further site of action at the level of antigen

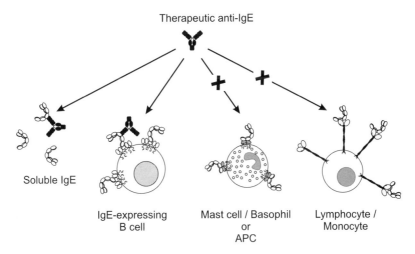

Therapeutic anti-IgE

Soluble IgE

IgE-expressing
B cell

Mast cell / Basophil
or
APC

Lymphocyte /
Monocyte

Fig. 4 Potential effects of an anti-IgE therapeutic agent. From the left: sequestering free IgE; interaction with mIgE (shown with Ig-α and β chains) on B-cells, either cross-linking mIgE or disrupting interactions required for signalling to suppress IgE synthesis; inhibition of IgE binding to FcεRI on mast cells, basophils or antigen presenting cells; inhibition of IgE binding to CD23 on antigen presenting cells. (After Fig. 1 in Chang[33].)

presentation. Both FcεRI[38,39] and CD23[6] have been implicated in this process, and since the binding sites for both receptors are known to overlap in the Cε3 domain, simultaneous inhibition of both interactions is feasible. Not only may IgE-dependent allergen presentation be inhibited in this way, but it has also been proposed that the IgE–anti-IgE complexes may serve a beneficial role. Their relatively long half-life of approximately 14 days may enable them to mop up free allergen and clear it from the system *via* IgG-dependent mechanisms[33]. It has even been suggested that this short-term shift towards a non-IgE-dependent response may lead to longer-term alteration in the response of patients undergoing anti-IgE therapy[33].

The future for this therapeutic antibody, which has already completed Phase III clinical trials for allergic rhinitis and asthma, is therefore very promising. Administration is i.v., must be repeated regularly and may be costly, but it will certainly have application to the more severe allergic conditions. However, if prolonged treatment causes a permanent shift in the patient's response to allergen, away from IgE-mediated mechanisms, then this is a very exciting prospect indeed.

Receptor-based inhibitors

The crystal structure of the extracellular domains of FcεRIα (see Fig. 5A) was solved in 1998[40], but earlier molecular modelling of the two Ig-like

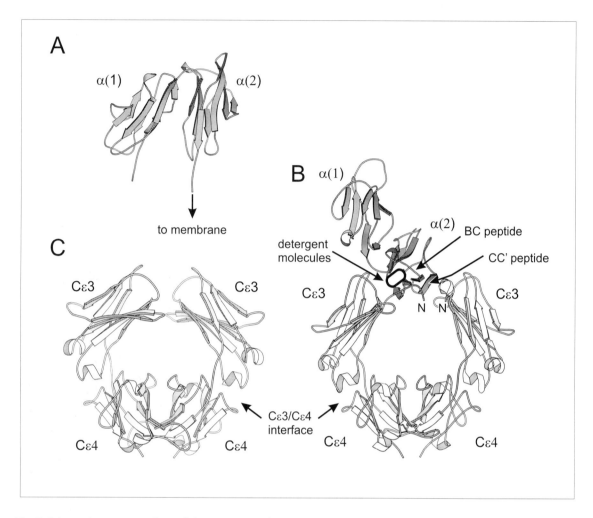

Fig. 5 Schematic representations of the structures of: (**A**) the FcεRI α-chain domains; (**B**) the complex between IgE Fc Cε3–Cε4 domains and FcεRIα; (**C**) the uncomplexed IgE Fc Cε3–Cε4. The locations of two inhibitory peptides, and the binding site of detergent molecules found in the crystal structure of the complex, are shown. N denotes the N-termini of the two Cε3 domains.

domains had provided a basis for the design of peptide inhibitors that incorporated amino-acids identified by mutagenesis to be critical for IgE binding. A peptide of 11 residues, constrained by a disulphide bridge between additional terminal cysteine residues to mimic the native conformation of the CC′ β-strands and intervening loop, inhibited IgE binding and mast cell degranulation *in vitro*[41]. Subsequent analysis of the peptide by nuclear magnetic resonance spectroscopy showed that the β-structure had indeed formed, and the crystal structure of the IgE/FcεRIα complex[8] now reveals that this region of the α(2) domain is critically involved. Another (linear) peptide from the adjacent BC loop region was found to inhibit IgE binding to FcεRI[42], and it too can now be seen to include residues at the interface[8]. However, even peptides constrained in structure to mimic a part of the IgE-Fc/FcεRIα interface may not compete effectively with such a high affinity interaction, and more success has been obtained using larger fragments. The whole sFcεRIα fragment has been investigated in several *in vitro* and *in vivo* animal model studies (see Sutton & Gould[26] for a review), which showed that it could prevent IgE binding to mast cell receptors if administered before allergen challenge. Furthermore, a suppressive effect on IgE synthesis, as a result of binding of sFcεRIα to mIgE, was demonstrated *in vitro* with human B-cells[36]. As mentioned above in relation to rhuMab-E25, the mechanism of this effect is not clear. sFcεRIα is obviously monomeric, yet earlier studies with an anti-IgE concluded that a bivalent molecule was required for suppression, presumably to cross-link mIgE[24]. A bivalent form of the soluble receptor, a fusion protein with IgG Fc in which two sFcεRIα fragments replace the Fab arms of IgG, has been generated and shown to be effective in inhibition of mast cell degranulation *in vitro* and the passive cutaneous anaphylaxis reaction in a rodent model[43]. However, there have been no reports of the effect of this molecule upon IgE synthesis, or its mechanism of action, but it might be predicted to be more effective than sFcεRIα.

FcεRIα has been the subject of extensive mutagenesis studies to identify key residues in IgE binding, and it has proved possible to modestly enhance the affinity[44,45]. Knowledge of the crystal structure of the complex[8] now provides a basis for designing more effective mutations. Thus soluble receptor fragments in either monovalent or bivalent form might yet prove to be valuable therapeutic agents, with the ability not only to inhibit mast cell sensitisation, but also suppress IgE synthesis.

Ironically, a soluble form of the low affinity receptor, sCD23, has also been proposed as means to inhibit IgE binding to the high affinity receptor FcεRI. A modified version of sCD23 with an isoleucine zipper motif (which promotes α-helical trimer formation) fused to the stalk[46], displays greater stability as a trimer and higher affinity for IgE than natural sCD23 or mCD23, presumably through an avidity effect. The construct is 10,000-fold better at inhibiting IgE binding to mast cells than sCD23, and can, therefore, in principle compete with FcεRI.

The IgE-FcεRI complex as a basis for inhibitor design

A landmark in the study of IgE was the determination of the crystal structure of the complex between IgE Fcε3–4 (the Fc region consisting of the Cε3 and Cε4 domains), and the extracellular region of FcεRIα[8].

This structure is represented in Figure 5B, which shows how the α(2) domain and linker region to α(1) of the receptor make contact with the N-terminal regions of both Cε3 domains of IgE. While the structure confirms many of the conclusions drawn from mutagenesis studies about the location and nature of the interface[23,44,45], it is also instructive to rationalise how mutations outside the binding interface, such as at the Cε3/Cε4 interface in IgE[47,48], also exert an effect on binding. These allosteric effects provide clues to effective ways of inhibiting the interaction, as will be discussed below. It is fascinating to note the crucial involvement of the N-terminal linker region of Cε3 that includes precisely those residues proposed 25 years earlier by sequence comparisons[19], and that the CC' and BC loop peptides predicted to be important on the receptor[41,42], are indeed central to the interface.

The binding interface is extensive, and dominated by hydrophobic residues on the receptor, but intriguingly in the crystal structure, immediately adjacent to the interface, molecules of detergent from the crystallisation medium are seen to bind[8]. One of these molecules interacts with amino-acid residues from one of the Cε3 domains, and seems to mimic the interaction occurring between the receptor and the same amino-acids on the other Cε3 domain. The authors suggest that the structure of this molecule could be extended in such a way as to disrupt the interaction; in effect it provides a lead compound for the design of a small molecule inhibitor.

Another lead towards designing an inhibitor comes from the discovery that the binding of receptor to the Cε3 domains involves a substantial conformational change in the IgE Fc. The structure of the free Fcε3–4 fragment was also determined[49] (see Fig. 5C) and, when compared with the structure of the Fcε3–4 in the complex, a change in the angle of the Cε3 domains relative to the Cε4 domains was seen. In Figure 5, comparison of B and C clearly shows how both Cε3 domains 'open up' to accommodate the receptor. This change involves relative movement of amino-acids at the Cε3/Cε4 interface region (indicated in Fig. 5B,C), and thus explains why amino-acid substitutions in this region have been found to affect receptor binding[47,48]. If this conformational change can be prevented, perhaps by designing a molecule to bind to the Cε3/Cε4 interface, receptor binding could be blocked by this 'allosteric' mechanism. The targeting of molecules to the homologous interdomain region of IgG has already been the subject of a detailed analysis[50]. Comparison of the structure of the free receptor molecule[40] with that of the complex, reveals that there is also conformational change in the C' β-strand of the receptor upon binding. Clearly, there is induced fit of both partners upon interaction, a surprise for such a high affinity interaction (since conformational change incurs an energy cost), but an aspect that can perhaps be exploited in inhibitor design. Over the years, a number of small molecules have been reported to inhibit IgE binding to FcεRI, including oligonucleotides[51] and tetracyclic aromatic compounds[52]; it would be instructive now to investigate whether they bind directly to the interface or act allosterically.

Finally, it must be remembered that two IgE Fc domains are missing from the crystal structure of the complex. The expected location of the Cε2 domains may be inferred from the positions of the N-terminal residues of Cε3 (indicated in Fig. 5B), and clearly there may even be direct interaction between Cε2 and FcεRIα. Although it has been shown that the presence or absence of the Cε2 domains does not appreciably affect the overall affinity of the interaction[53], the kinetics are substantially affected, such that both on-rate and off-rate are slower when they are present[44]. In fact, the Cε2 domains have the effect of slowing the dissociation rate 20-fold (compared with Fcε3–4), thus contributing significantly to the long half-life of bound IgE and its ability to sensitise mast cells and basophils. It may, therefore, be possible, by targeting Cε2, to promote dissociation of IgE from the receptor. Since the bound detergent molecules in the crystal structure of the complex[8] may occupy some of the space required by the Cε2 domains, they may provide a lead here too. Targeting what may be a relatively weak interaction to affect the dissociation kinetics, rather than attempting to block a high affinity interaction, may be a more tractable proposition.

Conclusion

The extensive network of interactions between IgE, its receptors and their counter-receptors offers numerous opportunities for molecular intervention. Few of these are sufficiently well understood at present, but the most studied and best characterised interaction of all is that between IgE and FcεRI, and we may shortly see a truly novel therapeutic agent for allergy that inhibits this interaction, the anti-IgE antibody, in clinical use. As a large protein molecule, it may suffer from limitations in the mode of administration and high cost, but it proves the feasibility of the approach and looks very promising indeed. The precise molecular details of the IgE/FcεRI interaction have also been revealed by X-ray crystallography, providing for the first time a firm structural basis for rational design of small molecule inhibitors. The emerging picture of a flexible IgE molecule undergoing conformational change upon receptor binding, suggests ways of allosterically inhibiting the interaction that had not been anticipated. The exploitation of these new structural data is for the future, but in principle small molecules can be produced more cheaply, may be delivered in a variety of ways, and may thus find application to a wider range of allergic conditions. Understanding of CD23 and its interactions lags behind that of FcεRI, and precise structural data are still lacking, but it clearly plays a role in the regulation of IgE levels, and its interactions with IgE and CD21 may in due course provide new targets for therapeutic intervention.

Acknowledgements

The authors wish to acknowledge the support of the MRC, BBSRC, Wellcome Trust and National Asthma Campaign (UK) for their work in this field.

References

1   Sutton BJ, Gould HJ. The human IgE network. *Nature* 1993; **366**: 421–8
2   Aubry J-P, Pochon S, Graber P, Jansen KU, Bonnefoy J-Y. CD21 is a ligand for CD23 and regulates IgE production. *Nature* 1992; **358**: 505–7
3   Bonnefoy J-Y, Plater-Zyberk C, Lecoanet-Henchoz S, Gauchat J-F, Aubry J-P, Graber P. A new role for CD23 in inflammation. *Immunol Today* 1996; **17**: 418–20
4   Sutton BJ, Gould HJ. IgE and IgE Receptors. In: Kay AB. (ed) *Allergy and Allergic Diseases*. Oxford: Blackwell, 1997; 81–95
5   Kinet J-P. The high-affinity IgE receptor (FcεRI); from physiology to pathology. *Annu Rev Immunol* 1999; **17**: 931–72
6   Mudde GC, Bheekha R, Bruijnzeel-Koomen CAFM. Consequences of IgE/CD23-mediated antigen presentation in allergy. *Immunol Today* 1995; **16**: 380–3
7   Gould HJ, Beavil RL, Reljic R *et al*. IgE homeostasis: is CD23 the safety switch? In: Vercelli D. (ed) *IgE Regulation: Molecular Mechanisms*. Chichester: Wiley, 1997: 37–59
8   Garman SC, Wurzburg BA, Tarchevskaya SS, Kinet J-P, Jardetzky TS. Structure of the Fc fragment of human IgE bound to its high-affinity receptor FcεRIα. *Nature* 2000; **406**: 259–66
9   Flores-Romo L, Shields J, Humbert Y *et al*. Inhibition of an *in vivo* antigen-specific IgE response by antibodies to CD23. *Science* 1993; **261**: 1038–41
10   Dasic G, Juillard P, Graber P *et al*. Critical role of CD23 in allergen-induced bronchoconstriction in a murine model of allergic asthma. *Eur J Immunol* 1999; **29**: 2957–67
11   Nakamura T, Kloetzer WS, Brams P *et al*. *In vitro* IgE inhibition in B-cells by anti-CD23 monoclonal antibodies is functionally dependent on the immunoglobulin Fc domain. *Int J Immunopharmacol* 2000; **22**: 131–41
12   Marolewski AE, Buckle DR, Christie G *et al*. CD23 (FcεRII) release from cell membranes is mediated by a membrane-bound metalloprotease. *Biochem J* 1998; **333**: 573–9
13   Sarfati M, Bettler B, Letellier M *et al*. Native and recombinant soluble CD23 fragments with IgE suppressive activity. *Immunology* 1992; **76**: 662–7
14   Frémeaux-Bacchi V, Fischer E, Lecoanet-Henchoz S, Mani J-C, Bonnefoy J-Y, Kazatchkine MD. Soluble CD21 (sCD21) forms biologically active complexes with CD23: sCD21 is present in normal plasma as a complex with trimeric CD23 and inhibits soluble CD23-induced IgE synthesis by B-cells. *Int Immunol* 1998; **10**: 1459–66
15   Christie G, Barton A, Bolognese B *et al*. IgE secretion is attenuated by an inhibitor of proteolytic processing of CD23 (FcεRII). *Eur J Immunol* 1997; **27**: 3228–35
16   Shakib F, Schulz O, Sewell H. A mite subversive: cleavage of CD23 and CD25 by Der p1 enhances allergenicity. *Immunol Today* 1998; **19**: 313–6
17. Zheng Y, Shopes B, Holowka D, Baird B. Conformations of IgE bound to its receptor FcεRI and in solution. *Biochemistry* 1991; **30**: 9125–32
18   Beavil AJ, Young RJ, Sutton BJ, Perkins SJ. Bent domain structure of recombinant human IgE-Fc in solution by X-ray and neutron scattering in conjunction with an automated curve fitting

procedure. *Biochemistry* 1995; **34**: 14449–61

19 Hamburger RN. Peptide inhibition of the Prausnitz-Küstner reaction. *Science* 1975; **189**: 389–90

20 Bennich H, Ragnarsson U, Johansson SGO *et al*. Failure of the putative IgE pentapeptide to compete with IgE for receptors on basophils and mast cells. *Int Arch Allergy Appl Immunol* 1977; **53**: 459–68

21 Helm B, Marsh P, Vercelli D, Padlan E, Gould HJ, Geha R. The mast cell binding site on human immunoglobulin E. *Nature* 1988; **331**: 180–3

22 Helm B, Kebo D, Vercelli D *et al*. Blocking of passive sensitization of human mast cells and basophil granulocytes with IgE antibodies by a recombinant human ε-chain fragment of 76 amino acid residues. *Proc Natl Acad Sci USA* 1989; **86**: 9465–9

23 Henry AJ, Cook JPD, McDonnell JM *et al*. Participation of the N-terminal region of Cε3 in the binding of human IgE to its high affinity receptor FcεRI. *Biochemistry* 1997; **36**: 15568–78

24 Stampfli MR, Miescher S, Aebischer I, Zurcher AW, Stadler BM. Inhibition of human IgE synthesis by anti-IgE antibodies requires divalent recognition. *Eur J Immunol* 1994; **24**: 2161–7

25 Haba S, Nisonoff A. Inhibition of IgE synthesis by anti-IgE: role in long-term inhibition of IgE synthesis by neonatally administered soluble IgE. *Proc Natl Acad Sci USA* 1990; **87**: 3363–7

26 Sutton BJ, Gould HJ. Regulation of IgE-mediated inflammation by soluble fragments of the high affinity IgE receptor. In: Bousquet J. (ed) *Immunotherapy of Asthma*. New York: Marcel Dekker, 1999; 411–29

27 Davis FM, Gossett LA, Chang TW. An epitope on membrane-bound but not secreted IgE: implications in isotype-specific regulation. *Biotechnology* 1991; **9**: 53–6

28 Stanworth DR, Jones VM, Lewin IV, Nayyar S. Allergy treatment with a peptide vaccine. *Lancet* 1990; **336**: 1279–81

29 Zuercher AW, Miescher SM, Vogel M, Rudolf MP, Stadler MB, Stadler BM. Oral anti-IgE immunization with epitope-displaying phage. *Eur J Immunol* 2000; **30**: 128–35

30 Hellman L. Profound reduction in allergen sensitivity following treatment with a novel allergy vaccine. *Eur J Immunol* 1994; **24**: 415–20

31 Corne J, Djukanovic R, Thomas L *et al*. The effect of intravenous administration of a chimeric anti-IgE antibody on serum IgE levels in atopic subjects: efficacy, safety and pharmacokinetics. *J Clin Invest* 1997; **99**: 879–87

32 Jardieu PM, Fick RB. IgE inhibition as a therapy for allergic disease. *Int Arch Allergy Immunol* 1999; **118**: 112–5

33 Chang TW. The pharmacological basis of anti-IgE therapy. *Nat Biotechnol* 2000; **18**: 157–62

34 MacGlashan DW, Bochner BS, Adelman DC *et al*. Down-regulation of FcεRI expression on human basophils during *in vivo* treatment of atopic patients with anti-IgE antibody. *J Immunol* 1997; **158**: 1438–45

35 Shields RL, Whether WR, Zioncheck K *et al*. Inhibition of allergic reactions with antibodies to IgE. *Int Arch Allergy Immunol* 1995; **107**: 308–12

36 Yanagihara Y, Kajiwara K, Ikizawa K, Koshio T, Okumura, Ra C. Recombinant soluble form of the human high-affinity immunoglobulin E (IgE) receptor inhibits IgE production through its specific binding to IgE-bearing B-cells. *J Clin Invest* 1994; **94**: 2162–5

37 MacGlashan D, White-McKenzie J, Chichester K *et al*. Up-regulation of FcεRI on human basophils by IgE antibody is mediated by interaction of IgE with FcεRI. *J Allergy Clin Immunol* 1999; **104**, 492–8

38 Bieber T. FcεRI-expressing antigen-presenting cells: new players in the atopic game. *Immunol Today* 1997; **18**: 311–3

39 Maurer D, Fiebiger E, Reininger B *et al*. Fcε receptor I on dendritic cells delivers IgE-bound multivalent antigens into a cathepsin S-dependent pathway of MHC class II presentation. *J Immunol* 1998; **161**: 2731–9

40 Garman SC, Kinet J-P, Jardetzky TS. Crystal structure of the human high-affinity IgE receptor. *Cell* 1998; **95**: 951–61

41 McDonnell JM, Beavil AJ, Mackay GA *et al*. Structure based design and characterization of peptides that inhibit IgE binding to its high-affinity receptor. *Nat Struct Biol* 1996; **3**: 419–26

42 Rigby LJ, Trist H, Snider J *et al*. Monoclonal antibodies and synthetic peptides define the active site of FcεRI and a potential receptor antagonist. *Allergy* 2000; **55**: 609–19

43 Haak-Frendscho M, Ridgway J, Shields R, Robbins K, Gorman C, Jardieu P. Human IgE receptor α-chain IgG chimera blocks passive cutaneous anaphylaxis reaction *in vivo*. *J Immunol* 1993; **151**: 351–8

44 Cook JPD, Henry AJ, McDonnell JM, Owens RJ, Sutton BJ, Gould HJ. Identification of contact residues in the IgE binding site of human FcεRIα. *Biochemistry* 1997; **36**: 15579–88

45 Hulett MD, Brinkworth RI, McKenzie IFC, Hogarth PM. Fine structure analysis of interaction of FcεRI with IgE. *J Biol Chem* 1999; **274**: 13345–52

46 Kelly AE, Chen B-H, Woodward EC, Conrad DH. Production of a chimeric form of CD23 that is oligomeric and blocks IgE binding to the FcεRI. *J Immunol* 1998; **161**: 6696–704

47 Presta L, Shields R, O'Connell L *et al*. The binding site on human immunoglobulin E for its high affinity receptor. *J Biol Chem* 1994; **269**: 26368–73

48 Helm BA, Sayers I, Higginbottom A *et al*. Identification of the high affinity receptor binding region in human immunoglobulin E. *J Biol Chem* 1996; **271**: 7494–500

49 Wurzburg BA, Garman SC, Jardetzky TS. Structure of the human IgE-Fc Cε3-Cε4 reveals conformational flexibility in the antibody effector domains. *Immunity* 2000; **13**: 375–85

50 DeLano WL, Ultsch MH, de Vos AM, Wells JA. Convergent solutions to binding at a protein–protein interface. *Science* 2000; **287**: 1279–83

51 Wiegand TW, Williams PB, Dreskin SC, Jouvin M-H, Kinet J-P, Tasset D. High-affinity oligonucleotide ligands to human IgE inhibit binding to Fcε receptor I. *J Immunol* 1996; **157**: 221–30

52 Cheng Y-SE, Liu Y, Chu J *et al*. Inhibition of the binding of human IgE to its receptor by tetracyclic compounds for the alleviation of IgE-mediated immune response. United States Patent 1999; No. 5,965,605

53 Keown MB, Henry AJ, Ghirlando R, Sutton BJ, Gould HJ. Thermodynamics of the interaction of human immunoglobulin E with its high-affinity receptor FcεRI. *Biochemistry* 1998; **37**: 8863–9

Specific immunotherapy

Mark Larché

Allergy & Clinical Immunology, Imperial College School of Medicine, National Heart and Lung Institute, London, UK

The prevalence of atopic allergic disease increased substantially towards the end of the 20th century and is set to rise further. This group of diseases now constitutes the most common cause of chronic ill health in industrialised countries. Despite considerable attention from the pharmaceutical industry, little progress has been made in the development of disease-modifying therapies. In contrast, recent activity has focused almost exclusively on treatment of symptoms (palliation) rather than cause. The failure of palliative approaches to address the issue of increasing incidence of disease is in evidence in the case of allergic diseases and is a continuing focus of concern. At present, the most frequently employed non-palliative form of disease-modifying therapy is specific allergen immunotherapy (SIT) in which increasing doses of whole allergen extract are administered in increasing dose in order to desensitise the allergic subject.

Specific allergen immunotherapy

Desensitising immunotherapy was initially described by Noon and Freeman working at St Mary's Hospital in London at the beginning of the last century[1,2]. The technique involved administering increasing doses of crudely prepared, whole allergen extract to sensitised subjects until symptoms were ameliorated. The first controlled trial of specific allergen immunotherapy was performed by Frankland (also at St Mary's Hospital) in 1954[3]. Since that time, SIT has been widely evaluated and modified and has been shown to be efficacious in venom hypersensitivity, seasonal or perennial allergic rhinitis and mild allergic asthma. The role of allergen immunotherapy in the treatment of allergic disease, together with guidelines for its use were recently summarised in a WHO Position Paper[4]. Double-blind studies have shown that SIT with allergen extracts for grass pollen- and cat-induced rhinitis/asthma can be highly efficacious[3-5]. However, questions continue to be raised about safety, particularly in relation to immediate IgE-mediated anaphylactic reactions.

Although widely practised in mainland Europe and in the US, SIT is only given in the UK on a routine basis in patients with seasonal allergic rhinitis due to grass pollen (hayfever) who have failed to respond adequately to anti-allergic drugs and in patients with anaphylaxis due to

Correspondence to:
Dr Mark Larché, Allergy & Clinical Immunology, Imperial College School of Medicine, National Heart and Lung Institute, Dovehouse Street, London SW3 6LY, UK

wasp or bee venom hypersensitivity. Only high quality standardized allergen extracts licensed under the provision of the UK Medicines Act and associated European Directives are recommended[6].

The immune response to allergen

Allergen challenge in the clinical laboratory, in both the skin and the lung, has provided a useful model for investigating allergic inflammation. We have employed allergen inhalation challenge in asthmatic subjects in order to study the cellular mechanisms underlying allergic asthma. Allergen inhalation challenge of atopic asthmatics results in an early asthmatic reaction (EAR) followed by a late asthmatic reaction (LAR). The EAR is rapid, peaking at 15 min, and is dependent on the IgE-mediated release of mast cell-derived mediators such as histamine and leukotrienes[7–9]. In contrast, the LAR reaches a maximum at 6–9 h and is believed to represent, at least in part, the cellular inflammatory component of the asthmatic response. In this sense it has served as a useful model of chronic asthma. The LAR is characterised by infiltration of the airway with activated eosinophils and CD4 T-cells, with increased numbers of T-cells

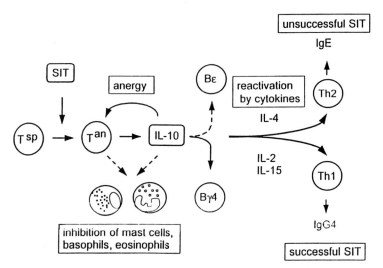

Fig. 1 Immunological mechanisms of specific immunotherapy. Continuous treatment with high doses of allergen establishes a state of allergen-specific anergy in peripheral T-cells (Tan), which is characterised by suppressed proliferative and cytokine responses, together with an increase in IL-10 production. IL-10 suppresses specific T-cells (Tsp) in an autocrine fashion. It also suppresses IgE production and enhances IgG$_4$. Subsequent activation, priming and survival of allergic inflammatory effector cells are down-regulated. The anergic T cell can be re-activated by cytokines from the tissue micro-environment. In successful SIT, anergic T-cells recover by the influence of micro-environmental IL-2 and/or IL-15 to produce Th0/Th1 cytokines. In an atopic individual, IL-4 may reconstitute a Th2 cytokine pattern and re-activate an allergic response. Figure courtesy of Dr K. Blaser, Davos, Switzerland.

expressing mRNA for the Th2-type (IL-4 and IL-5) and eosinophil-active cytokines (IL-3, IL-5 and GM-CSF)[10,11]. The ability of diverse agents such as antihistamines, anti-IgE monoclonal antibodies, leukotriene receptor antagonists and cyclosporin A to partially inhibit the decreased airway function which characterises the LAR, suggests that a number of mechanisms may contribute to late phase allergic inflammation.

The effects of SIT

Evidence suggests that SIT may exert effects on several aspects of the immune system including modulation of the allergen-specific antibody response and modification of T-cell function. SIT may induce a form of 'immune deviation' from a Th2 to a Th1 phenotype by down-regulation of IL-4 and/or up-regulation of IFN-γ. Alternatively, induction of tolerance, anergy, activation-induced cell death or hyporesponsiveness, and/or the production of cells with active suppressor function may have a role in the efficacy attributed to this form of therapy.

Modulation of the IgE-dependent early-phase response to allergen

Atopic allergic disorders are diagnosed on the basis of elevated allergen-specific IgE and an accompanying history of relevant symptomatology. Interleukin (IL)-4 and IL-13 are required for isotype switch to Cϵ and Cγ4 in addition to contact dependent signalling through CD40 and CD40 ligand[12]. Furthermore, at later stages, antigen-specific IgE antibody production by memory B cells also depends on IL-4 and IL-13.

Successful immunotherapy is accompanied by a variety of changes in the quality of the allergen-specific immune response (Fig. 1). One of the most notable is the increase in the specific IgG_4 to IgE ratio. It has been proposed that specific IgG_4 may compete with IgE for allergen, thus preventing interaction of the latter with mast cells and basophils. Recent studies have demonstrated that the majority of IgG_4 in multiply sensitised allergic individuals is bi-specific as a result of recombination of individual IgG_4 chains[13]. The mono-specific molecules generated may be important in the mode of action of IgG_4 in successful immunotherapy. Although there is an initial elevation in serum IgE concentrations during conventional immunotherapy with a gradual decrease to normal over a period of months, target organ sensitivity may decrease in the face of these elevations in serum IgE as a result of the more rapid increase in IgG_4. Thus, although serum levels of both isotypes increase during the early phase of treatment the ratio of specific IgE to IgG_4 decreased by 10–100-

fold[14]. The presence of high levels of bee venom phospholipase A_2-specific IgG_4 in hyperimmune, non-allergic bee keeper has been linked to high levels of expression of IL-10[15].

IL-10 has been shown to play a key role in the regulation of allergen-specific IgG_4 and IgE. IL-10 was shown to decrease epsilon transcripts induced by IL-4, in B cell cultures *in vitro* when added during the first 3 days of culture. Paradoxically, when added later, IL-10 enhanced IgE production. Interestingly, independently of the time of addition to cultures, IL-10 enhanced IgG_4 production probably by increasing IL-4-dependent class switching to gamma 4[16]. In bee venom hypersensitivity, IL-10 was a potent suppressor of both total and phospholipase A (PLA)-specific IgE, while simultaneously increasing IgG_4 formation[14]. The issue of whether or not intact B-cell epitopes are required for the induction of allergen-specific IgG_4 has been raised with regard to peptide immunotherapy. Data from Muller and colleagues suggest that peptides alone, perhaps through the induction of IL-10, are capable of inducing IgG_4[17]. Increases in serum allergen-specific IgG concentrations after immunotherapy may be related to increases in IL-10 and IL-12 both of which are increased after SIT. Thus, suggested mechanisms by which IgG may down-regulate the allergic response include: (i) competition with IgE for allergen binding (classical blocking antibody theory); (ii) prevention of aggregation of FcεRI-bound IgE through steric hindrance; and (iii) interference with antigen trapping and focusing by IgE bound to antigen-presenting cells[18].

Successful immunotherapy reduces both the early and late-phase response to allergen. The decrease in the magnitude of the immediate response is likely to be due, at least partially, to a reduction in the numbers of tissue mast cells[19] and the previously described alteration in the ratio of IgG_4 to IgE. Additionally, SIT characteristically inhibits, often dramatically, the late-phase reaction (LPR) and this in turn is associated with decreases in the numbers of mast cells, basophils and eosinophils both in blood and target organs[19-22].

Modulation of T-cell responses following SIT

T lymphocytes are present in increased numbers at the site of allergic inflammation and their numbers increase further following allergen challenge. *In vitro* experiments have shown that immunotherapy inhibited IL-4-dependent proliferation and production of IFN-γ by peripheral blood T-cells but that addition of IL-2 or IL-15 to cultures restored proliferation and IFN-γ production but not IL-4 production[23]. These data suggest that T cell anergy was induced in this model.

Data from a number of studies suggest that immunotherapy is associated with profound modulation of T cell function with either immune deviation from a Th1 to Th2 phenotype, induction of anergy or both. There is some evidence, mostly from experimental animals, that CD8[+] T-cells with suppressor activity may also be induced by SIT[24]. SIT results in a decrease in antigen-induced recruitment to tissues of CD4[+] T-cells and eosinophils with concomitant increases in cells expressing HLA-DR and CD25[21]. This may be the result of augmentation of HLA-DR and CD25 by IFN-γ derived from Th1 cells. Thus immunotherapy is associated with a decrease in recruitment of CD4 cells, possible enhancement of CD8[+] cell function, down-regulation of IL-4 and IL-5, and increases in IL-10 and IL-12.

In addition to its role in the regulation of IgG_4 and IgE synthesis, IL-10 has been demonstrated to exert a variety of effects on T-cells and effector leukocytes in the late-phase allergic response. IL-10 inhibits T cell proliferation and cytokine responses of both Th1 and Th2 cells and also blocks co-stimulatory pathways in T-cells. *In vitro*, IL-10 induces a long-term antigen-specific anergic state in human CD4[+] T-cells, and can give rise to a regulatory, IL-10 producing population termed Tr1 cells[25]. IL-10 may play a critical role in decreasing mast cell numbers and reactivity as well as down-regulating eosinophil function[15,26]. Furthermore, IL-10 inhibits GM-CSF production and CD40 expression by activated eosinophils[26].

Novel forms of immunotherapy

Antigen dose has been demonstrated to be an important factor in the commitment of T-cells to produce cytokines of a Th1 or Th2 phenotype in murine models[28,29], and also in the induction of T-cell non-responsiveness. Thus increasing antigen concentrations favour a Th1 phenotype whereas IL-4 was decreased at high antigen doses. This indicates that in certain situations, Th1/Th2 cells do not represent stable phenotypes but may be modulated by the dose of antigen. Therefore, in specific immunotherapy the concentration of antigen may be critical in determining IgE or IgG formation resulting in either hypersensitivity or immunity.

An important feature of the efficacy associated with SIT is the delivery of relatively high doses of allergen (compared to natural exposure), which may exert its effect through the mechanism described above such as the induction of a Th1 cytokine phenotype. Indeed the common monthly maintenance dose for aero-allergen immunotherapy is 5–20 μg, a figure several orders of magnitude higher than those encountered during natural exposure.

Delivery of high doses of allergen carries with it the risk of IgE-mediated events including systemic anaphylaxis, resulting from wide-spread mast cell degranulation, which may be life-threatening. A variety of approaches have been initiated by which the ability of material used for immunotherapy to interact with IgE has been reduced. A further feature of these approaches is that attempts are also made to retain regions of the molecule, particularly linear epitopes, which interact with T cell receptors. Some of these strategies, such as the generation of allergoids, have been clinically evaluated and shown to be efficacious. Others, such as recombinant allergens, naturally occurring allergen isoforms and allergen-derived peptides are currently at an earlier stage of development and require further analysis in controlled trials.

Allergoids

Modification of antibody-binding epitopes on the outer surface of native allergen molecules to generate 'allergoids' has most frequently been achieved with formaldehyde which modifies lysine residues and results in crosslinking of amino acid side chains, destroying three dimensional epitopes in the process[30]. Clinical evaluation of a variety of allergoid preparations has been performed, including ragweed[31,32], grass pollen[33–37], Parietaria[38] and mite allergens[39,40]. Routes of administration and treatment regimens have varied in line with unmodified allergen immunotherapy and have included RUSH protocols[33–36] and sublingual/oral administration[40].

Naturally occurring allergen isoforms

Isolation, by purification or recombinant expression, of allergens derived from plants and trees has identified naturally occurring isoforms of allergens which have a reduced capacity to bind IgE[41]. The relative lack of interaction with IgE generally results from amino acid substitutions or deletions within the IgE binding site or at sites which induce conformational changes in the molecule, preventing or substantially reducing IgE binding. These observations have led to suggestions that immunotherapy performed with hypoallergenic isoforms may allow higher doses to be used for immunotherapy, thereby providing a more effective method of modulating the T cell response to allergens. Induction of IgE responses in previously naïve individuals has, however, been observed during SIT[42,43], which may limit the effectiveness of allergen isoforms in immunotherapy.

Recombinant allergens

A number of groups have employed recombinant DNA technology to clone, sequence and express allergen proteins in the laboratory. Detailed analysis of IgE-binding epitopes has resulted in mapping of IgE binding site for a number of the major allergens. More recently, these findings together with the prior observations concerning the relative lack of immunogenicity associated with some allergen isoforms, have been exploited by the use of *in vitro* mutagenesis to create allergen proteins in which single amino acids have been modified, or deletions introduced, to produce molecules with substantially reduced IgE binding capacity[44-48].

Allergen engineering and the identification of low-IgE-binding allergen isoforms offer the prospect of purified, standardised allergen reagents for the diagnosis and therapy of allergic diseases. However, the large numbers of isoforms occurring naturally, particularly for plant and tree allergens may make such approaches unfeasible.

DNA vaccines

In contrast to strategies employing whole proteins or peptides to modify the immune response to allergens, recent interest has focused on direct immunisation with DNA encoding allergen proteins. A number of variations on the theme of DNA vaccination have been investigated. Unmethylated CpG motifs (ACGT) have been used to induce Th1 immune responses either alone or in combination with allergen proteins. Additionally, plasmid vectors encoding whole protein allergen genes have been injected directly into animals either before or after allergen challenge[49].

Palindromic nucleotide sequences containing the motif ACGT are found in microbial DNA and have previously been shown to induce the production of interferons in human peripheral blood mononuclear cells[50], activate B cells[51] and stimulate the production of Th1-enhancing cytokines such as IL-12, IFN-γ and TNF-α in mice[52,53].

Recently, oligonucleotides containing CpG motifs have been evaluated in murine models of asthma. Inhibition of IL-5 resulted in failure to release eosinophils from the bone marrow and was characterised by an inhibition of airways eosinophilia which was accompanied by modulation of airways inflammation and hyper-responsiveness[54,55]. Mice were sensitised with recombinant Der p 5 following immunisation with plasmid DNA encoding the allergen under the control of a CMV promoter (or empty vector control). Allergen-specific IgE levels were found to be 90% lower in mice immunised with the Der p 5 construct. In addition, Der p 5 specific CD8 T-cells were shown to produce high levels of IFN-γ and could adoptively transfer suppression of IgE responses[56]. In a rat model of asthma, immunisation with plasmid constructs encoding a house dust mite allergen prevented IgE synthesis, histamine release in the lung and airways hyper-responsiveness induced

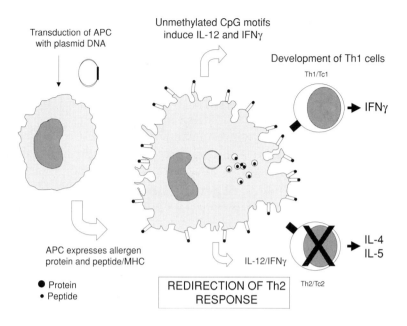

Fig. 2 Mechanisms of immune deviation by plasmid DNA vaccination. Following intradermal or subcutaneous administration of plasmid DNA containing unmethylated CpG motifs (immunostimulatory sequences; ISS) and encoding an antigen or antigen peptide (or in certain cases, cytokine), antigen presenting cells (APC) are transduced. APC become activated and produce IL-12, IL-18, IFN-α and IFN-γ in response to ISS sequences. Proteins (peptides or cytokines) encoded by the plasmid insert are transcribed and translated. Peptide fragments bind to MHC molecules and are presented to specific T-cells at the APC surface. Cytokines induced by ISS encourage Th1/Tc1 development and antagonise Th2/Tc2 development and effector function.

by allergen challenge[57]. In addition to immunisation with plasmid vectors encoding allergen proteins, inhibition of mucosal Th2-type immune responses has also been achieved following cytokine gene transfer. Li and colleagues expressed IFN-γ in the airway epithelium of mice following gene transfer and observed inhibition of both allergen and T cell-induced airways eosinophilia[58].

Thus, strategies to abrogate Th2-type cytokine production via immunisation with DNA motifs or plasmids encoding allergen and cytokine genes, hold promise for therapy of allergic disease including asthma (Fig. 2). However, the majority of data collected in this area to date has come from murine models of disease. A cautionary note has recently been sounded by Li and colleagues who demonstrate distinct, strain-dependent antibody isotype responses to plasmid encoded Ara h 2[59]. On the basis of their findings, the authors highlight the importance of selecting appropriate animal strains for investigation of DNA vaccines ultimately intended for human use.

Peptide immunotherapy

Anergy/tolerance

CD4[+] T cell activation is dependent upon presentation of peptide fragments of processed antigen by MHC class II on antigen presenting cells, to specific T cell receptors (TcR)[60]. Productive T cell responses also require co-stimulation through such pathways as CD28–CD80/CD86[61,62]. Much attention has focused on functional inactivation of such T cell responses leading to 'tolerance'. Presentation of antigen to high affinity TcR during thymic maturation leads to cell death by thymic deletion or central tolerance. Peripheral T cell tolerance may result from deletion following activation-induced cell death (AICD) or, equally, failure to receive TcR-mediated stimulation, inhibition of migration and active suppression. The absence of co-stimulation leads to T cell unresponsiveness ('anergy') to re-challenge[63,64]. In murine models injection of peptides produces T cell anergy or non-responsiveness through as yet unexplained mechanisms[65]. For example, production of IgG and IL-2 by lymphocytes from Fel d 1 primed mice was decreased after multiple injections of a peptide fragment of the priming allergen[65], and intranasal administration of peptides from Der p 1, could prevent sensitisation and could also inhibit lymphocyte responses in previously sensitised mice[66]. There is good evidence for peptide-induced non-responsiveness of human CD4 cells *in vitro*[67,68].

Clinical trials

Despite reservations regarding the use of peptides to treat allergic diseases in outbred human populations, peptide-based immunotherapy has recently been evaluated in subjects with allergic disease induced by either cat or ragweed allergens. Two relatively large peptides from the major cat allergen Fel d 1, termed IPC-1 and IPC-2, were evaluated by Norman and colleagues[69]. Following four injections of peptide in three dose groups, clinical efficacy was observed only at the highest dose of peptide (4 x 750 µg). Both nasal and lung symptom scores improved in response to peptide therapy, although treatment was associated with a significant incidence of adverse events which occurred a few minutes to several hours after peptide injection. Further studies from the same group[70] demonstrated reduced IL-4 production in IPC-1/IPC-2-specific T cell lines following therapy. A similar reduction in IL-4 production was reported by Pène and colleagues[71]. Peripheral blood mononuclear cells were stimulated with cat dander extract before and after treatment with IPC-1/IPC-2. A significant reduction (compared to background levels) of IL-4 production was observed in the high dose group (1500–4500 µg) but not in the lower dose groups. A reduction in allergen PD_{20} was also observed in response to both high and medium (150–450 µg) dose regimens when compared to baseline, but not when compared to placebo. Simons *et al* also observed late onset symptoms of rhinitis, asthma and pruritis following treatment of cat allergic subjects with 4-weekly doses of 250 µg of IPC-1/IPC-2[72]. In this placebo-controlled study of 42 individuals, the authors found no change in cytokine secretion patterns of PBMC before and after therapy. Furthermore, no changes in early and late-phase skin responses to whole allergen were observed at several time points after treatment. In a multicentre study of 133 patients, Maguire and colleagues reported an improvement in pulmonary function in subjects receiving 8 injections of 750 µg IPC-1/IPC-2, who had diminished baseline FEV1 but only at a single time point (3 weeks) post-therapy[73]. A large number of adverse events were reported in this study including some that required the use of adrenaline. In keeping with other studies evaluating IPC-1/IPC-2, late onset adverse reactions diminished with successive doses of peptide suggesting the induction of hyporesponsiveness. Thus, a relatively modest improvement in symptom scores combined with frequent adverse reactions resulted in cat and ragweed vaccines being withdrawn from clinical trials.

More recently, Muller and colleagues have identified three T-cell peptide epitopes in the bee venom phospholipase A_2 (PLA_2) molecule and have used these peptides to desensitize five allergic subjects[74]. Peptides were well tolerated and despite the differing MHC backgrounds of the subjects, T cell responses to all three peptides were observed suggesting that the problems of using peptide immunotherapy in an outbred population such as man, may not present as much of a problem as has been envisaged in the past.

T-cell tolerance is preceded by T-cell activation

In addition to rapid onset reactions, Norman[69] also observed asthma-like symptoms commencing several hours after administration of IPC1/IPC2. We hypothesised that these reactions were the result of direct, MHC-restricted activation of allergen-specific T-cells.

To determine whether T cell peptides, which do not crosslink IgE, can induce an isolated LAR, we designed three Fel d 1 chain 1-derived peptides (FC1P) of 16/17 residues and administered them, by intradermal injection, into cat allergic asthmatic subjects. Furthermore, by repeated administration of peptides, we tested the hypothesis that specific hyporesponsiveness could be induced.

We established that the peptides, by virtue of their small size, did not release histamine from basophil-enriched mononuclear cells[75].

Following intradermal injection of 80 µg of FC1P, 9 out of 40 subjects cat-allergic asthmatic subjects experienced a fall in FEV_1 which started at 3–4 h and reached a plateau by 6 h[75]. In none of the 40 subjects were immediate lung reactions observed. We hypothesised that these responses represented isolated Th2 cell-dependent LARs. Recognition of antigenic peptides by T-cells requires that the peptide be presented to the T-cell in the context of an appropriate MHC molecule, or 'restriction element'. Since not all individuals developed a response, the HLA DRB1 haplotype of all subjects was determined[75]. Using allergen-specific T-cell lines derived from the study subjects prior to peptide injection and L cells transfected with appropriate HLA-DR alleles, it was determined that peptide FC1P3 could be presented to T-cells by both HLA-DRB1*0101 and two microvariants of DR13 (HLA-DRB1*1301 and HLA-DRB1*1302)[75] leading to proliferation and secretion of IL-5. Additionally, another of the three peptides (FC1P2), could be presented by HLA-DRB1*0405 to T cell derived from an autologous (HLA-DRB1*0405) subject and interestingly, to an individual expressing HLA-DRB1*0408.

MHC-based allergen peptide vaccine

The recognition of the two peptides in the context of more than one MHC molecule suggests that these peptides are capable of promiscuous binding. This observation may be of some significance, since one argument against the use of peptides for disease-modulating immunotherapy in humans, is that since the human population differ widely in their MHC haplotypes, a very large (and therefore impractical) number of peptides will have to be employed in any therapeutic preparation. In fact, what our findings suggest is that individual peptides are capable not only of binding promiscuously to more than one MHC molecule, but that there is also a degree of plasticity at the level of the T-cell receptor, since a T-cell receptor from a HLA-DRB1*0408 individual can recognise FC1P2 when it is presented in the context of HLA-DRB1*0405. Based on these early observations, therefore, it appears that a relatively small number of carefully selected peptides from an allergen may be efficacious in the treatment of allergic disease. This concept has recently been supported by data from Texier and colleagues[76].

Thus, it was possible to account for FC1P-mediated induction of LAR by virtue of the nine individuals expressing a DR1, DR4 or DR13 allele. These findings strongly support the hypothesis that direct, MHC-restricted activation of Th2 lymphocytes by allergen-derived peptides leads to the development of the LAR suggesting that both the Th2

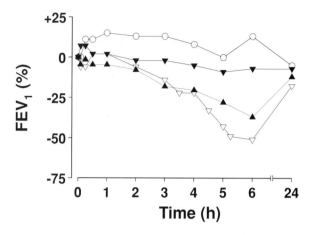

Fig. 3 Repeat challenge with a second injection of FC1P demonstrates transient attenuation of the LAR. The first dose (80 μg) induced a LAR (open down triangle) which was attenuated on the second dose (80 μg; closed down triangle). Re-challenge with the same dose after 12 months (closed up triangles) resulted in a LAR of similar magnitude to the initial challenge. Open circles indicate a control day in which FEV₁ was monitored after injection of 30 BU of whole cat dander extract which would not be expected to cause a LAR.

component of asthma and strategies to down regulate this response are founded firmly in MHC restricted Th2 cell recognition of allergen epitopes.

During the course of these investigations, three subjects displaying an isolated LAR were given a further dose of peptide and this was followed by a markedly reduced or absent response[75], suggesting that T cell hyporesponsiveness had been induced by the initial injection, strongly supporting the hypothesis. Interestingly, following a further peptide injection more than one year after the first, LAR of similar magnitude to the initial response were observed (Fig. 3)[75]. These findings suggested that hyporesponsiveness lasted for more than several weeks but less than one year. Collectively, these observations were further investigated with a larger mixture of overlapping peptides from the same allergen.

Data obtained with FC1P indicated that in order to elicit peptide LAR and subsequent non-responsiveness in the majority of cat-allergic asthmatics, administration of synthetic peptides covering the entire sequence of the Fel d 1 molecule would be required, since recognition of individual regions of the molecule was restricted by MHC haplotype. Thus 16 overlapping peptides were designed spanning both chains of the Fel d I molecule. Four of the 16 proved to be poorly soluble in aqueous solution and were, therefore, excluded from the mixture of peptides, termed MOP (multiple overlapping peptides) which were subsequently administered to cat allergic asthmatic subjects.

Initially, dose-response experiments were undertaken to establish the relationship between peptide dose and both the magnitude and frequency of isolated LAR. Isolated LAR in cat-asthmatic volunteers could be induced at doses as low as 1 µg of each of the 12 peptides as a mixture. Furthermore, at 1 µg of peptide, 1 out of 8 individuals experienced an isolated LAR. At a dose of 2.5 µg, 2 out of 8 individuals developed reactions which were of greater magnitude than at 1 µg. Finally, at a dose of 5 µg, 50% of individuals (4/8) developed LAR which were generally of greater magnitude than the reactions observed with lower doses. In common with the earlier FC1P peptide preparation, MOP induced isolated LAR on initial administration to cat allergic asthmatic individuals which was followed by a markedly reduced or absent response upon re-challenge with the same dose. By varying the time interval between the first and second administrations of MOP, it was established that hyporesponsiveness to peptide re-challenge lasts for several months after the initial, single injection and that full reactivity did not return until more than 1 year. We hypothesise that by using an incremental dosing regime involving a number of injections, it may be possible to effect hyporesponsiveness for a period of 1 year or more.

The cellular mechanisms which underlie the peptide-induced, MHC-restricted reactions and subsequent hyporesponsiveness described in this review remain to be elucidated. Recently, much attention has focused on T-cells that may regulate the immune response. A number of such regulatory T-cell populations has been described in animal studies[25,77–79]. The mechanisms by which these cells modulate Th1 or Th2 responses require further clarification, but cytokines such as IL-10 and TGF-β are likely to be important factors in this 'regulation'. Linked suppression is a phenomenon, demonstrated in animal models, in which administration of a single epitope from a protein modifies responses of non-tolerant T-cells specific for other epitopes within the same protein and in some models epitopes derived from other proteins ('bystander suppression')[80]. The mechanism(s) of linked suppression vary from model to model[81,82]. Induction of non-responsiveness to whole proteins following administration of a single peptide epitope has been demonstrated in a number of models[65,83–87]. Hoyne and colleagues have demonstrated linked suppression in T-cell responses to epitopes within the same allergen protein after inhalation challenge of a single immunodominant epitope[88]. The phenomenon of linked suppression has not been demonstrated *in vivo* in a human model. However, since both the FC1P and MOP preparations do not span the entire Fel d I molecule, it will be possible within this model to investigate whether T cell responses (*in vitro*) to peptides not injected into patients, are down-regulated at the same time as those to injected peptides. If this can be demonstrated, it will be the first demonstration of linked suppression in a human *in vivo* situation.

Conclusions

Specific immunotherapy has been successfully performed on sensitised individuals for 90 years. Whilst efficacious, this form of therapy is associated with the risk of adverse, IgE-mediated events including systemic anaphylaxis. The mechanisms underlying successful SIT include modulation of the specific immune response to allergen which are manifest by a relative decrease in Th2-type responses and a concomitant increase in Th1-type parameters. Additionally, increases in the allergen-specific IgG_4 to IgE ratio have been consistently observed which may be dependent upon cytokines such as IL-10 from T-cells, B-cells and monocytes.

Attempts to reduce the interaction between allergen preparations and IgE have lead to the development of effective therapies such as allergoids and also, more recently, to experimental strategies including naturally occurring hypoallergenic allergen isoforms, engineered allergens with reduced IgE binding capacity and the use of T cell peptide epitopes. Experience from our own laboratory with peptides derived from the major cat allergen Fel d 1, suggest that peptides can be used to induce profound and long-lasting hyporesponsiveness *in vivo*, in the absence of adverse events, thus providing an exciting opportunity to effectively modify existing disease and to go some way towards redressing the continuing increase in the prevalence of allergic diseases.

Acknowledgements

I would like to thank my colleagues Professor AB Kay, Drs BM Haselden, W Oldfield, DS Robinson, S Ying and Ms K Shirley for their important contributions to this work together with the following collaborators: Dr Meinir Jones, Professor Robert Lechler, Dr Giovanna Lombardi, Professor Jonathan Lamb, Dr Carolyn Katovich-Hurley, Dr John Richert, Dr Amanda Bennett and Professor Martin Church.

References

1   Noon L. Prophylactic inoculation against hay fever. *Lancet* 1911; i: 1572
2   Freeman J. Vaccination against hay fever: report of results during the first three years. *Lancet* 1914; i: 1178
3   Frankland AW, Augustin R. Prophylaxis of summer hayfever and asthma. A controlled trial comparing crude grass pollen extracts with the isolated main protein component. *Lancet* 1954; i: 1055–7
4   World Health Organization. Allergen immunotherapy: therapeutic vaccines for allergic diseases. *Allergy* 1998; **53** (Suppl): 1–42
5   Durham SR, Till SJ. Immunologic changes associated with allergen immunotherapy. *J Allergy Clin Immunol* 1998; **102**: 157–64

6   Anon. Position paper on allergen immunotherapy. Report of a BSACI working party. *Clin Exp Allergy* 1993; **3 (Suppl)**: 1–44

7   Metzger WJ, Zavala D, Richerson HB *et al*. Local allergen challenge and bronchoalveolar lavage of allergic asthmatic lungs. Description of the model and local airway inflammation. *Am Rev Respir Dis* 1987; **135**: 433–40

8   Sedgwick JB, Calhoun WJ, Gleich GJ *et al*. Immediate and late airway response of allergic rhinitis patients to segmental antigen challenge. Characterization of eosinophil and mast cell mediators. *Am Rev Respir Dis* 1991; **144**: 1274–81

9   Liu MC, Hubbard WC, Proud D *et al*. Immediate and late inflammatory responses to ragweed antigen challenge of the peripheral airways in allergic asthmatics. Cellular, mediator, and permeability changes. *Am Rev Respir Dis* 1991; **144**: 51–8

10 Bentley AM, Meng Q, Robinson DS, Hamid Q, Kay AB, Durham SR. Increases in activated T lymphocytes, eosinophils, and cytokine mRNA expression for interleukin-5 and granulocyte/macrophage colony-stimulating factor in bronchial biopsies after allergen inhalation challenge in atopic asthmatics. *Am J Respir Cell Mol Biol* 1993; **8**: 35–42

11 Ying S, Humbert M, Barkans J *et al*. Expression of IL-4 and IL-5 mRNA and protein product by CD4+ and CD8+ T-cells, eosinophils, and mast cells in bronchial biopsies obtained from atopic and non atopic (intrinsic) asthmatics. *J Immunol* 1997; **158**: 3539–44

12 Vercelli D. Molecular regulation of the IgE immune response. *Clin Exp Allergy* 1995; **25 (Suppl 2)**: 43–5

13 Schuurman J, Van Ree R, Perdok GJ, Van Doorn HR, Tan KY, Aalberse RC. Normal human immunoglobulin G4 is bispecific: it has two different antigen-combining sites. *Immunology* 1999; **97**: 693–8

14 Akdis CA, Blesken T, Akdis M *et al*. Induction and differential regulation of bee venom phospholipase A$_2$-specific human IgE and IgG4 antibodies *in vitro* requires allergen-specific and non-specific activation of T and B cells. *J Allergy Clin Immunol* 1997; **99**: 345–53

15 Akdis CA, Blesken T, Akdis M, Wüthrich B, Blaser K. Role of interleukin 10 in specific immunotherapy. *J Clin Invest* 1998; **102**: 98–106

16 Jeannin P, Lecoanet S, Delneste Y, Gauchat JF, Bonnefoy JY. IgE versus IgG4 production can be differentially regulated by IL-10. *J Immunol* 1998; **160**: 3555–61

17 Muller U, Akdis CA, Fricker M *et al*. Successful immunotherapy with T-cell epitope peptides of bee venom phospholipase A$_2$ induces specific T-cell anergy in patients allergic to bee venom. *J Allergy Clin Immunol* 1998; **101**: 747–54

18 Stingl G, Maurer D. IgE-mediated allergen presentation via Fc epsilon RI on antigen-presenting cells. *Int Arch Allergy Immunol* 1997; **113**: 24–9

19 Durham SR, Varney VA, Gaga M *et al*. Grass pollen immunotherapy decreases the number of mast cells in the skin. *Clin Exp Allergy* 1999; **29**: 1490–6

20 Nish WA, Charlesworth EN, Davis TL *et al*. The effect of immunotherapy on the cutaneous late phase response to antigen. *J Allergy Clin Immunol* 1994; **93**: 484–93

21 Varney VA, Hamid QA, Gaga M *et al*. Influence of grass pollen immunotherapy on cellular infiltration and cytokine mRNA expression during allergen-induced late-phase cutaneous responses. *J Clin Invest* 1993; **92**: 644–51

22 Furin MJ, Norman PS, Creticos PS *et al*. Immunotherapy decreases antigen-induced eosinophil cell migration into the nasal cavity. *J Allergy Clin Immunol* 1991; **88**: 27–32

23 Akdis CA, Akdis M, Blesken T *et al*. Epitope-specific T cell tolerance to phospholipase A$_2$ in bee venom immunotherapy and recovery by IL-2 and IL-15 *in vitro*. *J Clin Invest* 1996; **98**: 1676–83

24 Renz H, Lack G, Saloga J *et al*. Inhibition of IgE production and normalization of airways responsiveness by sensitized CD8 T-cells in a mouse model of allergen-induced sensitization. *J Immunol* 1994; **152**: 351–60

25 Groux H, O'Garra A, Bigler M *et al*. A CD4+ T-cell subset inhibits antigen-specific T-cell responses and prevents colitis. *Nature* 1997; **389**: 737–42

26 Akdis CA, Blaser K. IL-10-induced anergy in peripheral T cell and reactivation by microenvironmental cytokines: two key steps in specific immunotherapy. *FASEB J* 1999; **13**: 603–9

27 Borish L. IL-10: evolving concepts. *J Allergy Clin Immunol* 1998; **101**: 293–7

28 Hosken NA, Shibuya K, Heath AW, Murphy KM, O'Garra A. The effect of antigen dose on CD4⁺ T helper cell phenotype development in a T cell receptor-alpha beta-transgenic model. *J Exp Med* 1995; **182**: 1579–84

29 Constant SL, Bottomly K. Induction of Th1 and Th2 CD4⁺ T cell responses: the alternative approaches. *Annu Rev Immunol* 1997; **15**: 297–322

30 Marsh DG, Lichtenstein LM, Campbell DH. Studies on 'allergoids' prepared from naturally occurring allergens. I. Assay of allergenicity and antigenicity of formalinized rye group component. *Immunology* 1970; **18**: 705–22

31 Norman PS, Lichtenstein LM, Marsh DG. Studies on allergoids from naturally occurring allergens. IV. Efficacy and safety of long-term allergoid treatment of ragweed hay fever. *J Allergy Clin Immunol* 1981; **68**: 460–70

32 Norman PS, Lichtenstein LM, Kagey-Sobotka A, Marsh DG. Controlled evaluation of allergoid in the immunotherapy of ragweed hay fever. *J Allergy Clin Immunol* 1982; **70**: 248–60

33 Bousquet J, Hejjaoui A, Skassa-Brociek W *et al*. Double-blind, placebo-controlled immunotherapy with mixed grass-pollen allergoids. I. Rush immunotherapy with allergoids and standardized orchard grass-pollen extract. *J Allergy Clin Immunol* 1987; **80**: 591–8

34 Bousquet J, Maasch H, Martinot B, Hejjaoui A, Wahl R, Michel FB. Double-blind, placebo-controlled immunotherapy with mixed grass-pollen allergoids. II. Comparison between parameters assessing the efficacy of immunotherapy. *J Allergy Clin Immunol* 1988; **82**: 439–46

35 Bousquet J, Maasch HJ, Hejjaoui A *et al*. Double-blind, placebo-controlled immunotherapy with mixed grass-pollen allergoids. III. Efficacy and safety of unfractionated and high-molecular-weight preparations in rhinoconjunctivitis and asthma. *J Allergy Clin Immunol* 1989; **84**: 546–56

36 Bousquet J, Hejjaoui A, Soussana M, Michel FB. Double-blind, placebo-controlled immunotherapy with mixed grass-pollen allergoids. IV. Comparison of the safety and efficacy of two dosages of a high-molecular-weight allergoid. *J Allergy Clin Immunol* 1990; **85**: 490–7

37 Pastorello EA, Pravettoni V, Incorvaia C *et al*. Clinical and immunological effects of immunotherapy with alum-absorbed grass allergoid in grass-pollen-induced hay fever. *Allergy* 1992; **47**: 281–90

38 Tari MG, Mancino M, Ghezzi E, Frank E, Cromwell O. Immunotherapy with an alum-adsorbed *Parietaria*-pollen allergoid: a 2-year, double-blind, placebo-controlled study. *Allergy* 1997; **52**: 65–74

39 Pecoud A, Nicod L, Badan M, Agrell B, Dreborg S, Kolly M. Effects of one-year hyposensitization in allergic rhinitis. Comparison of two house dust mite extracts. *Allergy* 1990; **45**: 386–92

40 Passalacqua G, Albano M, Fregonese L *et al*. Randomised controlled trial of local allergoid immunotherapy on allergic inflammation in mite-induced rhinoconjunctivitis. *Lancet* 1998; **351**: 629–32

41 Ferreira F, Hirtenlehner K, Jilek A *et al*. Dissection of immunoglobulin E and T lymphocyte reactivity of isoforms of the major birch pollen allergen Bet v 1: potential use of hypoallergenic isoforms for immunotherapy. *J Exp Med* 1996; **183**: 599–609

42 Breiteneder H, Ferreira F, Hoffmann-Sommergruber K *et al*. Four recombinant isoforms of Cor a I, the major allergen of hazel pollen, show different IgE-binding properties. *Eur J Biochem* 1993; **212**: 355–62

43 Schenk S, Hoffmann-Sommergruber K, Breiteneder H *et al*. Four recombinant isoforms of Cor a 1, the major allergen of hazel pollen, show different reactivities with allergen-specific T-lymphocyte clones. *Eur J Biochem* 1994; **224**: 717–22

44 Ferreira F, Ebner C, Kramer B *et al*. Modulation of IgE reactivity of allergens by site-directed mutagenesis: potential use of hypoallergenic variants for immunotherapy. *FASEB J* 1998; **2**: 231–42

45 Stanley JS, King N, Burks AW *et al*. Identification and mutational analysis of the immunodominant IgE binding epitopes of the major peanut allergen Ara h 2. *Arch Biochem Biophys* 1997; **342**: 244–53

46 Smith AM, Chapman MD. Reduction in IgE binding to allergen variants generated by site-directed mutagenesis: contribution of disulfide bonds to the antigenic structure of the major house dust mite allergen Der p 2. *Mol Immunol* 1996; **33**: 399–405

47 Takai T, Yokota T, Yasue M et al. Engineering of the major house dust mite allergen Der f 2 for allergen-specific immunotherapy. Nat Biotechnol 1997; 15: 754–8

48 Schramm G, Kahlert H, Suck R et al. 'Allergen engineering': variants of the timothy grass pollen allergen Phl p 5b with reduced IgE-binding capacity but conserved T cell reactivity. Immunology 1999; 162: 2406–14

49 Tighe H, Corr M, Roman M, Raz E. Gene vaccination: plasmid DNA is more than just a blueprint. Immunol Today 1998; 19: 89–97

50 Yamamoto T, Yamamoto S, Katakota T, Komura K, Kohase M, Tokungaga T. Synthetic oligonucleotides with certain palindromic sequences stimulate interferon production of human peripheral blood lymphocytes in vitro. Jpn J Cancer Res 1994; 85: 775–9

51 Krieg AM, Yi AK, Matson S et al. CpG motifs in bacterial DNA trigger direct B cell activation. Nature 1995; 374: 546–9

52 Halpern MD, Kurlander RJ, Pisetsky DS. Bacterial DNA induces murine interferon-gamma production by stimulation of interleukin-12 and tumor necrosis factor-alpha. Cell Immunol 1996; 167: 72–8

53 Klinsman DM, Yi AK, Beaucage SL, Conover J, Krieg AM. CpG motifs present in bacterial DNA rapidly induce lymphocytes to secrete interleukin 6, interleukin 12 and interferon-γ. Proc Natl Acad Sci USA 1996; 93: 2879–83

54 Kline JN, Waldschmidt TJ Businga TR et al. Modulation of airway inflammation by CpG oligodeoxynucleotides in a murine model of asthma. J Immunol 1998; 160: 2555–9

55 Broide D, Schwarze J, Tighe H et al. Immunostimulatory DNA sequences inhibit IL-5, eosinophilic inflammation and airway hyperresponsiveness in mice. J Immunol 1998; 161: 7054–62

56 Hsu CH, Chua KY, Tao MH, Huang SK, Hsieh KH. Inhibition of specific IgE response in vivo by allergen-gene transfer. Int Immunol 1996; 8:1405–11

57 Hsu CH, Chua KY, Tao MH et al. Immunoprophylaxis of allergen-induced immunoglobulin E synthesis and airway hyperresponsiveness in vivo by genetic immunization. Nat Med 1996; 2: 540–4

58 Li XM, Chopra RK, Chou TY, Schofield BH, Wills-Karp M, Huang SK. Mucosal IFN-gamma gene transfer inhibits pulmonary allergic responses in mice. J Immunol 1996; 157: 3216–9

59 Li X, Huang CK, Schofield BH et al. Strain-dependent induction of allergic sensitization caused by peanut allergen DNA immunization in mice. J Immunol 1999; 162: 3045–52

60 Jorgensen JL, Reay PA, Ehrich EW, Davis MM. Molecular components of T-cell recognition. Annu Rev Immunol 1992; 10: 835–73

61 Schwartz RH. Co-stimulation of T lymphocytes: the role of CD28, CTLA-4, and B7/BB1 in interleukin-2 production and immunotherapy. Cell 1992; 71: 1065–8

62 Larché M, Till SJ, Haselden B-M et al. Co-stimulation through CD86 is involved in airway presenting cell and T cell responses to allergen in atopic asthmatics. J Immunol 1998; 161: 6375–82

63 Schwartz RH. T cell clonal anergy. Curr Opin Immunol 1997; 9: 351–7

64 Lamb JR, Skidmore BJ, Green N, Chiller JM, Feldmann M. Induction of tolerance in influenza virus-immune T lymphocyte clones with synthetic peptides of influenza hemagglutinin. J Exp Med 1983; 157: 1434–47

65 Briner TJ, Kuo MC, Keating KM, Rogers BL, Greenstein JL. Peripheral T-cell tolerance induced in naive and primed mice by subcutaneous injection of peptides from the major cat allergen Fel d I. Proc Natl Acad Sci USA 1993; 90: 7608–12

66 Hoyne GF, O'Hehir RE, Wraith DC, Thomas WR, Lamb JR. Inhibition of T cell and antibody responses to house dust mite allergen by inhalation of the dominant T cell epitope in naive and sensitized mice. J Exp Med 1993; 178: 1783–8

67 O'Hehir RE, Garman RD, Greenstein JL, Lamb JR. The specificity and regulation of T-cell responsiveness to allergens. Annu Rev Immunol 1991; 9: 67–95

68 Higgins JA, Lamb JR, Marsh SG et al. Peptide-induced non-responsiveness of HLA-DP restricted human T-cells reactive with Dermatophagoides spp. (house dust mite). J Allergy Clin Immunol 1992; 90: 749–56

69 Norman PS, Ohman Jr JL, Long AA et al. Treatment of cat allergy with T-cell reactive peptides. Am J Respir Crit Care Med 1996; 154: 1623–8

70 Marcotte GV, Braun CM, Norman PS et al. Effects of peptide therapy on ex vivo T-cell responses. J Allergy Clin Immunol 1998; 101: 506–13

71 Pene J, Desroches A, Paradis L et al. Immunotherapy with Fel d 1 peptides decreases IL-4 release by peripheral blood T-cells of patients allergic to cats. J Allergy Clin Immunol 1998; 102: 571–8

72 Simons FE, Imada M, Li Y, Watson WT, HayGlass KT. Fel d 1 peptides: effect on skin tests and cytokine synthesis in cat-allergic human subjects. Int Immunol 1996; 8: 1937–45

73 Maguire P, Nicodemus C, Robinson D, Aaronson D, Umetsu DT. The safety and efficacy of ALLERVAX CAT in cat allergic patients. Clin Immunol 1999; 93: 222–31

74 Muller U, Akdis CA, Fricker M et al. Successful immunotherapy with T-cell epitope peptides of bee venom phospholipase A$_2$ induces specific T-cell anergy in patients allergic to bee venom. J Allergy Clin Immunol 1998; 101: 747–54

75 Haselden BM, Kay AB, Larché M. IgE-independent MHC-restricted T cell peptide epitope-induced late asthmatic reactions. J Exp Med 1999; 189: 1885–94

76 Texier C, Pouvelle S, Busson M et al. HLA-DR restricted peptide candidates for bee venom immunotherapy. J Immunol 2000; 164: 3177–84

77 Weiner HL, Inobe J, Kuchroo V, Chen Y. Induction and characterisation of TGFβ secreting Th3 cells. FASEB J 1996; 10: A1444

78 Powrie F, Carlino J, Leach MW, Mauze S, Coffman RL. A critical role for transforming growth factor-β but not IL-4 in the suppression of T helper type 1-mediated colitis by CD45RB(low) CD4$^+$ T-cells. J Exp Med 1996; 183: 2669–74

79 Bridoux F, Badou A, Saoudi A et al. Transforming growth factor beta (TGF-beta)-dependent inhibition of T helper cell 2 (Th2)-induced autoimmunity by self-major histocompatibility complex (MHC) class II-specific, regulatory CD4(+) T cell lines. J Exp Med 1997; 185: 1769–75

80 Davies JD, Leong LYW, Mellor A, Cobbold SP, Waldmann H. T cell suppression in transplantation tolerance through linked suppression. J Immunol 1996; 156: 3602–7

81 Lombardi G, Sidhu S, Batchelor R, Lechler R. Anergic T-cells as suppressor cells in vitro. Science 1994; 264: 1587–1589

82 Chen Y, Kuchroo VK, Inobe J, Hafler DA, Weiner HL. Regulatory T cell clones induced by oral tolerance: suppression of autoimmune encephalomyelitis. Science 1994; 265: 1237–40

83 Gaur A, Wiers B, Liu A, Rothbard J, Fathman GC. Amelioration of experimental autoimmune encephalomyelitis by myelin basic protein synthetic peptide-induced anergy. Science 1992; 258: 1491–4

84 Ku G, Kronenberg M, Peacock DJ et al. Prevention of experimental autoimmune arthritis with a peptide fragment of type II collagen. Eur J Immunol 1993; 23: 591–9

85 Vaysburd M, Lock C, McDevitt H. Prevention of insulin-dependent diabetes mellitus in non-obese diabetic mice by immunogenic but not tolerated peptides. J Exp Med 1995; 182: 897–902

86 Staines NA, Harper N, Ward FJ, Malmstrom V, Holmdahl R, Bansal S. Mucosal tolerance and suppression of collagen-induced arthritis (CIA) induced by nasal inhalation of synthetic peptide 184–198 of bovine type II collagen (CII) expressing a dominant T cell epitope. Clin Exp Immunol 1996; 103: 368–75

87 Clayton JP, Gammon GM, Ando DG, Kono DH, Hood L, Sercarz EE. Peptide-specific prevention of experimental allergic encephalomyelitis. J Exp Med 1989; 169: 1681–91

88 Hoyne GF, Jarnicki AG, Thomas WR, Lamb JR. Characterization of the specificity and duration of T cell tolerance to intranasally administered peptides in mice: a role for intramolecular epitope suppression. Int Immunol 1997; 9: 1165–73

Future treatments of allergic diseases and asthma

R G Stirling and **K F Chung**

National Heart & Lung Institute, Imperial College School of Medicine and Royal Brompton Hospital, London, UK

Recent advances in the understanding of the inflammatory and immunological mechanisms of allergic diseases have illuminated many potential therapeutic strategies that may prevent or even reverse the abnormalities of allergic inflammation. As the roles of effector cells, and of signalling and adhesion molecules are better understood, the opportunities to inhibit or prevent the inflammatory cascade have increased. In addition, there have been advances in the synthesis of proteins, monoclonal antibodies and new small molecule chemical entities, which provide further valuable flexibility in the therapeutic approach to asthma. Such new approaches are aimed at prevention of T-cell activation; redressing the imbalance of T helper cell populations thus inhibiting or preventing Th-2-derived cytokine expression; and the inhibition or blockade of the downstream actions of these cytokines such as effects on IgE and eosinophils. Approaches such as these allow both broad and highly specific targeting, and may pave the way towards the prevention and reversal of the immunological and inflammatory processes driving asthma, allergic rhinitis and atopic dermatitis. The development of effective agents with effects beyond those provided by current therapies coupled with lesser side-effects will further address the unmet needs of allergic disease.

Chronic allergic inflammation as manifest in asthma, allergic rhinitis and atopic dermatitis is characterised by cellular tissue infiltration by diverse effector cells, including T lymphocytes, eosinophils, monocytes/macrophages and mast cells[1–3]. Co-ordination of the mobilisation, activation and trafficking of these effector cells to sites of inflammation is controlled by a complex milieu of cytokines and chemokines chiefly derived from activated CD4[+] T helper (Th) cells and resident cells. Key to this process are T helper cells of type 2 variety (Th-2), so defined by the secretion of a specific pattern of Th-2 cytokines, which follows cognate stimulation of the T-cell by antigen presenting cells, such as the dendritic cell in the airway and the Langerhans cell in the skin.

Additionally, chronically inflamed tissue may undergo structural changes labelled as remodelling and these too may be determined by the

*Correspondence to:
Professor Fan Chung,
Department of Thoracic
Medicine, National Heart
& Lung Institute,
Dovehouse Street,
London SW3 6LY, UK*

expression of soluble mediators such as cytokines and chemokines. Features of remodelling include thickening of the airway smooth muscle and subepithelial basement membrane, myofibroblast activation, collagen deposition, angiogenesis and increase in epithelial goblet cell numbers[4]. The precise significance of chronic inflammation as opposed to remodelling in the clinical presentation of asthma is unclear, but may be of central importance to our understanding of disease determinants such as bronchial hyper-responsiveness (BHR), airway narrowing and the acute exacerbations that characterise the disease.

Control of chronic inflammation is, therefore, a key goal in allergic disease, an idea supported by the potent actions of topical cortico-steroids in controlling the eosinophilic and lymphocytic inflammation of asthma, while effectively improving lung function and bronchial hyper-responsiveness[5].

The identification of the key immunological and inflammatory precedents to functional abnormalities and symptoms remains to be elucidated. Given that the vast majority of asthmatics and rhinitics have an atopic background, the inflammatory process of asthma may well be largely driven by exposure to common aero-allergens to which previous sensitisation has occurred. However, in non-atopic asthma too, the inflammatory process bears many similarities to those observed in the allergic process including the presence of eosinophils, activated CD4[+] T-cells, and the expression of Th-2-derived cytokines[6].

This article focuses primarily on immunological approaches to the treatment of asthma using non-(allergen) specific methods.

Prevention of T-cell activation

Three main thrusts of research into new therapies have developed: (i) preventing T-cell activation; (ii) prevention or reversal of Th-2 polarisation; and (iii) ablation of the effects of Th-2 cytokines and downstream mediators (Table 1).

T-cell immunomodulators

Cyclosporin-A and the functionally related tacrolimus (FK506) are powerful immunosuppressant agents used widely to prevent immune rejection in organ transplantation. They inhibit T-cell growth by blocking the G_0 phase through inhibition of T-cell growth factors such as IL-2. Both agents strongly inhibit mitogen-stimulated IL-5 release. Cyclosporin A and FK506 also have effects on other cells and markedly reduce basophil histamine release. Cyclosporin-A by inhalation provides significant

Table 1 Novel strategies for the inhibition and prevention of allergic asthma

Target	Agent
Prevention of T-cell activation	Anti-CD4
	CTLA-4
	Cyclosporin
	FK506
	Methotrexate
	Azathioprine
	Mycophenolate mofetil
	Suplatast tosilate
Prevention or reversal of Th-2 expression	
Inhibition of Th-2 cytokines/phenotype	Soluble IL-4Rα
	rhu IL-4 mutant proteins
	STAT6 inhibition
	Anti IL-5 monoclonal antibody
	GATA3 inhibition
	Soluble IL-13 Rα
Promotion of Th-1 cytokines/phenotype	IFN-γ
	IL-12
	IL-18
Inhibition of downstream mediators	
Anti-inflammatory cytokines	IL-10
	IL-1Ra
Inhibition of eosinophil migration and activation	CCR3 antagonist/antisense
	VLA4 inhibitor
	ICAM-1 inhibitor
	met-RANTES
	met-Ckbeta7
IgE inhibition	Monoclonal anti-IgE (E25)

inhibition of the allergen-induced late allergic reaction[7]. In corticosteroid-dependent asthma, low-dose cyclosporin-A improved lung function[8] allowing for a 62% reduction in oral steroid dose requirement[9], albeit at the expense of adverse effects which would not prove tolerable in mild disease. Methotrexate, a folate antagonist, has well recognised anti-inflammatory effects in rheumatoid arthritis and is used as a steroid-sparing agent in asthma. Meta-analysis of controlled trials confirms steroid-sparing effect, but show no significant evidence of benefit on lung function or symptoms[10]. In clinical practice, these immunomodulators are only modestly effective in a proportion of patients.

Suplatast tosilate is a novel immunomodulator developed in Japan which selectively prevents the release of IL-4 and IL-5 from Th-2 cells and can reduce bronchial eosinophilia in animal models of bronchial hyper-responsiveness. It has the added advantage of providing improvement in pulmonary function and symptom control, and decrease in the dose of inhaled corticosteroid[11] and has been launched for treatment of asthma in Japan.

Azathioprine, tacrolimus, cyclosporin and mycophenolate mofetil (MMF) have all been used systemically in the treatment of severe atopic dermatitis with marked benefits on dermatitis severity scores and quality of life markers. Oral MMF therapy was also associated with a reduction in IgE levels, decreased IL-10 and increased IFN-γ expression[12]. The use of topical tacrolimus in ointment form provides the added benefit of protection from systemic exposure and has demonstrated marked to excellent clearance of dermatitis after 12 months[13].

Selective T-cell depletion: anti-CD4 monoclonal antibody

Depletion of CD4+ T-cells in murine sensitised and allergen-challenge models using recombinant monoclonal antibodies results in ablation of airway hyper-responsiveness and airway eosinophilia, while antibody-mediated CD8+ T-cell depletion augments BHR and eosinophilic inflammation. A single dose of anti-CD4 monoclonal antibody that reduces circulating CD4+ T-cells in severe corticosteroid dependent asthma[14] led to an improvement in morning and evening peak expiratory flows but did not significantly impact on asthma symptoms. One uncertainty regarding the approach of CD4 depletion relates to the induction of CD4 lymphopenia and immunosuppression and the resultant risk of opportunistic infection and neoplasia[15]. It is also likely that other T-cell subsets may also be important in asthma. Recent investigations have highlighted the existence of CD8+ T-cells (*i.e.* T_{C2}), which secrete Th-2 type cytokines and their influence on the mediation of allergic airways disease is as yet to be established[16].

Inhibition of T-cell co-stimulation: CTLA4-Ig

The potential for disruption of antigen presentation by specific inhibition of co-stimulatory molecule interaction has been recognised and studied in murine models. A recombinant fusion protein consisting of the extracellular domain of CTLA4 linked to the constant region of IgG_1, known as CTLA4–Ig, binds B7 molecules with an affinity similar to membrane CTLA4. It therefore acts as a powerful inhibitor of B7/CD28 mediated co-stimulation. T-cell activation following B7/CD28 signalling may be blocked by CTLA4-Ig, and this can reduce bronchial hyper-responsiveness, BAL eosinophilia and specific IgE responses when given either prior to sensitisation or to allergen challenge[17]. CTLA4-Ig reduced IL-4 and IgE levels while IFN-γ and IgG_{2a} were unchanged, suggesting down-regulation of Th-2 response without up-regulation of the Th-1 response[18]. CTLA4-Ig may have powerful immunomodulatory

Table 2 Summary of Th-1 and Th-2 type cytokine effects as predicted by cytokine stimulation and ablation studies (animal and human data included)

| | THelper Polarisation | | BHR | IgE | Eosinophils | | | Mucus hyperplasia | Mast cell activation | Mediator release | Surface markers |
	Th-1	Th-2			Blood	Airway	Survival				
IL-4	↓	↑	↑	↑							↑ VCAM ↑ MHC II
IL-5					↑	↑	↑				
IL-9			↑	↑		↑		↑	↑		
IL-10					↓	↓	↓				↓ MHC II
IL-13	↓						↑	↑			↑ VCAM
IFN-γ	↑	↓		↓	↓	↓				↑ TNF-α ↑ IL-1β	
IL-12	↑	↓	↓	↓	↓	↓				↑ IFN-γ ↓ IL-10	
IL-18	↑		↓	↓↑			↓			↑ IFN-γ ↑ Chemokines ↓ IL-10	

effects with the potential for the suppression of Th-2 based allergen responses.

Modulation of Th-1/Th-2 differentiation

Specific attempts to alter Th-1/Th-2 balance by enhancing Th-1, or abrogation of Th-2 responses have been the major thrust of immune approaches to the prevention and treatment of allergies and of asthma. The most direct approaches include administration of cytokines that will induce activation of Th-1 pathways (*e.g.* IFN-γ, IL-12 and IL-18) or blocking antibodies that inhibit the effect of Th-2-related cytokines (*e.g.* anti-IL-4, anti-IL-5, anti-IL-9, and anti-IL-13) as summarised in Table 2.

Inhibition of allergy and asthma by Th-1 related cytokines

Interferon-γ

IFN-γ, released from CD4+ (Th-1) and CD8+ (T$_{C2}$) cells, is a critical factor regulating the balance of Th-1/Th-2 development, exerting an inhibitory effect on Th-2 cells[19]. IFN-γ is also a powerful and relatively specific inhibitor of IL-4-induced IgE and IgG$_4$ synthesis by B-cells. IFN-γ also reduced lung Th-2 cytokine levels, attenuated allergen-induced BHR with concomitant reduction in BAL eosinophilia, while an IFN-γ blocking antibody led to an increase in airway CD4+ T-cells and BHR in murine and rat models[20]. Inhalation of IFN-γ by non-asthmatic humans increases epithelial lining and BAL fluid IFN-γ levels but does not affect serum IFN-γ levels and, therefore, may avoid toxicity associated with systemic administration[21]. Subcutaneous IFN-γ therapy in steroid-dependent asthma has also been evaluated, but had no effect on lung function or treatment requirement although significantly reducing circulating eosinophil numbers[22].

Interleukin-12

IL-12 is produced by antigen-presenting cells and enhances the growth of activated T and NK cells, stimulating them to produce IFN-γ[23]. IL-12 also promotes the differentiation of IFN-γ producing T-cells and inhibits the differentiation of T-cells into IL-4 secreting cells[23]. Thus, IL-12 can regulate Th-1 cell differentiation while suppressing the expansion of Th-2 cell clones by early priming of undifferentiated Th-0 cells for IFN-γ secretion. In murine asthma models, administration of IL-12 leads to a reduction in allergen specific IgE levels, ablation of airway hyper-responsiveness and inhibition of eosinophil recruitment[24]. In therapeutic trials, IL-12 levels increased during corticosteroid therapy[25] and during specific immunotherapy[26]. In a Phase I trial of IL-12 in asthma, a significant reduction of peripheral eosinophils and trend to reduction in airway eosinophils was observed without effect on allergen-induced early or late phase responses[27]. Significant toxicity including arrhythmias, liver function abnormalities and flu-like illness will limit its potential utility in asthma.

Interleukin-18

IL-18 (IFN-γ inducing factor) is a potent inducer of IFN-γ production by T, NK and B-cells and plays an important part in the induction of Th-1 responses[28]. IL-18 receptors are expressed selectively on murine Th-1 but not Th-2 cells. Recombinant human IL-18 potently induces IFN-γ production by mitogen-stimulated peripheral blood mononuclear cells and enhances natural killer (NK) cell cytotoxicity, increases GM-CSF and reduces IL-10 production[29]. IL-18 and IL-12 have synergistic effects on Th-1 development, which may be due to reciprocal up-regulation of their receptors. IL-18 may be important in the control of allergen-induced BHR by vaccination. Vaccination using heat-killed *Listeria monocytogenes* caused marked inhibition of allergen-induced BHR and airway inflammation, associated with conversion to the Th-1 phenotype in mice[30]. This effect was IL-12-dependent and associated with marked up-regulation of IL-18 mRNA expression. These studies also demonstrated that administration of adjuvant after allergen, was able to reverse established BHR.

Inhibition of Th-2 related cytokines

Interleukin-4

IL-4 induces polarisation of the Th-0 cell to the Th-2 phenotype[31] as well as isotype-switch from IgM to IgE synthesis by B-cells[32]. It up-regulates IgE receptors and VCAM1 expression on vascular endothelium thereby facilitating endothelial passage and accumulation of eosinophils and basophils. Anti-IL-4 monoclonal antibody treatment of mice prior to allergic sensitisation markedly reduces IgE synthesis[33], but does not appear to inhibit airway eosinophilia or BHR[34]. A recombinant soluble IL-4 receptor (sIL-4R) has been designed as a mimic of the cell-surface receptor, which thus binds and sequesters free IL-4, but lacking transmembrane and cytoplasmic domains, they act effectively as an IL-4 receptor blocker. In murine studies, sIL-4R reduces allergen-specific IgE responses, airway hyper-responsiveness, VCAM-1 expression and eosinophil accumulation[35]. Single doses of sIL-4R improved lung function and reduced rescue β_2-agonist requirement in asthma[36], with a trend to reduction in serum ECP levels and exhaled NO levels. A recombinant mutant human protein that binds the IL-4 receptor α- but not γc-chain (BAY 16-9996) antagonises receptor transduction and substantially reversed allergen-induced bronchial hyper-responsiveness with a reduction in airway inflammation in a primate model[37].

Another approach to inhibition of IL-4 production is to target the control of transcription factors of the IL-4 gene. STAT-6 responsive elements are found in the promoter region of IL-4 inducible genes and are expressed at abnormally high levels in the epithelium of severe asthmatics[38]. STAT-6 knockout mice demonstrate a defect in IL-4 and IL-13 mediated signal transduction[39]. The potential utility of STAT-6 targeted therapies is high-lighted by the ability of STAT-6 directed antisense oligonucleotides to markedly down-regulate germline Cϵ mRNA levels, reflecting inhibition of IL-4-dependent IgE isotype switching[40].

Interleukin-5

Eosinophil mobilisation and trafficking, their maturation and maintenance are largely promoted by the Th-2 cytokine, IL-5, making it an attractive therapeutic target in eosinophilic conditions such as asthma and rhinitis. Ablation of the effects of IL-5 has been accomplished with antisense oligonucleotides in rodent models or with blocking anti-IL-5 antibody in many species accompanied by reduction in allergen-induced eosinophilia and variable effects on BHR[41]. Two humanised forms of anti-IL-5 (SB-240563 and Sch 55700) have been studied[42,43]. In mild asthmatics, SB-240563 had inhibitory effects on both allergen-induced sputum and peripheral blood eosinophil numbers[44], but without significant effect on bronchial responsiveness or the late phase response to allergen challenge. Phase-I trials in severe persistent asthma have provided similar results[45]. None of these studies have shown conclusively that chronic dosing with anti-IL-5 depletes tissues of eosinophils and/or their granule products.

IL-5 receptor signalling is complex and various IL-5 dependent functions are mediated by distinct secondary messenger systems. Thus, targeting such pathways may lead to inhibition of IL-5 effector functions. IL-5 has anti-apoptotic effects on eosinophils and these are dependent on the activation of lyn, Jak2 and Raf-1 kinase, while of these, only Raf-1 is necessary for eosinophil activation and degranulation[46,47]. Lyn-kinase dependent signalling may be specifically inhibited by a peptide inhibitor, resulting in inhibition of lyn-dependent IL-5 signalling without affecting Janus kinase-2 dependent IL-5 signalling. This inhibitor blocks allergen-driven airway eosinophilia[48]. The transcription factor GATA-3 is critical for IL-5 expression in Th-2 cells. Increased GATA-3 gene expression in association with IL-5 mRNA positivity has been shown in airway cells isolated from asthmatics supporting a causal association between augmented GATA-3 expression and dysregulated IL-5 expression in asthma[49]. Importantly, the specific inhibition of GATA-3 expression using antisense technology in a murine model has been demonstrated to reduce Th-2 cell expression although effects on the asthma phenotype are yet to be demonstrated[50].

Interleukin-9

IL-9 has been identified in the airways of asthmatics and can induce BHR, elevated serum IgE, mucin gene transcription and epithelial CC chemokine release[51–54]. Specific blockade of IL-9 activity by intratracheal instillation of monoclonal anti-IL-9 antibody inhibited BHR, airway eosinophilia, serum IgE, airway inflammatory cell infiltration and mucin production induced by allergen. As yet there are no clinical trials adopting IL-9 as a therapeutic target.

Interleukin-13

This cytokine shares 70% sequence homology with IL-4 and despite a degree of functional redundancy due to sharing of the IL-4Rα subunit, a specific role in inflammatory activation has been demonstrated in murine models. Notably, IL-13 does not share the IL-4 effect on specific induction of the Th-2 phenotype from naïve Th-0 cells. Blockade of IL-13 activity has been achieved using a soluble form of the IL-13Rα chain of the IL-13 receptor, known to bind IL-13 exclusively. This agent caused a significant reduction in airway hyper-reactivity, airway eosinophilia and mucus hyperplasia in mice. However, when administered after the initial allergen sensitisation, this agent had no effect on serum IgE levels[55].

Th-1/Th-2 modulation by vaccination

An indirect way of modulating Th-1/Th-2 balance has been to boost innate immunity by the use of vaccines, particularly for the redirection of the Th-2 response in favour of Th-1 response. Several approaches are currently under investigation, raising the possibility of prevention of the development of asthma and allergic diseases. The beneficial effects of specific immunotherapy may result from increasing Th-1 immune responses and the development of peptide immunotherapy may lead to a more effective and safer treatment for allergies against defined allergens.

Mycobacterium spp.

The potential benefit of BCG vaccination in atopic diseases was first raised by a study in Japanese schoolchildren, in whom an association between BCG vaccination and diminished incidence of atopy and allergic disease was observed. This suggested a role for early mycobacterial exposure in subsequent development of atopic responsiveness[56]. Experimental models have supported this concept using the non-pathogenic mycobacterial products of *Mycobacterium bovis* and *Mycobacterium vaccae*. Mice vaccinated with BCG prior to allergen sensitisation had increased IFN-γ and decreased IL-4 and IL-5 expression along with reduced levels of airway T-cells, eosinophils and BHR[57]. *M. vaccae* is ubiquitously present in the soil as a saprophyte and can evoke a strong production of IFN-γ. A suppression of Th-2 activation has been demonstrated using heat-killed *M. vaccae* in mice[58], and these studies have opened the way to clinical studies in human asthma.

Potential drawbacks of manipulating Th-1/Th-2 balance

The mounting evidence for Th-2 cell activation in allergic asthma suggests down-regulation or ablation of the Th-2 response to be an appropriate aim in treating asthma and allergic disorders. However, the consequences of such a strategy are as yet unclear. Two potential outcomes need consideration: (i) the consequences of Th-2 ablation; and (ii) those of allowing a Th-1 dominated immune activation. Parasite exposure induces Th-2 type cytokine synthesis, and mice with Th-2 cytokine deletions demonstrate impaired parasite clearance. Indeed, although early Th-1 expression may be a more important response to acute phase parasitemia, subsequent parasite clearance appears more Th-2 cytokine dependent. Autoimmune diseases, including experimental allergic encephalomyelitis, myasthenia gravis and hypothyroidism may be derived from an exuberance of Th-1 activity. Associations between IFN-γ, IFN-β and IL-12 exposure and the development or exacerbation of autoimmune processes have been reported.

Th-1 cells may contribute to asthmatic inflammation. In adoptive transfer studies of Th-1 cells in mice, a prolonged enhancement of cell-mediated immune responses was observed, and passive transfer of Th-1 cells with Th-2 cells induces enhanced tissue eosinophilia compared to when Th-2 cells alone were administered. However, in other studies in mice and rats, transfer of allergen-specific Th-1 cells inhibited the effects of allergen-specific Th-2 cells, namely broncho-alveolar lavage eosinophilia and BHR in rats, without itself inducing any inflammation[59]. Nevertheless, IFN-γ produced by Th-1 cells may activate epithelial cells to induce the production of pro-inflammatory cytokines and chemokines.

Two further observations appear important to the contribution of Th-1 type processes to asthma. First, the prominent expression of the Th-1 dependent transcription factor, STAT1, in stable asthma and second, the association between respiratory viral infections and asthma. Viral infections induce Th-1 expression with up-regulation of TNF-α and VCAM1 expression supporting a role for Th-1 mediated processes in asthma exacerbation. Caution, therefore, appears prudent as we investigate resetting the Th-1/Th-2 balance in the treatment of asthma and allergic diseases.

Anti-IgE antibody

Studies of the recombinant human anti-IgE antibody (rhu MAb-E25, Xolair) are now in Phase IV in asthma and allergic rhinitis. E25 binds to free IgE at the high affinity receptor-binding site (FcϵR$_1$), preventing the crosslinking of IgE bound to effector mast cells and basophils. This strategy ensures that the antibody is non-anaphylactoid. The antibody may be delivered by subcutaneous injection on a 2–4 weekly schedule, based on weight and serum IgE levels. Tolerability and adverse effect profiles are thus far acceptable with no reports of serum sickness, hypersensitivity reaction or the development of anti-E25 antibodies. E25 induces a dose-dependent reduction in serum free IgE associated with a reduction in basophil $Fc\varepsilon R_1$ expression and histamine release. A significant improvement in both early and late phase bronchoconstrictor responses to allergen challenge and a reduction in methacholine-induced hyper-responsiveness, with reduction in sputum eosinophil numbers have been reported following E25 administration. Results of several clinical trials show subjective improvement and significant effects on corticosteroid reduction in moderate to severe asthma[60], and allergic rhinitis[61]. This treatment should become available in the near future, and its initial role is likely to be in severe atopic asthma, although effects in non-atopic asthma and mild asthma are as yet to be demonstrated.

Inhibition of eosinophil activation and chemo-attraction

Although IL-5 is involved in the maturation and mobilisation of eosinophils, other factors are more important in the chemo-attraction and tissue activation of eosinophils.

Chemokine receptor antagonists

Chemokines are inducible pro-inflammatory proteins whose key function is leukocyte chemo-attraction and activation. Three families are currently described, distinguished on a structural basis into the C, CC and CXC families. Chemokine effects are mediated by chemokine receptors and differential cell receptor profiles allows cell-specific attraction. Thus, the CC chemokine eotaxin has an eosinophil specific role in recruitment due to restriction of the eotaxin receptor CCR3 to the eosinophil, although these agents are also involved in recruitment of monocytes, dendritic cells, T-lymphocytes, natural killer cells, B-lymphocytes and basophils. High-affinity chemokine receptor antagonists obtained by modification of endogenous chemokines such as met-RANTES and met-Ckβ7 are potent CCR3 specific antagonists which inhibit CCR3 receptor signalling and consequent eosinophil migration. To date, several small-molecular weight CCR3 antagonists have been developed and await clinical evaluation. One possibility is combining the inhibition of IL-5 and of eotaxin, a double-pronged approach that would reduce mobilisation, chemo-attraction and activation of eosinophils more effectively given that co-operativity between IL-5 and eotaxin has been demonstrated in *in vivo* models[62].

Blocking adhesion molecules and integrins (VLA-4/LFA-1)

Eosinophil migration to sites of allergic inflammation is mediated by interactions between endothelium, epithelium and eosinophil adhesion molecules including the α4-integrin VLA4. *In vivo* studies have shown that peptidomimetic small molecule VLA4 inhibitors administered prior to allergen challenge prevent increases in VLA4+ leukocytes (eosinophils, lymphocytes and macrophages) in lung tissue while significantly inhibiting early and late phase allergic responses[63]. Similar approaches inhibiting interactions between LFA-1 and ICAM-1 have also proven effective in blocking eosinophil adhesion and transmigration.

Inhibition of pro-inflammatory cytokines and pathways

The pro-inflammatory cytokines TNF-α and IL-1β have been shown to be endogenously overexpressed in asthma, while exogenous or environmental pro-inflammatory mediators such as endotoxin (present in house dust) have been shown to further augment the activation of pro-inflammatory cytokines. Activation of the transcription factor, NFκB, which can regulate the production of a range of pro-inflammatory cytokines including IL-1, IL-6, IL-8 and TNF-α and of adhesion molecules ICAM-1 and VCAM-1, has been shown in the airway epithelium and macrophages of patients with mild asthma. Similarly increased expression of the transcription factor AP-1, has also been reported.

Tumour necrosis factor-α

TNF-α increases airway responsiveness in Brown-Norway rats and in humans, together with an increase in sputum neutrophils. TNF-α also potently stimulates airway epithelial cells to produce cytokines including RANTES, IL-8 and GM-CSF, and increases the expression of the adhesion molecule, ICAM-1. TNF-α synergises with IL-4 and IFN-γ, increasing VCAM-1 expression on endothelial cells. TNF-α may be an important mediator in initiating chronic inflammation in the airways. Several approaches to inhibition of TNF-α synthesis and effects are now under investigation in asthma, including monoclonal antibodies to TNF and soluble TNF receptors. An anti-TNF-α antibody retarded the progression of severe rheumatoid arthritis with clinical amelioration[64], but has not yet been evaluated in asthma, particularly severe asthma. Inhibitors of TNF-α converting enzyme (TACE), or of the cysteine protease caspase-1 (IL-1 converting enzyme, ICE) are also potential anti-inflammatory compounds currently under development. A further exciting approach entails the disruption of post receptor intracellular signalling cascades such as inhibitors of p38 MAP kinase already shown to inhibit the synthesis of pro-inflammatory cytokines *in vivo*[65].

Interleukin-1

IL-1 co-induces CD4+ T-cell proliferation and IL-2 secretion following interaction of T-cells with antigen presenting cells, and is an important growth factor for antigen primed Th-2 cells. IL-1 also potently induces the synthesis and release of multiple pro-inflammatory cytokines and chemokines. The IL-1 receptor antagonist (IL-1Ra) polypeptide shows significant homology with IL-1α and IL-1β and binds the IL-1 receptor[66]. IL-1Ra has been isolated from multiple tissues including alveolar macrophages, and inhibits most activities of IL-1. IL1-Ra blocks Th-2 but not Th-1 clonal proliferation *in vitro* and in the guinea pig reduces allergen induced BHR and pulmonary eosinophilia. Manipulation of this endogenous control mechanism may, therefore, impact on asthma and needs to be evaluated in the clinical setting.

Interleukin-10

Although in mice IL-10 is predominantly a Th-2-derived cytokine, in man it is produced by both Th-2 and Th-1 cells and has anti-inflammatory properties that could be used to control asthmatic inflammation. IL-10 is derived largely from mononuclear cells, alveolar macrophages and both naive and committed T-cells. It reduces MHC and co-stimulatory molecule expression, reduces pro-inflammatory cytokine release and increases IL-1Ra expression. T-cell and macrophage IL-10 synthesis is significantly reduced in asthmatic subjects compared with non-asthmatics but IL-10 expression in alveolar macrophages is increased by corticosteroid therapy, suggesting *in vivo* relevance of this cytokine. A polymorphism in the promoter sequence of IL-10 associated with attenuated IL-10 expression has been identified with increased frequency in severe asthma, while promoter polymorphisms have been demonstrated in asthma probands and associate with elevated IgE levels. This latter observation is of particular interest given a proposed suppressive effect of IL-10 on IL-4-induced IgE isotype switching by B-cells. IL-10 administration to mice reduces airway eosinophilia and allergen-induced late responses. When given to normal volunteers, IL-10 reduced circulating CD3, CD4 and CD8 lymphocyte number and proliferative response and reduced TNF-α and IL-1 production[67].

Conclusions

Recent advances in techniques for synthesis and manufacture of monoclonal antibodies, synthetic peptides and peptidomimetic small molecules has broadened our potential for the creation of specific inhibitors of immune processes during allergic inflammation. These agents have enabled specific intervention in inflammatory cascades and allow clearer understanding of the roles of specific agents in this cascade, while at the same time provide the possibility of therapeutic intervention. In the first instance, it is likely that these strategies will be aimed at those with severe difficult-to-treat disease, particularly asthma, as it is here that the failings of conventional therapy are most evident. While preliminary data for many of these agents appear most promising, these agents await rigorous evaluation of efficacy, long-term safety and cost-effectiveness. Several agents targeted to specific immunological or cytokine pathways may become available and may be more effective in disease subtypes in which newer techniques such as pharmacogenetic profiling may help identify the best responders to particular types of specific drugs[68]. The identification of appropriate therapeutic targets is only a preliminary step and the development of such new approaches and agents provides an exciting, yet daunting, future.

References

1 Azzawi M, Bradley B, Jeffery PK *et al*. Identification of activated T lymphocytes and eosinophils in bronchial biopsies in stable atopic asthma. *Am Rev Respir Dis* 1990; 142: 1407–13

2 Leung DY. Pathogenesis of atopic dermatitis. *J Allergy Clin Immunol* 1999; 104: S99–108

3 Durham SR. Mechanisms of mucosal inflammation in the nose and lungs. *Clin Exp Allergy* 1998; 28 (Suppl 2): 11–6

4 Bousquet J, Jeffery PK, Busse WW, Johnson M, Vignola AM. Asthma. From bronchoconstriction to airways inflammation and remodeling. *Am J Respir Crit Care Med* 2000; 161: 1720–45

5 Barnes PJ. Efficacy of inhaled corticosteroids in asthma. *J Allergy Clin Immunol* 1998; 102: 531–8

6 Humbert M, Menz G, Ying S *et al*. The immunopathology of extrinsic (atopic) and intrinsic (non-atopic) asthma: more similarities than differences. *Immunol Today* 1999; 20: 528–33

7 Sihra BS, Kon OM, Durham SR, Walker S, Barnes NC, Kay AB. Effect of cyclosporin A on the allergen-induced late asthmatic reaction. *Thorax* 1997; 52: 447–52

8 Alexander AG, Barnes NC, Kay AB. Trial of cyclosporin in corticosteroid-dependent chronic severe asthma. *Lancet* 1992; 339: 324–8

9 Lock SH, Kay AB, Barnes NC. Double-blind, placebo-controlled study of cyclosporin A as a corticosteroid-sparing agent in corticosteroid-dependent asthma. *Am J Respir Crit Care Med* 1996; 153: 509–14

10 Davies H, Olson L, Gibson P. Methotrexate as a steroid sparing agent for asthma in adults. *Cochrane Database Syst Rev* 2000; 2: CD000391. 2: CD000391

11 Tamaoki J, Kondo M, Sakai N *et al*. Effect of Suplatast tosilate, a TH$_2$ cytokine inhibitor, on steroid-dependent asthma: a double blind randomised study. *Lancet* 2000; 356: 273–8

12 Neuber K, Schwartz I, Itschert G, Dieck AT. Treatment of atopic eczema with oral mycophenolate mofetil. *Br J Dermatol* 2000; 143: 385–91

13 Reitamo S, Wollenberg A, Schopf E *et al*. Safety and efficacy of 1 year of tacrolimus ointment monotherapy in adults with atopic dermatitis. The European Tacrolimus Ointment Study Group. *Arch Dermatol* 2000; 136: 999–1006

14 Kon OM, Sihra BS, Compton CH, Leonard TB, Kay AB, Barnes NC. Randomised, dose-ranging, placebo-controlled study of chimeric antibody to CD4 (keliximab) in chronic severe asthma. *Lancet* 1998; 352: 1109–13

15 Laurence J. T-cell subsets in health, infectious disease, and idiopathic CD4$^+$ T lymphocytopenia. *Ann Intern Med* 1993; 119: 55–62

16 Vukmanovic-Stejic M, Vyas B, Gorak-Stolinska P, Noble A, Kemeny DM. Human Tc1 and Tc2/Tc0 CD8 T-cell clones display distinct cell surface and functional phenotypes. *Blood* 2000; 95: 231–40

17 Van Oosterhout AJ, Hofstra CL, Shields R *et al*. Murine CTLA4-IgG treatment inhibits airway eosinophilia and hyperresponsiveness and attenuates IgE upregulation in a murine model of allergic asthma. *Am J Respir Cell Mol Biol* 1997; **17**: 386–92

18 Krinzman SJ, De Sanctis GT, Cernadas M *et al*. Inhibition of T-cell co-stimulation abrogates airway hyperresponsiveness in a murine model. *J Clin Invest* 1996; **98**: 2693–9

19 Chung KF, Barnes PJ. Cytokines in asthma. *Thorax* 1999; **54**: 825–57

20 Huang TJ, MacAry PA, Wilke T, Kemeny DM, Chung KF. Inhibitory effects of endogenous and exogenous interferon-gamma on bronchial hyperresponsiveness, allergic inflammation and T-helper 2 cytokines in Brown-Norway rats. *Immunology* 1999; **98**: 280–8

21 Jaffe HA, Buhl R, Mastrangeli A *et al*. Organ specific cytokine therapy. Local activation of mononuclear phagocytes by delivery of an aerosol of recombinant interferon-gamma to the human lung. *J Clin Invest* 1991; **88**: 297–302

22 Boguniewicz M, Schneider LC, Milgrom H *et al*. Treatment of steroid-dependent asthma with recombinant interferon-gamma. *Clin Exp Allergy* 1993; **23**: 785–90

23 Macatonia SE, Hosken NA, Litton M *et al*. Dendritic cells produce IL-12 and direct the development of Th1 cells from naive CD4⁺ T-cells. *J Immunol* 1995; **154**: 5071–9

24 Gavett SH, O'Hearn DJ, Li X, Huang SK, Finkelman FD, Wills-Karp M. Interleukin 12 inhibits antigen-induced airway hyperresponsiveness, inflammation, and Th2 cytokine expression in mice. *J Exp Med* 1995; **182**: 1527–36

25 Naseer T, Minshall EM, Leung DY *et al*. Expression of IL-12 and IL-13 mRNA in asthma and their modulation in response to steroid therapy. *Am J Respir Crit Care Med* 1997; **155**: 845–51

26 Hamid QA, Schotman E, Jacobson MR, Walker SM, Durham SR. Increases in IL-12 messenger RNA⁺ cells accompany inhibition of allergen-induced late skin responses after successful grass pollen immunotherapy. *J Allergy Clin Immunol* 1997; **99**: 254–60

27 O'Connnor B, Hansel T, Holgate S, Barnes P. Effects of recombinant human IL-12 on allergen induced airway inflammation and the late response. *Am J Respir Crit Care Med* 2000; **161**: A592

28 Tomura M, Maruo S, Mu J *et al*. Differential capacities of CD4⁺, CD8⁺, and CD4⁻CD8⁻ T-cell subsets to express IL-18 receptor and produce IFN-gamma in response to IL-18. *J Immunol* 1998; **160**: 3759–65

29 Fehniger TA, Shah MH, Turner MJ *et al*. Differential cytokine and chemokine gene expression by human NK cells following activation with IL-18 or IL-15 in combination with IL-12: implications for the innate immune response. *J Immunol* 1999; **162**: 4511–20

30 Yeung VP, Gieni RS, Umetsu DT, DeKruyff RH. Heat-killed *Listeria monocytogenes* as an adjuvant converts established murine Th2-dominated immune responses into Th1-dominated responses. *J Immunol* 1998; **161**: 4146–52

31 Maggi E, Parronchi P, Manetti R *et al*. Reciprocal regulatory effects of IFN-gamma and IL-4 on the *in vitro* development of human Th1 and Th2 clones. *J Immunol* 1992; **148**: 2142–7

32 Lebman DA, Coffman RL. Interleukin 4 causes isotype switching to IgE in T-cell-stimulated clonal B cell cultures. *J Exp Med* 1988; **168**: 853–62

33 Zhou CY, Crocker IC, Koenig G, Romero FA, Townley RG. Anti-interleukin-4 inhibits immunoglobulin E production in a murine model of atopic asthma. *J Asthma* 1997; **34**: 195–201

34 Tanaka H, Nagai H, Maeda Y. Effect of anti-IL-4 and anti-IL-5 antibodies on allergic airway hyperresponsiveness in mice. *Life Sci* 1998; **62**: L169–74

35 Henderson WRJ, Chi EY, Maliszewski CR. Soluble IL-4 receptor inhibits airway inflammation following allergen challenge in a mouse model of asthma. *J Immunol* 2000; **164**: 1086–95

36 Borish LC, Nelson HS, Lanz MJ *et al*. Interleukin-4 receptor in moderate atopic asthma. A phase I/II randomized, placebo-controlled trial. *Am J Respir Crit Care Med* 1999; **160**: 1816–23

37 Harris P, Lindell D, Fitch N, Gundel R. The IL-4 receptor antagonist (BAY 16-9996) reverses airway hyperresponsiveness in a primate model of asthma. *Am J Respir Crit Care Med* 2000; **159**: A230

38 Mullings RE, Wilson SJ, Djukanovic R *et al*. Increased Stat6 expression in bronchial epithelium of severe asthmatic subjects. *Am J Respir Crit Care Med* 2000; **63**: A46

39 Heim MH. The Jak-STAT pathway: cytokine signalling from the receptor to the nucleus. *J Recept Signal Transduct Res* 1999; **19**: 75–120

40   Hill S, Herlaar E, Le Cardinal A, van Heeke G, Nicklin P. Homologous human and murine antisense oligonucleotides targeting Stat6. Functional effects on germline c-epsilon transcript. *Am J Respir Cell Mol Biol* 1999; **21**: 728–37

41   Karras JG, McGraw K, McKay RA *et al*. Inhibition of antigen-induced eosinophilia and late phase airway hyperresponsiveness by an IL-5 antisense oligonucleotide in mouse models of asthma. *J Immunol* 2000; **164**: 5409–15

42   Zhang J, Kuvelkar R, Murgolo NJ *et al*. Mapping and characterization of the epitope(s) of Sch 55700, a humanized mAb, that inhibits human IL-5. *Int Immunol* 1999; **11**: 1935–44

43   Zia-Amirhosseini P, Minthorn E, Benincosa LJ *et al*. Pharmacokinetics and pharmacodynamics of SB-240563, a humanized monoclonal antibody directed to human interleukin-5, in monkeys. *J Pharmacol Exp Ther* 1999; **291**: 1060–7

44   Leckie M, ten Brinke A, Lordan J *et al*. IL-5 monoclonal antibody, SB-240563, single dose therapy: initial safety and activity in patients with asthma. *Am J Respir Crit Care Med* 1999; **159**: A624

45   Kips JC, O'Connor BJ, Langley SJ *et al*. Results of a phase I trial with SCH55700, a humanised anti-IL-5 antibody, in severe persistent asthma. *Am J Respir Crit Care Med* 2000; **161**: A505

46   Adachi T, Choudhury BK, Stafford S, Sur S, Alam R. The differential role of extracellular signal-regulated kinases and p38 mitogen-activated protein kinase in eosinophil functions. *J Immunol* 2000; **165**: 2198–204

47   Adachi T, Alam R. The mechanism of IL-5 signal transduction. *Am J Physiol* 1998; **275**: C623–33

48   Adachi T, Pazdrak K, Stafford S, Alam R. The mapping of the Lyn kinase binding site of the common beta subunit of IL-3/granulocyte-macrophage colony-stimulating factor/IL-5 receptor. *J Immunol* 1999; **162**: 1496–501

49   Nakamura Y, Ghaffar O, Olivenstein R *et al*. Gene expression of the GATA-3 transcription factor is increased in atopic asthma. *J Allergy Clin Immunol* 1999; **103**: 215–22

50   Zhang DH, Yang L, Cohn L *et al*. Inhibition of allergic inflammation in a murine model of asthma by expression of a dominant-negative mutant of GATA-3. *Immunity* 1999; **11**: 473–82

51   Shimbara A, Christodoulopoulos P, Soussi-Gounni A *et al*. IL-9 and its receptor in allergic and nonallergic lung disease: increased expression in asthma. *J Allergy Clin Immunol* 2000; **105**: 108–15

52   Longphre M, Li D, Gallup M *et al*. Allergen-induced IL-9 directly stimulates mucin transcription in respiratory epithelial cells. *J Clin Invest* 1999; **104**: 1375–82

53   Dong Q, Louahed J, Vink A *et al*. IL-9 induces chemokine expression in lung epithelial cells and baseline airway eosinophilia in transgenic mice. *Eur J Immunol* 1999; **29**: 2130–9

54   McLane MP, Haczku A, van de Rijn M *et al*. Interleukin-9 promotes allergen-induced eosinophilic inflammation and airway hyperresponsiveness in transgenic mice. *Am J Respir Cell Mol Biol* 1998; **19**: 713–20

55   Wills-Karp M, Luyimbazi J, Xu X *et al*. Interleukin-13: central mediator of allergic asthma. *Science* 1998; **282**: 2258–61

56   Shirakawa T, Enomoto T, Shimazu S, Hopkin JM. The inverse association between tuberculin responses and atopic disorder. *Science* 1997; **275**: 77–9

57   Erb KJ, Holloway JW, Sobeck A, Moll H, Le Gros G. Infection of mice with *Mycobacterium bovis*-Bacillus Calmette-Guerin (BCG) suppresses allergen-induced airway eosinophilia. *J Exp Med* 1998; **187**: 561–9

58   Camporota L, Corkhill A, Long H *et al*. Effects of intradermal injection of SRL-172 (killed *Mycobacterium vaccae* suspension) on allergen induced airway responses and IL-5 generation by PBMC in asthma. *Am J Respir Crit Care Med* 2000; **161**: A477

59   Cohn L, Homer RJ, Niu N, Bottomly K. T helper 1 cells and interferon gamma regulate allergic airway inflammation and mucus production. *J Exp Med* 1999; **190**: 1309–18

60   Milgrom H, Fick RBJ, Su JQ *et al*. Treatment of allergic asthma with monoclonal anti-IgE antibody. rhuMAb-E25 Study Group. *N Engl J Med* 1999; **341**: 1966–73

61   Adelroth E, Rak S, Haahtela T *et al*. Recombinant humanized mAb-E25, an anti-IgE mAb, in birch pollen-induced seasonal allergic rhinitis. *J Allergy Clin Immunol* 2000; **106**: 253–9

62   Collins PD, Marleau S, Griffiths-Johnson DA, Jose PJ, Williams TJ. Cooperation between interleukin-5 and the chemokine eotaxin to induce eosinophil accumulation *in vivo*. *J Exp Med* 1995; **182**: 1169–74

63 Abraham WM, Ahmed A, Sielczak MW, Narita M, Arrhenius T, Elices MJ. Blockade of late-phase airway responses and airway hyperresponsiveness in allergic sheep with a small-molecule peptide inhibitor of VLA-4. *Am J Respir Crit Care Med* 1997; **156**: 696–703

64 Elliott MJ, Maini RN, Feldmann M *et al*. Repeated therapy with monoclonal antibody to tumour necrosis factor alpha (cA2) in patients with rheumatoid arthritis. *Lancet* 1994; **344**: 1125–7

65 Underwood DC, Osborn RR, Kotzer CJ *et al*. SB 239063, a potent p38 MAP kinase inhibitor, reduces inflammatory cytokine production, airways eosinophil infiltration, and persistence. *J Pharmacol Exp Ther* 2000; **293**: 281–8

66 Hannum CH, Wilcox CJ, Arend WP *et al*. Interleukin-1 receptor antagonist activity of a human interleukin-1 inhibitor. *Nature* 1990; **343**: 336–40

67 Chernoff AE, Granowitz EV, Shapiro L *et al*. A randomized, controlled trial of IL-10 in humans. Inhibition of inflammatory cytokine production and immune responses. *J Immunol* 1995; **154**: 5492–9

68 Drazen JM, Yandava CN, Dube L *et al*. Pharmacogenetic association between ALOX5 promoter genotype and the response to anti-asthma treatment. *Nat Genet* 1999; **22**: 168–70

Heterogeneity of therapeutic responses in asthma

Jeffrey M Drazen[1], Edwin K Silverman[1] and Tak H Lee[2]

[1]Department of Medicine, Brigham and Women's Hospital and Harvard Medical School, Boston, USA and [2]Department of Respiratory Medicine and Allergy, Guy's, King's and St Thomas' School of Medicine, Guy's Hospital, London, UK

Asthma is a complex clinical syndrome with multiple genetic and environmental factors contributing to its phenotypic expression. This aetiological heterogeneity adds to the complexity when addressing variation in the response to anti-asthma treatment. Currently, there are three main lines of treatment available: (i) inhaled glucocorticoids which have multiple mechanisms of action; (ii) β_2-agonists which are very effective bronchodilators and act predominantly on airway smooth muscle; and (iii) cysteinyl-leukotriene inhibitors. Analysis of the repeatability (r) of the treatment response, defined as the fraction of the total population variance which results from among-individual differences, shows values of r between 60–80% indicating that a substantial fraction of the variance of the treatment response could be genetic in nature. Among the sources of variability that could contribute to the observed heterogeneity in the response to treatment are the degree of underlying inflammation, such as in glucocorticoid resistance, and polymorphisms in the genes encoding the drug target, such as β_2-adrenoceptor and 5-lipoxygenase.

Bronchial asthma is a disease which is characterised clinically by episodic symptoms of wheeze, dyspnoea and chest tightness. Physiological abnormalities include a variable reduction in airflow which is secondary to increased airway resistance and bronchial hyper-responsiveness (BHR) to specific and non-specific agents such as allergen and histamine, respectively. Pathologically, even in the mildest of asthma cases, there is evidence for airway inflammation with a cellular infiltrate of mononuclear cells and eosinophils into the airway mucosa. These cells are present in increased numbers and are activated to secrete pro-inflammatory cytokines that may be pertinent to the pathophysiology of the asthmatic process.

Currently, there are three main asthma treatments available: (i) inhaled glucocorticoids; (ii) β_2-agonists; and (iii) leukotriene inhibitors. Bronchial asthma is a heterogeneous disorder, but even in patients with an apparently identical clinical phenotype, response to drug treatment may be remarkably variable. It is common for some patients to respond in

Correspondence to:
Prof. TH Lee, Department of Respiratory Medicine and Allergy, 5th Floor Thomas Guy House, Guy's Hospital, London SE1 9RT, UK

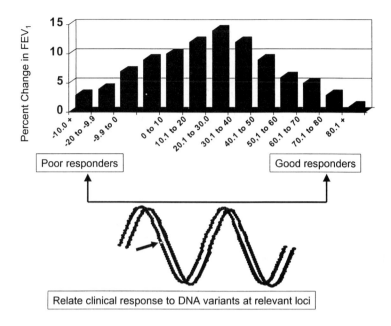

Fig. 1 Data from asthma drug treatment trials which show high repeatability (see text) are stratified by the magnitude of response. DNA from patients with a salutary clinical response (good responders) and a poor clinical response is genotyped at loci related to the treatment pathway of interest and related by contingency table analysis. A pharmacogenetic locus is one in which there is a strong association between the presence of a given DNA sequence variant and a clinical response. The relationship between drug response and DNA sequence variants discovered by this process needs to be confirmed by prospective clinical studies.

a salutary fashion to a given treatment while others fail to manifest such a response. The basis for this variable treatment response is not known with certainty, but there is good reason to believe that a significant component of the variability is genetic in nature. The basis for this statement derives from evaluation of the repeatability of the asthma treatment response. Repeatability is an upper limit estimate of the heritability of the treatment response (h^2) that can be made from data available from treatment trials of unrelated individuals[1,2]. The essence of this approach is to estimate the within-individual variance in the treatment response, assumed to be due to environmental variance and measurement error, and compared it with the total population variance in the treatment response, assumed to be due to genetic, environmental, and measurement errors[3]. Since the variance within a given subject of the most commonly used measurement of lung function, *i.e.* FEV_1, is relatively small[4,5] repeatability can be defined by the relationship $r = (V_G + V_{Eg})/V_P$ where V_G is the genetic variance, V_{Eg} is the general environmental variability which is defined[1] as the 'environmental variance contributing to the between-individual component and arising from permanent or non-localised circumstances' and V_p is the total variance. The repeatability thus sets an upper limit to the degree of genetic determination. We used the data available from asthma treatment trials to estimate 'r' in the treatment response to inhaled β_2-agonists, to inhaled steroids, and to leukotriene modifiers (Fig. 1).

We estimated the percentage of variation in the FEV_1 response to salbutamol, that was attributable to between individual differences, which corresponds to the maximal possible percentage attributable to genetic causes, *i.e.* 'r'; it constituted 60.6% of the total variance. We estimated the among-patient variability and within-population variability from the final percent of the predicted FEV_1 achieved after 6 weeks of treatment with inhaled triamcinolone acetonide and found a value of 'r' of 86.1%, thus providing evidence that a clinically significant component of the treatment response to inhaled corticosteroids is likely heritable. Finally, we estimated 'r' from a data set obtained in a clinical trial of ABT-761, a 5-lipoxygenase (ALOX5) inhibitor, in which 110 patients were treated with high-dose ABT-761 for 12 weeks. The within-patient variability and within-population variability were estimated as noted above for β_2-agonists, leading to a value of 'r' of 61.2%. Thus, our findings indicate the potential for a substantial component of the treatment response being inheritable in nature. Our analysis of existing treatment trials indicates that at least half of the observed variance of the treatment response to inhaled β_2-agonists, to inhaled steroids, and to leukotriene modifiers can be ascribed to among-patient differences. This value represents an upper limit of the genetic variability and indicates that a clinically significant fraction of the total population variance is potentially genetic in origin. With this as a background it makes sense to examine evidence for association between the drug treatment response and known genetic variation in treatment outcomes.

Glucocorticoid therapy – variable treatment responses

Although glucocorticoids (GCs) are the mainstay of treatment for bronchial asthma, there has been increasing recognition of a group of asthmatic patients who do not appear to benefit from glucocorticoid therapy, *i.e.* the GC-resistant (GCR) asthmatic[6]. GC responsiveness is probably a continuous spectrum with individuals who demonstrate GC resistance falling at one end of a unimodal distribution. For clinical purposes, a common definition of GC resistance is the failure of an asthmatic patient to improve FEV_1 by 15% from a baseline of ≤75% predicted after an adequate dose (*e.g.* ≥40 mg prednisolone) for an adequate duration of time (*e.g.* 1–2 weeks), despite demonstrating greater than 15% reversibility to an inhaled β_2-agonist and provided compliance was ensured.

This is a pragmatic definition, which nevertheless is useful because it defines a sufficiently high dose of glucocorticoid and a duration of usage after which physicians would feel uncomfortable in maintaining patients on continuous systemic GCs. GCR asthma was first described by Schwartz and colleagues in 1967[7]. In 1981, Carmichael described 58 subjects with chronic asthma who were clinically resistant to prednisolone therapy[8]. Compared with GCS subjects, these patients had a longer duration of asthma, a more frequent family history of asthma, poorer morning lung function, and a greater degree of bronchial reactivity. These early clinical studies suggested that both genetic (family history of asthma) and environmental (longer duration of asthma) factors may play a role in the pathogenesis of this condition.

Cellular abnormalities in glucocorticoid resistant asthma

In view of the lack of evidence for any gross biochemical abnormality in these patients, subsequent studies focused on the role played by peripheral blood mononuclear cells in GCR asthma. Many studies have now demonstrated that GCR asthma is associated with impaired *in vitro* and *in vivo* responsiveness of monocytes and T lymphocytes to the suppressive effects of GCs[9].

Corrigan has shown enhanced interleukin-2 (IL-2) and HLA-DR receptor expression on peripheral T lymphocytes in GCR as opposed to GCS asthma[10]. In addition, he has shown that PHA-induced T cell proliferation and the elaboration of IFN-γ and IL-2 from mitogen-stimulated T lymphocytes was inhibited by dexamethasone in GCS, but not in GCR subjects[11]. Interestingly, cyclosporin-A was seen to partially reverse this *in vitro* resistance, suggesting a potentially therapeutic role for this treatment in GCR asthma.

Leung has examined the effects of a 1 week course of prednisolone on BAL cells obtained from patients with GCR asthma[12]. It was shown that GCR subjects had elevated cell numbers expressing IL-2 and IL-4 before prednisolone treatment as compared to the GCS subjects. In contrast to GCS subjects, prednisolone failed to suppress IL-4 and IL-5 expression in the GCR subjects. Therefore, the airway cells from patients with GCR compared with GCS asthma have different patterns of cytokine gene expression and distinct responses to GC therapy.

Tissue specificity of glucocorticoid resistance in asthma

We have examined whether the lack of clinical response to GCs seen in GCR bronchial asthma is reflected in abnormalities of endogenous cortisol secretion and in the sensitivity of the hypothalamic-pituitary-adrenal (HPA) in GCR subjects by using a modification of the standard dexamethasone suppression test in response to 0.25 mg and 1 mg oral dexamethasone[13]. The data indicate that GCR asthma is not reflected in an altered secretory rate of endogenous cortisol or in a different sensitivity of the HPA axis to dexamethasone suppression. In order to assess whether GCR asthmatic patients are equally at risk from the side effects of GCs on bone metabolism, GCS and GCR asthmatic patients received prednisolone 40 mg orally for 5 days. Prednisolone suppressed osteocalcin equally in both the GCS and GCR groups[14]. These two studies indicate that 'non-immune' tissue responds normally to GCs in GCR asthma and that these subjects are, therefore, equally at risk of Cushingoid side effects. An explanation of these findings is that the presence of inflammation in these cells is a necessary prerequisite for the unmasking of the resistant profile.

Glucocorticoid bioavailability in glucocorticoid resistant asthma

Interest has also focused on whether impaired bioavailability of GCs can account for the differences in therapeutic responses in steroid dependent and steroid resistant asthma. May *et al* measured the pharmacokinetic profile of a single dose of 15 mg oral prednisolone in 12 steroid-dependent asthmatic subjects by radioimmunoassay (RIA) and found no inter-individual differences in these subjects with respect to C_{max}, plasma half life and area under the concentration/time curve: they concluded that differences in prednisolone bioavailability is not a factor in determining the dose required to control asthma[15]. Rose and colleagues observed that the plasma protein binding, distribution and clearance of prednisolone are not responsible for the large prednisolone requirement of steroid-dependent asthmatics. He extended the above studies to GC dependent and resistant asthmatic children and again found no difference in bioavailability parameters. We have examined the pharmacokinetic profile of an oral dose of 40 mg prednisolone in GCS and GCR asthmatic subjects[16]. We found that there was no significant difference in AUC, C_{max} and estimated clearance values between the normal group studied and each of the asthmatic groups. This implies that clinical GC resistance in asthmatic subjects is not reflected in any gross abnormality of the absorption or elimination of prednisolone. These data are in agreement with pharmacokinetic studies carried out in GCR asthma by other groups who observed no differences in estimated clearance values of a single dose of oral prednisolone between groups of well characterised GCR and GCS asthmatic subjects[11].

Glucocorticoid receptor characteristics in glucocorticoid resistant asthma

The mechanisms of glucocorticoid action are summarised in Figures 2–4. Competitive binding studies on nuclear extracts derived from peripheral blood monocytes using [^{3}H]-dexamethasone have demonstrated no difference in the K_d, R_o or nuclear translocation of the activated receptor complex between GCS and GCR asthmatics[17]. We have shown that GC resistance in bronchial asthma cannot be explained by abnormalities in receptor nuclear translocation, density or binding affinity. It is possible that the phenomenon of GC resistance may be heterogeneous. Indeed, a 4-fold reduction in receptor binding affinity has been described in T-cells. However, the authors concluded that such a small reduction in K_d was insufficient to explain the gross difference in GC responsiveness at the clinical level[11]. Similarly, Sher *et al* have described two patterns of ligand

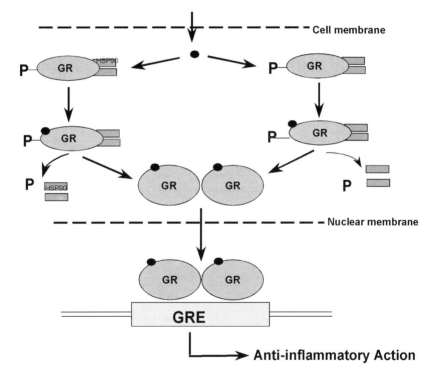

Fig. 2 Glucocorticoids mediate their effects via the glucocorticoid receptor (GR) which is present in the cytoplasm of all cells. Glucocorticoids enter the cell by passive diffusion where they bind to the GR non-covalently by hydrophobic and hydrogen ion interactions. This results in a conformational change in the GR described as activation. This process modifies the receptor allosterically, whereupon the GR undergoes dephosphorylation, dissociates into two 90 kDa associated heat shock proteins, forms dimers and translocates into the nucleus where it binds to sequences in DNA known as glucocorticoid response elements (GREs) in the promoter regions of the glucocorticoid responsive genes, leading to either induction of inflammatory genes or suppression of anti-inflammatory genes.

binding abnormalities in their group of GCR asthmatics termed type 1 and 2[18]. The more common type 1 defect was associated with 'Cushingoid side effects', reduced K_d, normal receptor numbers, localisation to T-cells, reversibility with serum deprivation and was IL-2 and IL-4-dependent. The less common type 2 defect was associated with reduced receptor density with a normal K_d, was irreversible and was seen in the total mononuclear cell population. The type 1 defect is acquired as a result of long-standing inflammation whereas the type 2 defect is more likely to be a genetic defect.

We have demonstrated a reduction in the binding of the activated glucocorticoid receptor complex to its GRE using gel retardation assays in nuclear extracts from mononuclear cells obtained from GCS, GCR and non-asthmatic control subjects[19]. Dexamethasone was seen to induce a significant rapid and sustained 2-fold increase in GRE binding in the mononuclear cells from the GCS subjects and non-asthmatic

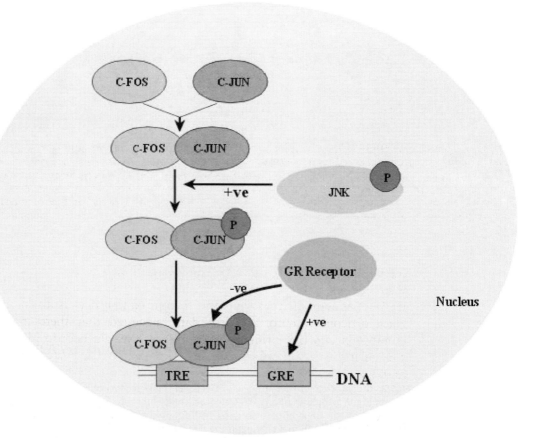

Fig. 3 Inducible AP-1 is formed by dimerisation of c-Fos and c-Jun following dephosphorylation of Jun N-terminal kinase (JNK). AP-1 binds to the TPA response element (TRE) to activate genes encoding for inflammatory cytokines. Glucocorticoid receptor inhibits AP-1 either by direct sequestration or by spatial interference. +ve indicates activism and –ve indicates inhibition.

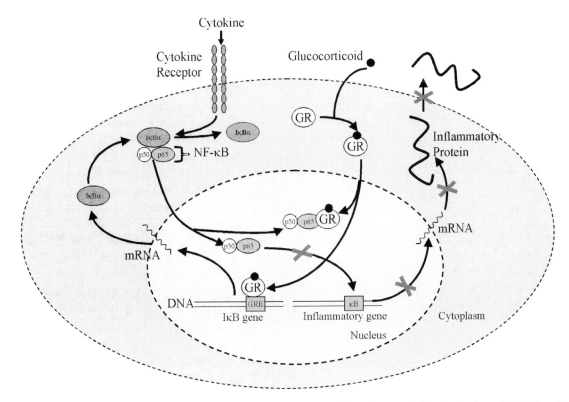

Fig. 4 Activation of NF-κB by, for example, cytokines can be blocked by glucocorticoids. Activation of NF-κB involves phosphorylation and subsequent proteolytic degradation of the inhibitory protein IκB by specific IκB kinases. The free NF-κB (p50 and p65 heterodimer) can then translocate to the nucleus where it binds to κB sites in the promoter genes of inflammatory proteins. Glucocorticoid receptor (GR) complexes bind to the p65 subunit of NF-κB preventing NF-κB activation of inflammatory genes. Synthesis of IκBα is promoted by the binding of glucocorticoid–GR complexes to a glucocorticoid responsive element in the promoter region of the IκBα gene.

control subjects that was significantly (P <0.005) reduced in the GCR subjects. These data have recently been confirmed by other investigators who have suggested that this defect may occur as a result of an IL-2- and IL-4-dependent increase in the pro-inflammatory isoform of the glucocorticoid receptor[20]. These data suggested that there may be a mutation(s) in the primary structure of the glucocorticoid receptor, particularly in its DNA-binding domain which could account for this functional abnormality.

We have tested whether the reduction in DNA binding of the glucocorticoid receptor is due to polymorphisms in its primary structure using the sensitive technique of chemical mutational analysis (CMA)[21]. Using this technique we did not detect any base pair mismatch between the 6 GCS and 6 GCR patients and the corresponding wild type glucocorticoid receptor, despite a 100% detection of control mutations indicating that in these patients the defect in GCR asthma does not lie in the structure of the glucocorticoid receptor. This was further confirmed by dideoxy sequencing using linear PCR elongation and chain termination[22]. Therefore, a defect in the primary structure of the glucocorticoid receptor does not account for the reduction of *in vitro* DNA binding and prompted us to further examine the binding characteristics of receptor-DNA interaction. Subsequent Scatchard analysis indicated that the defect in the GR subjects was underpinned by a reduction in the numbers of nuclear translocated glucocorticoid receptors available for DNA interaction. This was despite there being an equal amount of nuclear translocated receptors available on the basis of previous ligand binding experiments. These data indicated to us that the DNA binding sites of the glucocorticoid receptors were being competed out, possibly by pro-inflammatory transcription factors. These factors are bound by glucocorticoid receptor DNA binding sites and so prevent their subsequently activating pro-inflammatory cytokine genes. Thus the reduction in the 'read-out' of DNA binding of the GRE may reflect the presence of excess pro-inflammatory activity rather than a direct problem with gene transcription *per se*. It is, therefore, important to review the mechanisms of negative gene regulation by GCs.

Transcription factor interactions in glucocorticoid resistant asthma

We have examined whether the functional abnormality of reduced DNA binding of the glucocorticoid receptor in GCR asthma is caused by increased activity of pro-inflammatory transcription factors[23]. We examined the activities of AP-1, NF-κB and CREB using gel shift assays in nuclear extracts from unstimulated PBMCs obtained from GCR and GCS subjects and found that AP-1, but not NF-κB and CREB, DNA binding was significantly (P <0.01) increased approximately 2-fold in the GCR subjects. In order to further understand these mechanisms, we sequenced the c-jun and c-fos major components of AP-1 and found no evidence for polymorphism in their primary structure. We have recently shown that T lymphocytes and monocytes from GCR subjects generate a 2-fold excess of Fos protein which is secondary to an increase in the *c-fos* transcription rate[24]. We were able to suppress glucocorticoid receptor DNA binding in GCS subjects to levels seen in GCR subjects by a PMA inducible factor, which we have shown by co-immunoprecipitation studies to be c-Fos. Therefore, GCR subjects generate excess c-Fos which results excess AP-1 activity[25]. This would result in perpetuation of AP-1-mediated inflammation and would render the therapeutic effects of GCs less effective by sequestration of glucocorticoid receptors within the nucleus.

We then used the tuberculin-induced model of dermal inflammation to evaluate the effect of corticosteroids in regulating components of AP-1 *in vivo* on 9 GCS and 6 GCR asthmatic subjects for the regulatory components of AP-1 before and after 9 days of either of 40 mg prednisolone or placebo. Significantly greater expression of c-Fos, phosphorylated c-Jun and phosphorylated Jun amino terminal kinase (JNK) protein has been identified in GCR compared to GCS subjects. Corticosteroids suppressed phosphorylation of c-Jun and JNK in the GCS group, but enhanced phosphorylation of c-Jun and JNK in the GCR group[26].

Although we have yet to define a genetic mechanism, it is clearly established that there is excess AP-1 activity in GCR asthma. This molecular observation is consistent with the clinical observation that prolonged untreated asthma renders the subsequent response to GCs less effective . We speculate that this occurs as a result of chronic unopposed AP-1-mediated inflammation. If true, then early suppression of inflammation by GCs would predict a more favourable outcome in asthma by early suppression of AP-1-mediated inflammation.

β_2-Agonist therapy

β_2-Adrenoceptor agonists are used by virtually all patients as rescue bronchodilator[27,28]. Short and long-acting β_2-agonists exhibit protective effects against a variety of direct and indirect bronchoconstrictor stimuli. However, regularly scheduled treatment with β_2-agonists is associated with tachyphylaxis to the functional antagonism against bronchoconstrictor stimuli. There is evidence to show that inhaled corticosteroids and long-acting β_2-agonists given on a regular basis have additive effects in improving long-term asthma control. The debate about the safety of regular β-agonist use in asthma has evolved substantially over the past decade. In spite of epidemiological data suggesting an association between β-agonist use and asthma deaths and an early study suggesting decreased asthma control on regular fenoterol[29], the overwhelming message from subsequent, large clinical studies, has been reassuring[30,48].

β_2-Adrenoceptor polymorphism

One of the remaining issues in this debate is whether there might be a subgroup in the asthmatic population which does not benefit from regular β_2-agonist use, or which may be more vulnerable to rapid deterioration. One potential source of such an anomalous response could be DNA sequence variants within the β_2-adrenoceptor (β_2AR) gene. This intronless gene was cloned in 1987 and is situated on the long arm of chromosome 5 (5q 31-33). Nine polymorphisms have been described within the single coding region. Although five are degenerate, the four remaining polymorphisms result in single amino acid substitutions: glycine for arginine at amino acid 16, glutamate for glutamine at amino acid 27, methionine for valine at 34 and isoleucine for threonine at position 164. Amino acids 16 and 27 lie in the extracellular N-terminal domain, whereas amino acids 34 and 164 are in the transmembrane spanning regions. These polymorphisms have been found with equal frequency in normal and asthmatic populations[31] and are unlikely to be a cause of asthma *per se*, although they may influence the phenotype of the illness once it is expressed.

In vitro studies have shown that these polymorphisms have potential functional consequences. The relatively uncommon Ile-164 polymorphism results in a major decrease in agonist binding affinity and coupling to adenylate cyclase. Polymorphisms Gly-16 and Glu-27 did not affect receptor binding or coupling but markedly altered agonist-promoted receptor down-regulation and functional desensitisation; Gly-16 enhanced this down-regulation, whereas Glu-27 protected against it.

There are a number of recent clinical studies relating to the Gly-16 and Glu-27 polymorphisms, because the frequency of the minor allele is on the order of 40–50%; as would be expected there is strong linkage disequilibrium between these two sequence variants making it difficult to assign an effect to a single allele in association studies. A relatively early report suggested that homozygous Gly-16 was associated with a more severe asthma phenotype[31], but this has not been supported by more recent studies[32]. Gly-16 has also been associated with nocturnal asthma[33] and in children it has been reported to be associated with decreased broncho-dilator response to an inhaled β_2-agonist[34]. The potential protective Glu-27 polymorphism has indeed been reported to be associated with decreased airway reactivity in asthma[35] but it did not seem to influence nocturnal asthma[33] or bronchodilator responsiveness[34]. The Gln-27 allele, on the other hand, has been associated with elevated IgE levels and with an increase in self-reported asthma in children.

Lipworth et al[36] have recently reported that Gly-16 increased the propensity for bronchodilator desensitisation after the regular use of formoterol, although whether such tachyphylaxis actually occurs has been quite contro-versial, with most groups failing to find any drop-off in the bronchodilator effectiveness of β-agonists when they are used long-term in populations without genotype stratification. Lipworth *et al* pursued tachyphylaxis to bronchoprotection further and investigated the relationship of the common β_2AR polymorphisms to the fall-off in protection afforded by β_2-agonists against induced bronchoconstriction when in regular use (bronchoprotective subsensitivity or tachyphylaxis). β_2-agonist subsensitivity occurred irrespective of variations in β_2AR genotype. They found no association with the Glu-27 polymorphism although this may have been confounded by its linkage disequilibrium with Gly-16. At lower doses of formoterol, whereas the Gly-16 homozygotes showed uniform marked loss of protection, there was a much greater variability when Arg-16 allele was present.

Recently, Hancox and colleagues[37] reported the genotypes of the patients originally reported in 1990, where they studied the effects of regular *versus* as-needed fenoterol in a group of 64 asthmatics[29]. The earlier report showed a deterioration in 'asthma control' with regularly scheduled fenoterol treatment compared with as-needed. These investigators have now assessed β_2AR genotype at positions 16 and 27 in 61 of these subjects to determine whether changes in these variables in the earlier study were associated with β_2AR polymorphisms. During treatment with regularly scheduled fenoterol, subjects who were homozygous for Arg-16 had an increase in bronchial responsiveness to methacholine compared with their responsiveness when they did not receive regular treatment. This finding is consistent with patients who are homozygous for the Arg 16 form of the β_2-AR being predisposed to an adverse reaction to the regularly scheduled use of this β-agonist.

These findings have been corroborated by results obtained from the United States National Institutes of Health sponsored Asthma Clinical Research Network. They had previously shown, in a 16-week, randomised, placebo-controlled, double-blind, crossover trial in 255 patients with asthma, that, on average, regularly scheduled (2 puffs 4 times/day) salbutamol had no clinical or physiological deleterious effects compared with the use of salbutamol on an as-needed use schedule[38]. Although deleterious effects were not observed in the entire group, some individuals did display tachyphylaxis, particularly in the group allocated to regular salbutamol use. Genotyping at the 16th and 27th amino acids of the β_2AR was carried out with genomic DNA obtained from the patients after additional informed consent in 190 patients. Individuals with the Arg/Arg genotype receiving regularly scheduled salbutamol experienced a significant decline in morning PEFR over the course of the study ($P = 0.012$)[39]. This tachyphylaxis was not observed when treatment was given on an as-needed basis to patients with the same genotype. In contrast, those with the Gly/Gly genotype, even when receiving regularly scheduled albuterol, showed no tachyphylaxis. A similar pattern was observed with evening PEFR. The findings were not influenced by the position 27 genotype, race, sex, or initial lung function. These data are consistent with polymorphisms of the β_2AR at locus 16 being a significant genetic predictor of tachyphylaxis to the β-agonist salbutamol. Indeed, these results are consistent with the notion that the Gly-16 receptor is down-regulated maximally by endogenous catecholamines and thus cannot display additional down-regulation by salbutamol. On the other hand, the Arg-16 receptor is less down-regulated by endogenous catecholamines, but is down-regulated with chronic administration of salbutamol. This concept of dynamic regulation[40] is consistent with the results of Martinez *et al*[34], who showed a decreased initial response to salbutamol in patients homozygous for Gly-16.

Taken together, these data clearly indicate that genotype at the β_2AR can influence the response to a variety of treatment regimes with agents acting at this receptor. However, at present no clear picture has emerged about the relative importance of genotype on treatment outcomes and further study will be required before treatment recommendations stratified by genotype can be made.

Anti-leukotriene therapy

The newly released family of specifically targeted asthma treatments, namely agents that interfere with the synthesis or action of the leukotrienes, provide a previously unavailable method to identify a subset of patients in whom leukotrienes are key contributors to the expression of the asthma phenotype. These agents are produced when the 5-lipoxygenase (ALOX5) pathway, the name given to the series of biochemical reactions which result in the transformation of arachidonic acid, which is esterified in membrane phospholipids into leukotrienes[41], is activated.

There a number of observations suggesting that leukotrienes contribute to the pathogenesis of asthma. Firstly, they can induce many of the abnormalities seen in asthma, including airway obstruction, bronchovascular leak, mucus gland secretion, and granulocyte chemotaxis[42,43]. Secondly, they are, on a molar basis, among the most potent effector molecules known to cause airway obstruction. Thirdly, leukotriene E_4 (LTE_4), an end-product of leukotriene metabolism, can be recovered in increased amounts from the urine of individuals with allergic asthma after antigen challenge[44,45]. In addition, elevated levels of urinary LTE_4 are present in over two-thirds of patients presenting for the emergency treatment of asthmatic airway obstruction[42].

Leukotriene action may be pharmacologically modulated by antagonism at the receptor site or by biosynthesis inhibition. Both LTE_4 receptor antagonism and inhibition of ALOX5 biosynthesis have been shown to be effective anti-asthma treatments. There are several antileukotriene drugs which have been approved for the treatment of asthma. Zileuton is an inhibitor of ALOX5, while zafirlukast, pranlukast and montelukast are inhibitors of the action of LTD_4 at its receptor. A large number of clinical trials have been completed with these agents, establishing their efficacy in the treatment of spontaneous or induced asthma. All drugs have been shown to provide a superior effect, when compared to placebo, in the treatment of patients with mild-to-moderate asthma.

5-Lipoxygenase gene promoter polymorphisms

The failure of a patient with asthma to respond to antileukotriene treatment provides evidence consistent with the hypothesis that leukotrienes are not critical to the expression of the asthmatic phenotype in that patient. Among the pharmacogenetic causes of this clinical phenotype are genetic variants that down-regulate gene expression of ALOX5. A family of polymorphisms exists in the core promoter of the ALOX5 gene[46]. They consist of an alteration in the number of tandem Sp-1 and Egr-1 (early growth response protein) consensus binding sites, from the deletion of one or two or addition of one zinc finger binding sites in the region 176 to 147 base pairs up-stream from the ATG translation start site. The wild-type contains five such tandem repeats. 5-Lipoxygenase promoter reporter constructs containing these polymorphisms display less capacity for promoter binding and direct less gene transcription than constructs containing the wild-type ALOX5 core promoter. It seemed possible that such polymorphisms could explain a fraction of the heterogeneous therapeutic response to ALOX5 inhibition in asthmatic patients.

We reasoned that a patient harbouring any of the mutant forms of the ALOX5 core promoter would have decreased ALOX5 gene transcription and thus down-regulated ALOX5 expression. If ALOX5 products were among the several mediators contributing to the airway obstruction in asthma, and if patients harbouring the mutant genotypes had decreased leukotriene production, then these patients would have airway obstruction mediated by mechanisms other than the leukotrienes. As a consequence of this 'natural inhibition', patients harbouring the mutant genotypes would have a diminished response to exogenous ALOX5 inhibition. To test this idea, we examined data from a 12 week randomised, placebo-controlled and double-blind clinical trial of the effect of an ALOX5 inhibitor, ABT-761, stratified by genotype at the ALOX5 core promoter locus[47].

Patients with moderate asthma were treated with ABT-761 (high or low dose) or placebo for 12 weeks during which measurements of the FEV_1 were made at intervals; the FEV_1 was the primary outcome indicator. A total of 325 patients completed the entire protocol of whom about one-third received high dose ABT-761 therapy; this yielded enough patients to demonstrate superior efficacy of ABT-761 compared with placebo when FEV_1 was used as the outcome indicator. As expected from our previously published work[46], an allele frequency of 0.81 was found. Among the mutant alleles, most were deletion alleles S, that is alleles at this locus with fewer than 5 tandem repeats of the Sp-1 binding domain; the allele frequencies for alleles with 3 and 4 tandem Sp-1 binding motifs were 0.038 and 0.172, respectively.

Among the individuals receiving active treatment, patients with two wild-type alleles had a significantly greater FEV_1 at the completion of the trial than patients with no wild-type alleles (Fig. 5). The average change in the FEV_1 at the end of the active-treatment period was 18.8 ± 3.6% in wild-type patients and −1.1 ± 2.9% in mutant patients; the degree of change was significantly ($P = 2.5 \times 10^{-5}$) greater in the former group than

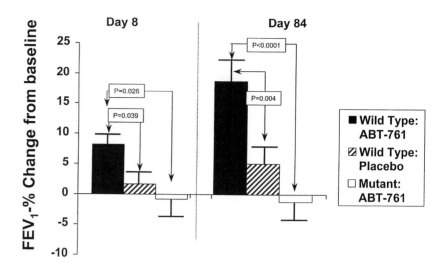

Fig. 5 Percent change in the FEV$_1$ from baseline for patients who had the wild-type genotype at the ALOX5 core promoter locus and were treated with either ABT-761 (green) or placebo (yellow) and for patients with no wild-type alleles at this locus (red) treated with ABT-761. Data are shown for the first, 29th, and final day of active treatment. The dose of ABT-761 was escalated from 150 mg/day to 300 mg/day after the measurement on day 29 was taken. Reprinted from[47] with permnission from the publisher.

in the latter. Although there were patients in whom a salutary therapeutic response was not observed who harboured the wild-type genotype, patients without wild-type alleles failed to manifest a salutary therapeutic response. This suggests that there are multiple ways for a patient to manifest a failed therapeutic response, of which a mutation in this core promoter genotype is one. It seems likely that a panel of DNA sequence variants at various loci in the ALOX5 pathway will be needed to explain all the observed variance in this novel form of asthma treatment.

Summary

Our understanding of asthma and its therapy has changed markedly over the last few years, particularly with the application of molecular and cell biology and the discovery of new and more specific pharmacological tools. It is timely to use these novel technologies to elucidate the mechanism(s) of heterogeneity of responsiveness to drug therapy, as this may provide insight into optimal targeting of drug therapy to subgroups of asthmatic patients. This may, in turn, provide greater understanding of underlying pathogenetic mechanisms.

References

1 Falconer DS, Mackay TFC. *Introduction to Quantitative Genetics.* Harlow: Addison Wesley Longman, 1996

2 Lynch M, Walsh B. *Genetics and Analysis of Quantitative Traits.* 1998

3 Lesells CM, Boag PT. Unrepeatable repeatabilities: a common mistake. *Auk* 1987; **104**: 116–21

4 Enright PL, Connett JE, Kanner RE, Johnson LR, Lee WW. Spirometry in the Lung Health Study II: determinants of short-term intra-individual variability. *Am J Respir Crit Care Med* 1995; **151**: 406–11

5 Enright PL, Johnson LR, Connett JE, Voelker H, Buist AS. Spirometry in the Lung Health Study I: methods and quality control. *Am J Respir Crit Care Med* 1991; **143**: 1215–23

6 Lane SJ, Lee TH. Mechanism and detection of glucocorticoid insensitivity in asthma. *Allergy Clin Immunol Int* 1997; **9**: 165–73

7 Schwartz HJ, Lowell FC, Melby JC. Steroid resistance in bronchial asthma. *Ann Intern Med* 1968; **69**: 4493

8 Carmichael J, Paterson IC, Diaz P, Crompton GK, Kay AB, Grant IWB. Corticosteroid resistance in chronic asthma. *BMJ* 1981; **282**:1419–22

9 Lane SJ. Pathogenesis of steroid-resistant asthma. *Br J Hosp Med* 1997; **57**: 394–8

10 Corrigan CJ, Brown PH, Barnes NC, Tsai JJ, Frew AJ, Kay AB. Glucocorticoid resistance in chronic asthma – peripheral-blood lymphocyte-T activation and comparison of the lymphocyte-T inhibitory effects of glucocorticoids and cyclosporin-A. *Am Rev Respir Dis* 1991; **144**: 1026–32

11 Corrigan CJ, Brown PH, Barnes NC et al. Glucocorticoid resistance in chronic asthma – glucocorticoid pharmacokinetics, glucocorticoid receptor characteristics, and inhibition of peripheral blood T cell proliferation by glucocorticoids *in vitro. Am Rev Respir Dis* 1991; **144**: 1016–25

12 Leung DYM, Martin RJ, Szefler SJ et al. Dysregulation of interleukin-4, interleukin-5, and interferon-gamma gene-expression in steroid-resistant asthma. *J Exp Med* 1995; **181**: 33–40

13 Lane SJ, Atkinson BA, Swaminathan R, Lee TH. Hypothalamic-pituitary-adrenal axis in corticosteroid-resistant bronchial asthma. *Am J Respir Crit Care Med* 1996; **153**: 557–60

14 Lane SJ, Vaja S, Swaminathan R, Lee TH. Effects of prednisolone on bone turnover in patients with corticosteroid resistant asthma. *Clin Exp Allergy* 1996; **26**:1197–201

15 May CS, Caffin JA, Halliday JW, Bochner F. Prednisolone pharmacokinetics in asthmatic patients. *Br J Dis Chest* 1980; **74**: 91–2

16 Rose JQ, Nickelson JA, Ellis EF, Middleton E, Jusko WJ. Prednisolone disposition in steroid-dependent asthmatic children. *J Allergy Clin Immunol* 1981; **67**: 188–93

17 Lane SJ, Lee TH. Glucocorticoid receptor characteristics in monocytes of patients with corticosteroid-resistant bronchial-asthma. *Am Rev Respir Dis* 1991; **143**: 1020–4

18 Sher ER, Leung DYM, Surs W et al. Steroid-resistant asthma – cellular mechanisms contributing to inadequate response to glucocorticoid therapy. *J Clin Invest* 1994; **93**: 33–9

19 Adcock IM, Lane SJ, Brown CR, Peters MJ, Lee TH, Barnes PJ. Differences in binding of glucocorticoid receptor to DNA in steroid-resistant asthma. *J Immunol* 1995; **154**: 3500–5

20 Leung DYM, Hamid Q, Vottero A et al. Association of glucocorticoid insensitivity with increased expression of glucocorticoid receptor beta. *J Exp Med* 1997; **186**: 1567–74

21 Lane SJ, Arm JP, Staynov DZ, Lee TH. Chemical mutational analysis of the human glucocorticoid receptor cDNA in glucocorticoid-resistant bronchial asthma. *Am J Respir Cell Mol Biol* 1994; **11**: 42–8

22 Lane SJ. *Mechanism of Glucocorticoid Resistance in Chronic Bronchial Asthma.* PhD thesis: University of London, 1994

23 Adcock IM, Lane SJ, Brown CR, Lee TH, Barnes PJ. Abnormal glucocorticoid receptor activator protein-1 interaction in steroid-resistant asthma. *J Exp Med* 1995; **182**: 1951–8

24 Lane SJ, Adcock IM, Barnes PJ, Lee TH. Increased c-Fos synthesis in mononuclear-cells from patients with corticosteroid resistant asthma. *J Allergy Clin Immunol* 1996; **97**: 529

25 Lane SJ, Adcock IM, Richards D, Hawrylowicz C, Barnes PJ, Lee TH. Corticosteroid-resistant bronchial asthma is associated with increased c-Fos expression in monocytes and T lymphocytes. *J Clin Invest* 1998; **102**: 2156–64

26 Sousa AR, Lane SJ, Lee TH. *In vivo* resistance to corticosteroids in bronchial asthma is associated with enhanced phosphorylation of jun amino terminal kinase (JNK) and failure of prednisolone to inhibit JNK phosphorylation. *J Allergy Clin Immunol* 1999; **104**: 565–74

27 National Asthma Education and Prevention Programme. *Guidelines for the Diagnosis and Management of Asthma.* Expert Panel Report II. Bethesda, MD: National Institutes of Health publication. 1997

28 Anon. The British guidelines on asthma management. *Thorax* 1997; **52**: S1

29 Sears MR, Taylor DR, Print CG *et al*. Regular inhaled beta-agonist treatment in bronchial asthma. *Lancet* 1990; **336**: 1391–6

30 Taylor DR, Town GI, Herbison GP *et al*. Asthma control during long-term treatment with regular inhaled salbutamol and salmeterol. *Thorax* 1998; **53**: 744–52

31 Reihsaus E, Innis M, MacIntyre N, Liggett SB. Mutations in the gene encoding for the beta$_2$-adrenergic receptor in normal and asthmatic subjects. *Am Respir Cell Mol Biol* 1993; **8**: 334–9

32 Dewar JC, Wheatley AP, Venn A, Morrison JFJ, Britton J, Hall IP. Beta$_2$-adrenoceptor polymorphisms are in linkage disequilibrium but are not associated with asthma in an adult population. *Clin Exp Allergy* 1998; **28**: 442–8

33 Turki J, Pak J, Green SA, Martin RJ, Liggett SB. Genetic polymorphisms of the beta$_2$-adrenergic receptor in nocturnal and non-nocturnal asthma. *J Clin Invest* 1995; **95**: 1635–41

34 Martinez FD, Graves PE, Baldini M, Solomon S, Erickson R. Association between genetic polymorphisms of the beta$_2$-adrenoceptor and response to albuterol in children with and without a history of wheezing. *J Clin Invest* 1997; **100**: 3184–8

35 Hall IP, Wheatley A, Wilding P, Liggett SB. Association of the Glu-27 beta$_2$-adrenoceptor polymorphism with lower airway reactivity in asthmatic subjects. *Lancet* 1995; **345**: 1213–4

36 Lipworth BJ, Hall IP, Aziz I, Tan KS, Wheatley A. Beta$_2$-adrenoceptor polymorphism and bronchoprotective sensitivity with regular short and long-acting beta$_2$-agonist therapy. *Clin Sci* 1999; **96**: 253–9

37 Hancox RJ, Sears MR, Taylor DR. Polymorphism of the beta(2)-adrenoceptor and the response to long-term beta(2)-agonist therapy in asthma. *Eur Respir J* 1998; **11**: 589–93

38 Drazen JM, Israel E, Boushey HA *et al*. Comparison of regularly scheduled with as-needed use of albuterol in mild asthma. *N Engl J Med* 1996; **335**: 841–7

39 Israel E, Drazen JM, Boushey HA *et al*. The effects of polymorphisms of the beta$_2$-adrenergic receptor on the response to regular use of albuterol in asthma. *Am J Respir Crit Care Med* 2000; **162**: 75–80

40 Liggett SB, Green SA. Molecular biology of the β_2-adrenergic receptor: focus on interactions of agonist with receptor. In: Pauwels R, Lofdahl CG, O'Byrne P. (eds) *Beta$_s$-Agonists in Asthma Treatment*. New York: Marcel Dekker, 1996; 19–34

41 Samuelsson B. Leukotrienes: mediators of immediate hypersensitivity reactions and inflammation. *Science* 1983; **220**: 568–75

42 Drazen JM, O'Brien J, Sparrow D *et al*. Recovery of leukotriene-E$_4$ from the urine of patients with airway obstruction. *Am Rev Respir Dis* 1992; **146**: 104–8

43 Piper PJ. Leukotrienes and the airways. *Eur J Anaesthesiol* 1989; **6**: 241–55

44 Taylor GW, Taylor I, Black P *et al*. Urinary leukotriene E$_4$ after antigen challenge and in acute asthma and allergic rhinitis. *Lancet* 1989; **i**: 584–8

45 Sladek K, Dworski R, Fitzgerald GA *et al*. Allergen-stimulated release of thromboxane A$_2$ and leukotriene E$_4$ in humans. Effect of indomethacin. *Am Rev Respir Dis* 1990; **141**: 1441–5

46 In KH, Asano K, Beier D, Grobholz J *et al*. Naturally-occurring mutations in the human 5-lipoxygenase gene promoter that modify transcription factor binding and reporter gene transcription. *J Clin Invest* 1997; **99**: 1130–7

47 Drazen JM, Yandava C, Dube LM *et al*. Pharmacogenetic association between *ALOX5* promoter genotype and the response to anti-asthma treatment. *Nat Genet* 1999; **22**: 168–70

48 Dennis S, Sharpe S, Vickers M et al. The effects of regular inhaled salbutamol on asthma control: the main result of TRUST. *Lancet* 2000; **355**: 1675–9

Allergen avoidance: does it work?

Ashley Woodcock and **Adnan Custovic**

North West Lung Centre, Wythenshawe Hospital, Manchester, UK

The first recorded example of allergen avoidance in the treatment of allergic disorders dates from the 16th century. The Italian physician Gerolamo Cardano (1501–1576) was invited to Scotland by John Hamilton, Archbishop of St Andrews (and brother of the Regent), to give advice on the treatment of his asthma. Cardano recommended that the Archbishop should get rid of his feather bedding, which was followed by a 'miraculous' remission of otherwise troublesome symptoms. The first controlled attempts to treat asthma by environmental manipulation date to the beginning of 20th century. In 1925, the Leopold brothers treated patients with asthma and other allergic disorders by moving them into a dust free room[1]. Storm van Leeuwen created a 'climate' chamber in The Netherlands in 1927 and demonstrated that asthmatic patients improved when moved from their homes into the chamber[2]. One year later, Dekker observed that measures aimed at reducing the amount of dust in bedrooms had a beneficial effect on asthma symptoms in patients allergic to house dust[3]. Van Leeuwen wrote[2]: *'In our endeavours to find the cause of the attack...we utilised the known fact that the environment of the asthmatic patient is, as a rule, of primary importance in determining the intensity and frequency of his attacks'*. Nowadays, more than ever, it is essential to address the environmental influences on the increasing prevalence of asthma and allergic disorders.

The majority of people in the industrialised world spend most of their time inside one type of building or another, and the indoor environment has begun to attract deserved attention over the last several years. We are beginning to appreciate that living in a damp house may have more adverse effects on respiratory health than living next to a busy motorway. The indoor environment of modern homes contains many substances that can cause or exacerbate allergic disease in susceptible individuals. The major biological sources of allergens are acarids (*e.g.* house dust mites), insects (*e.g.* cockroaches), domestic animals (cats and dogs) and fungi, but also such sources as rodents and pollens derived from outside. In addition, environmental tobacco smoke (ETS), indoor air pollution (*e.g.* NO_2 and ozone) and endotoxin may have potential roles as the enhancers of both allergic sensitisation and disease.

*Correspondence to:
Prof. Ashley Woodcock,
Lung Function Unit,
North West Lung Centre,
Wythenshawe Hospital,
Southmoor Road,
Manchester M23 9LT, UK*

Avoidance of indoor allergens

The effectiveness of allergen reduction in the treatment of asthma was first suggested by studies in which patients were removed from their homes into a low allergen environment of high altitude sanatoria[4-6]. However, the real challenge is to create a low allergen environment in patients' homes. Although not easy, it is possible to achieve substantial reductions in allergen exposure. Effective control strategies should be tailored to individual allergens, flexible to suit individual needs and cost-effective.

Distribution and aerodynamic properties of indoor allergens-relevance to avoidance

Knowledge of the sources and aerodynamics of allergen-carrying particles is essential for the design of successful strategies to reduce personal exposure. Allergens from mites, cats, dogs and cockroaches have different aerodynamic properties (Table 1)[7-16]. Mite and cockroach allergens can be detected in the air in significant amounts only after vigorous disturbance, and are predominantly, but not exclusively, contained within relatively large particles (> 10 μm diameter)[7-12]. In contrast, airborne cat and dog allergens are readily measured in houses with pets (and in a quarter of the homes without pets), and ~25% of airborne Fel d 1 and Can f 1 is associated with small particles (< 5 μmm diameter)[13-16]. This underlies the difference in the clinical presentation of the disease. Mite and cockroach sensitive asthmatics are usually unaware of the relationship between allergen exposure at home and asthma symptoms (exposure is low grade and chronic). The large particles, however, may contain a large quantity of allergen, and even small numbers may cause a significant inflammatory response when impacted in the airways. In contrast, cat or dog allergic patients often develop symptoms within minutes of entering a home with a pet due to the inhalation of large amounts of airborne allergen on

Table 1 Aerodynamic characteristics of house dust mite, cat, dog and cockroach allergens

Allergen		Particle size	Airborne level	
Mite:	Group 1 Group 2	Large particles > 10 μm	**Undisturbed:** Undetectable with conventional assays (< 0.2 ng/m³ for mite allergens, < 0.02 ng/m³ for cockroach)	**Disturbed** Detectable after vigorous disturbance
Cockroach:	Bla g 1 Bla g 2			
Cat: Dog:	Fel d 1 Can f 1	Large particles >5 μm (~75%) Small particles <5 μm (~25%)	**Homes with animal** Detectable in all homes. Levels 4–5 times higher with animal in the room	**Homes without animal** Detectable in ~1/3 of the homes without artificial disturbance

small particles which can penetrate deep into respiratory tract inducing acute asthma. Application of this information in terms of avoidance strategies is important, implying, for example, that air filtration units have no place in mite or cockroach avoidance, but may be useful in removing cat and dog allergen from the air.

It is important to know where patients receive most of their exposure. The bed is the most important source of mite allergens and lowering exposure in the bedroom is the primary target of avoidance. In contrast, it is likely that the majority of exposure to allergens of domestic pets occurs in the living room area, and this must be taken into account when planning avoidance strategies.

Control of house dust mites and mite allergens

The most effective and probably most important avoidance measure is to cover mattress, pillows and duvet with covers that are impermeable to mite allergens. Development of water vapour-permeable fabrics which are both mite allergen impermeable and comfortable have considerably increased compliance. Allergen levels are dramatically reduced after the introduction of covers[17], which should be robust, easily fitted and easily cleaned, as their effectiveness is reduced if they are damaged. Mite allergens can accumulate on the covers and it is important that covers are wiped at each change of bedding. All exposed bedding should be washed at 55°C (the temperature that kills mites)[18]. The cold cycle of laundry washing reduces allergen levels, but most of the mites survive. Additives for detergents providing a concentration of 0.03% benzyl benzoate, or dilute solutions of essential oils in normal and low temperature washing provide alternative methods of mite control[19].

Carpets are an important microhabitat for mite colonisation and a possible source of allergen from which beds can be re-infested[20]. Fitted carpets should ideally be replaced with polished wood or vinyl flooring. Exposure of carpets to direct strong sunlight may be used in loosely fitted carpets in certain climatic areas[21]. Steam cleaning may be used as a method of killing mites and reducing allergen levels in carpets[22]. A number of different chemicals that kill mites (acaricides) have been identified, and shown to be effective under laboratory conditions[23]. However, data on whether these chemicals can be successfully applied to carpets and upholstered furniture are still conflicting, as the method of application of the benzyl-benzoate moist powder on carpets is very important[24]. The main problem of chemical treatment is not its ability to kill mites, but how to get the chemicals to penetrate deep into carpet and soft furnishing, the persistence of mite allergen until re-colonisation occurs, and the nuisance of frequent re-applications. Freezing with liquid nitrogen can also kill mites[25]. However, the technique can only be carried out by a trained operator, which limits its use, especially since treatment needs to be repeated regularly. When used, both acaricides and liquid nitrogen should be combined with intensive vacuum cleaning following administration.

The protein-denaturing properties of tannic acid are well recognised, and it has been recommended for the reduction of indoor allergen levels in house dust. However, high levels of proteins in dust (*e.g.* cat allergen in a home with a cat) block its effects[26].

Intensive vacuum cleaning may remove large amounts of dust from carpets, reducing the size of allergen reservoir. However, vacuum cleaners with inadequate exhaust filtration may increase airborne allergen levels during use[27]. Thus, atopic asthmatic patients should use HEPA-filter vacuum cleaners with double thickness vacuum cleaner bags, although the benefits have not been established in a clinical trial. Ducted systems offer similar advantages.

High levels of humidity in the microhabitats are essential for mite population growth, and reducing humidity may be an effective control method. However, detailed models of the humidity profile of domestic microclimates (*e.g.* in relation to humans in bed) are not yet available. Reducing central humidity alone may be ineffective in reducing humidity in mite microhabitats (*e.g.* in the middle of a mattress). Reducing humidity by mechanical ventilation heat recovery units or dehumidifiers should be used in areas where the climate is right, *i.e.* where winters are dry and cold[28–31].

Due to the aerodynamic characteristics of mite allergens, it makes little sense to use air filtration units and ionisers as the only way of reducing personal exposure.

Since mites live in different sites throughout the house, it is unlikely that a single measure can solve the problem of exposure, and an integrated approach including barrier methods, dust removal and removal of mite

Table 2 Measures for reducing house dust mite allergen exposure

Encase mattress, pillow and quilt in impermeable covers
Wash all bedding in the hot cycle (55–60°C) weekly
Replace carpets with linoleum or wood flooring
If carpets cannot be removed, treat with acaricides and/or tannic acid
Minimise upholstered furniture/replace with leather furniture
Keep dust accumulating objects in closed cupboards
Use a vacuum cleaner with integral HEPA filter and double thickness bags
Replace curtains with blinds or easily washable (hot cycle) curtains
Hot wash/freeze soft toys

microhabitats is needed (Table 2). One such approach was recently used and shown to be highly effective in achieving and maintaining a very low allergen environment in homes of children at high risk of allergic disease[32].

Pet allergen avoidance

Complete avoidance of pet allergens is all but impossible, as sensitised patients can be exposed to pet allergens not only in homes with pets, but also in homes without pets and in public buildings and public transport[33–35].

The major cat allergen Fel d 1 is produced primarily in the sebaceous glands and in the basal squamous epithelial cells of the skin. Its production is under hormonal control, and the castration of male cats results in a 3–5-fold reduction of Fel d 1 concentration in skin washing. Testosterone treatment restores the Fel d 1 levels to precastration values[36]. It has recently been suggested that Fel d 1 production is higher in male than in female cats[37]. However, the observed gender difference in Fel d 1 secretion is too small to suggest that patients allergic to cats could benefit by getting a female rather than male cat, or by castrating their male cats.

The best way to reduce exposure to cat or dog allergen is to remove the animal from the home. Even after permanent removal of the animal, it can take many months before reservoir allergen levels decrease[38]. Unfortunately, despite continued symptoms many pet allergic patients insist on keeping their pet. Asthma is often severe and difficult to control in pet sensitised asthmatics who continue to be exposed to high allergen levels because they refuse to get rid of the family pet[39].

Control of the airborne allergen levels with a pet in home

Airborne pet allergen levels increase by ~5-fold when a pet is in a room, indicating that the immediate presence of a pet contributes to airborne allergen levels[15]. Pets should be kept out of the bedroom, and preferably outdoors.

Several studies have investigated the effect of washing pets on allergen levels[40–42]. Washing dogs in a bath using a hand-held shower unit and shampoo and rinsing thoroughly produced a substantial, but short-lived, fall in recovered Can f 1[42]. Pet washing may reduce airborne allergen in an experimental room, but the effect in homes with pets is largely unknown[41,42]. De Blay et al reported a reduction in airborne Fel d 1 following washing one cat weekly over a 4 week period[41], and a similar reduction in airborne Can f 1 was observed in homes with dogs[42]. However, the main benefit of washing the pet regularly, probably twice

Table 3 Measures for reducing cat/dog allergen exposure

Remove cat/dog from the home
If the pet cannot be removed:
Keep the pet out of the main living areas and bedrooms
Install HEPA air cleaners in the main living areas and bedrooms
Have the pet washed twice a week
Thoroughly clean upholstered furniture/replace with leather furniture
Replace carpets with linoleum or wood flooring
Fit allergen-impermeable bedding covers
Use a vacuum cleaner with integral HEPA filter and double thickness bags

weekly, may be the reduction in the build-up of allergen in dust reservoirs (*e.g.* carpets and upholstered furniture), but this too is unproven.

Airborne pet allergens in homes with pets can be reduced by the use of a HEPA air cleaner[16,43]. Vacuum cleaners which contain integral HEPA filters and double thickness bags do not leak allergens into the air[44].

Since getting rid of the family pet is rarely a viable option, in patients who are allergic to cats or dogs and persist in keeping their pet we propose the set of measures listed in Table 3.

Avoidance of cockroach allergens

In areas where housing conditions sustain large cockroach populations, both physical and chemical control measures should be used[45]. Reducing access to food and water is critical, thus waste food should be removed and surface water should be contained by reducing leakage through faulty taps and pipework, and reducing condensation by improved ventilation. Cockroach access should be restricted by caulking and sealing cracks and holes in the plasterwork and flooring. Several chemicals are marketed for controlling cockroach infestation, including diazinon, chlorpyrifos and boric acid. The most useful for patients with allergic disease are bait stations, where the chemical (hydramethylnon, avermectin) is retained within a plastic housing. A paste formulation of hydramethylnon may be used on cockroach runways and underneath counters, *etc*. Bait stations are generally effective at reducing cockroach levels for 2–3 months.

The attempts to reduce cockroach allergen exposure rely on improving patient education and concerted attempts by pest control companies and public health departments to reduce cockroach infestation.

Fungi

Airborne fungal spore concentrations have been associated with adverse health outcomes in children (*e.g.* respiratory symptoms were associated with an increase in indoor *Cladosporium* exposure)[46]. Exposure to *Cladosporium* and *Penicillium* was found to be a risk factor for sensitisation to these genera, but also for allergy to other fungal extracts, and, in the case of *Penicillium* exposure, for allergy to house dust and dog[46]. It is thus possible that fungal exposure may have an allergen-specific effect on sensitisation, but also a non-specific effect on immune system facilitating sensitisation to other allergens (perhaps via mycotoxins and β-glucans). Therefore, reducing exposure to fungi may be important. Removing or cleaning mould-laden objects and maintaining a low humidity (less than 50%) may be beneficial in reducing fungal allergens. Using a dehumidifier and/or air conditioning unit can reduce both mould and bacteria. Care should be taken to make sure that dehumidifiers or air conditioning units do not become contaminated with moulds and thus form a new source of allergens or non-specific irritants. In tropical and subtropical climates, fungi might grow on the walls of the house due to water leakage and humidity. To avoid this, the walls could be tiled or cleaned as necessary.

Avoidance of outdoor allergens

The most important outdoor allergens which often induce symptoms in susceptible individuals are pollens and mould spores. However, the threshold levels which induce sensitisation and/or clinical reaction remain to be determined. Although outdoor pollens and moulds are impossible to avoid completely, closing windows and doors and remaining indoors (particularly when pollen and fungal spore counts are high) may reduce personal exposure and works at a symptomatic level in hay fever sufferers. The information about a patient's sensitivity to specific allergens may be useful for giving advice about the timing and location of the patient's travel.

Allergen avoidance: does it work?

Exposure to allergens has a profound effect on the development of IgE mediated sensitisation (primary sensitisation), progression from sensitisation to allergic disease (secondary exposure) and the severity of symptoms in the established disease (tertiary exposure). The potential benefits of allergen avoidance can be assessed in terms of: (i) prevention of allergic sensitisation (primary prevention by allergen avoidance); (ii) prevention of atopic disease in sensitised individuals (secondary avoidance); and (iii) effectiveness in the treatment of established disease.

There have been very few studies on primary or secondary avoidance. In contrast, there have been many studies of variable quality investigating allergen avoidance in the treatment of disease (reviewed by Custovic *et al*[45]).

Lessons from high altitude studies

In Europe, mite allergen levels are very low at high altitude where the ambient humidity is insufficient to support mite populations. Testing the hypothesis of a cause and effect relationship between exposure to dust mite allergens and sensitisation, Charpin *et al* compared the prevalence of asthma and positive skin test to mites in subjects living in the Alps and those living at sea level[47]. Briancon in the French Alps (altitude 1326 m) is the highest city in Europe, with a mean annual absolute outdoor humidity of 5.7 g/kg, thus making it unfavourable for mite population growth. Martigues (near Marseilles), on the contrary, is located on the French Mediterranean coast and has a mean annual absolute outdoor humidity of 9.3 g/kg, which is conducive for mite growth. The prevalence of mite allergy in a random sample of 18–65-year-old adults was found to be 4-fold higher in those living in Martigues (44.5%) compared to Briancon (10%). In a later study conducted by the same authors, a similar pattern of sensitisation was found in schoolchildren where the prevalence of skin test sensitivity to mite allergens was found to be 16.7% in Martigues compared with 4.1% in Briancon[48]. House dust mite allergen level in mattresses was found to be much lower in the Alps (0.36 mg/g of dust) than at sea level (15.8 mg/g of dust). The authors appropriately subtitled their paper *A paradigm of the influence of the environmental exposure on allergic sensitisation* and suggested that living in a mite-free environment reduce the risk of sensitisation and development of respiratory symptoms.

There are several sanatoria built in the Alps (*e.g.* Davos, Switzerland and Misurina, Italy), in which long-term residence can be beneficial for asthmatic children[49–56]. Dust mite sensitive asthmatic children had a progressive reduction in non-specific airway reactivity after a 1 year period spent in Davos[49,50]. Several studies from Misurina reported a reduction in asthma symptoms and significant decreases in mite allergen induced basophil histamine release, mite-specific serum IgE level and methacholine and allergen-induced airway reactivity. However, further studies also observed reversal of this trend towards improvement 15 days after returning to sea level. The result of high-altitude studies suggest that mite allergen avoidance leads to a decrease of airway inflammation with consequent improvement in specific and non-specific airway reactivity and symptoms and that re-exposure results in a rapid relapse. These studies were not controlled, and there is a possibility that other domestic factors (*e.g.* exposure to pets, environmental tobacco smoke, *etc.*) contributed to the observed improvement in asthma control. Nevertheless, mite avoidance is the most plausible reason for clinical success.

The high altitude studies suggest that:

- With low levels of allergen exposure in high altitude residents, rates of sensitisation and allergic disease are low

- To get clinical effect in established allergic disease, it is essential to achieve and maintain a major reduction in allergen levels

- Even with such a reduction in exposure, it may take many months for the effect on symptoms, medication use, pulmonary function, non-specific and specific airway reactivity and immunological parameters to become fully apparent.

High altitude studies provide an important proof of a principle: a substantial reduction in allergen exposure over a long period of time may result in clinical improvement in allergic asthmatic patients.

Clinical trials of mite allergen avoidance in patients' homes

Having explored various methods of allergen avoidance, the important question is whether allergen avoidance in homes by these techniques improves asthma control in sensitised patients. This is an area of controversy, mainly because of the inadequacies of the clinical studies on allergen avoidance. It is very difficult to conduct a placebo-controlled trial in this area: the combination of skin wheal and home visit is a potent stimulus for a change in behaviour, resulting in increased cleaning, removal of mite habitats and reduction in allergen levels even in a non-intervention group. Virtually every controlled study has observed a significant reduction in mite allergen levels and sometimes improved clinical symptoms in both the control group as well as the active group. Furthermore, as stressed previously, a successful trial would need to achieve and maintain a major reduction in allergen levels, be sufficiently long (*i.e.* probably not less that a year, with at least 6 weeks run-in period) and have adequate power.

The majority of studies on allergen avoidance in patients' homes have been small, poorly controlled and have often used measures that we now realise do not reduce mite allergen exposure. Consequently, many fail to show clinical benefits. We have recently reviewed 31 trials of mite allergen avoidance regimens in asthma in the literature[45,57–87]. Most of the studies have been small, poorly controlled and have used measures that failed to reduce mite allergen exposure. Of the 31 studies, only 9 showed significant reduction in mite counts and/or mite allergen levels.

In 3 of these 9, the period of treatment was too short, but nonetheless showed some effect. The final 6 controlled studies, all of which used bed covers, achieved both significant reduction in mites/allergen levels and were sufficiently long to show an effect on outcomes. Although these 6 studies had different endpoints, they all showed some evidence of clinical benefit. Whilst all trials of bed coverings suggest they are clinically effective, the impact of their widespread use by asthmatics has not been determined in a public health context. The Cochrane Airways Group have also recently published a meta-analysis on the effectiveness of mite allergen avoidance[88]. Of 23 studies, only 3 met the basic criteria of: (i) being randomised and controlled; (ii) demonstrating substantial reduction in mite allergen exposure; and (iii) lasting 6 months or longer. These 3 studies (1 in adults, 2 in children, total randomised subjects 123), although small and with diverse endpoints, again suggest some clinical benefit. Which patients benefit and whether treatment is cost-effective is unknown. Large-scale trials are underway to answer these questions. One such study on the effect of mite allergen avoidance by the use of allergen impermeable bedding on asthma control is currently being carried out in the UK. This is a randomised, parallel group, double blind, placebo controlled trial, due to randomise 1500 patients. During the first 6 months of the trial, patients will take their usual inhaled steroid therapy, and during the next 6 months patients will make a controlled reduction of inhaled steroids.

House dust mite allergen avoidance have been shown to be of some benefit in the treatment of atopic dermatitis and perennial allergic rhinitis[89-95].

Clinical trial of pet allergen avoidance

A recent study investigated the effectiveness of environmental allergen control using high efficiency particulate arrest (HEPA) air cleaners in the management of asthma and rhinitis in cat allergic patients who were sharing their home with one or more cats[96]. Although a small reduction in airborne Fel d 1 was observed in the active (but not in the control group), there was no difference between the groups in any of the outcome measures during the 3 months of a study. The reduction in cat allergen exposure afforded by the measures used in this trial was modest (~50%). It seems likely that a much more complex series of measures are needed if substantial reduction in exposure to airborne cat allergen is to be achieved. As outlined before, these could include keeping the pet out of the bedrooms and main living areas, installing HEPA air filtration units in the main living areas and bedrooms, washing the pet twice a week, thorough cleaning of the upholstered furniture (or replacing it with leather furniture), replacing carpets with linoleum or wood flooring and using a vacuum cleaner with integral HEPA filter and double thickness bags. Although such an integrated approach may have a desired clinical effect, it is essential that this is validated in a clinical trial.

Allergen avoidance in the primary prevention of atopy

Epidemiological studies suggest that in the areas with low levels of allergens in homes, the prevalence of sensitisation is low. Any primary allergen avoidance should be started early in infancy if maximum benefit is to be achieved. The Isle of Wight study has produced the first indication that even a modest reduction in house dust mite allergen levels in homes of infants at risk of allergy may reduce the prevalence of sensitisation to mites and recurrent wheezing during the first years of life[97,98]. The trial was unfortunately complicated by a multifaceted intervention strategy, including dietary advice to mothers during the pregnancy, as well as an attempt to reduce mite allergen exposure by the use of the acaricide benzyl benzoate (a relatively ineffective avoidance measure).

Recent studies have suggested that it may be necessary to start the environmental manipulation even before birth, *i.e.* early in pregnancy. There is an increasing body of evidence that the initial priming of the T cell system to environmental allergens may occur before birth, probably during late gestation, and that this process in infants at high risk of atopy may be skewed from Th1-like to Th2-like phenotype. This has been the subject of three recent review articles[99–101]. It has recently been suggested that maternal exposure to allergens from the 22nd week of pregnancy may play an important role in fetal T-cell priming. It is possible that allergen crossing the placenta may be involved in the subsequent development of atopy. Whilst this scenario may be applicable for food allergens, which are present at relatively high concentrations in the maternal circulation, it is considerably harder to explain how minute quantities of inhalant allergens (*e.g.* mite allergens with typical exposure in the order of 1 µg/year) could cross the placenta and sensitise the offspring. However, it would appear advisable to implement any trials of allergen avoidance during pregnancy (probably second and third trimester) in families at high risk of developing allergic disease.

Conclusions

Minimising the impact of identified environmental risk factors is a first step to reduce the severity of asthma. Although environmental control is difficult, we predict that it will be an integral part of the overall management of allergen sensitised patients. If the benefits attributable to allergen avoidance were instead attributed to a new drug, that drug would be the subject of trials involving thousands of patients. It is unfortunate that the perceived lack of commercial benefit has discouraged large-scale population-based trials.

The results of on-going large-scale trials of the widespread applicability of mite allergen avoidance and the effect on patient symptoms, exacerbation rate, use of medication and overall health costs study will conclusively show whether a simple intervention designed to reduce domestic mite allergen exposure can improve the clinical control of asthma, which subgroups of patients benefit, and whether the intervention is cost-effective. There is little data on benefits of primary and secondary prevention by environmental control, and several prospective studies are currently under way. The results of these trials will provide conclusive evidence of the effect of environmental control measures in prevention of sensitisation and development of allergic disease.

References

1 Leopold SS, Leopold CS. Bronchial asthma and allied allergic disorders. Preliminary report of a study under controlled conditions of environment, temperature and humidity. *JAMA* 1925; **84**: 731–5

2 Storm van Leeuwen W, Einthoven W, Kremer W. The allergen proof chamber in the treatment of bronchial asthma and other respiratory diseases. *Lancet* 1927; **i**: 1287–9

3 Dekker H. Asthma und milben. *Munch Med Wochenschr* 1928; **75**: 515–6

4 Piacentini GL, Martinati L, Fornari A *et al*. Antigen avoidance in a mountain environment: influence on basophil releasability in children with allergic asthma. *J Allergy Clin Immunol* 1993; **92**: 644–50

5 Peroni DG, Boner AL, Vallone G, Antolini I, Warner JO. Effective allergen avoidance at high altitude reduces allergen-induced bronchial hyperresponsiveness. *Am J Respir Crit Care Med* 1994; **149**: 1442–6

6 van Velzen E, van den Bos JW, Benckhuijsen JAW, van Essel T, de Bruijn R, Aalbers R. Effect of allergen avoidance at high altitude on direct and indirect bronchial hyperresponsiveness and markers of inflammation in children with allergic asthma. *Thorax* 1996; **51**: 582–4

7 Sakaguchi M, Inouye S, Yasueda H, Shida T. Concentration of airborne mite allergens (*Der* I and *Der* II) during sleep. *Allergy* 1992; **47**: 55–7

8 Custovic A, Taggart SCO, Niven RMcL, Woodcock A. Monitoring exposure to house dust mite allergens. *J Allergy Clin Immunol* 1995; **96**: 134–5

9 Swanson MC, Campbell AR, Klauck MJ, Reed CE. Correlation between levels of mite and cat allergens in settled and airborne dust. *J Allergy Clin Immunol* 1989; **83**: 776–83

10 Custovic A, Simpson B, Simpson A, Hallam C, Craven M, Woodcock A. Relationship between mite, cat and dog allergens in reservoir dust and ambient air. *Allergy* 1999; **54**: 612–6

11 De Lucca S, Sporik R, O'Meara T, Tovey ER. Mite allergen (Der p 1) is not only carried on mite feces. *J Allergy Clin Immunol* 1999; **103**: 174–5

12 Custovic A, Woodcock H, Craven M *et al*. Dust mite allergens are not carried only on large particles. *Pediatr Allergy Immunol* 1999; **10**: 258–60

13 Luczynska CM, Li Y, Chapman MD, Platts-Mills TAE. Airborne concentrations and particle size distribution of allergen derived from domestic cats (*Felis domesticus*): measurement using cascade impactor, liquid impinger and a two site monoclonal antibody assay for *Fel d* I. *Am Rev Respir Dis* 1990; **141**: 361–7

14 De Blay F, Heymann PW, Chapman MD, Platts-Mills TAE. Airborne dust mite allergens: comparison of Group II mite allergens with Group I mite allergen and cat allergen Fel d I. *J Allergy Clin Immunol* 1991; **88**: 919–26

15 Custovic A, Green R, Fletcher A *et al.* Aerodynamic properties of the major dog allergen, Can f 1: distribution in homes, concentration and particle size of allergen in the air. *Am J Respir Crit Care Med* 1997; **155**: 94–8

16 Custovic A, Smith A, Pahdi H, Green RM, Chapman MD, Woodcock A. Distribution, aerodynamic characteristics and removal of the major cat allergen Fel d 1 in British homes. *Thorax* 1998; **53**: 33–8

17 Owen S, Morgenstern M, Hepworth J, Woodcock A. Control of house dust mite in bedding. *Lancet* 1990; **335**: 396–7

18 McDonald LG, Tovey E. The role of water temperature and laundry procedures in reducing house dust mite populations and allergen content of bedding. *J Allergy Clin Immunol* 1992; **90**: 599–608

19 Bischoff ERC, Fischer A, Liebenberg B, Kniest FM. Mite control with low temperature washing. 1. Elimination of living mites on carpet pieces. *Clin Exp Allergy* 1996; **26**: 945–52

20 Custovic A, Green R, Smith A, Chapman MD, Woodcock A. New mattresses: how fast do they become significant source of exposure to house dust mite allergens? *Clin Exp Allergy* 1996; **26**: 1243–5

21 Tovey ER, Woodcock AJ. Direct exposure of carpets to sunlight can kill all mites. *J Allergy Clin Immunol* 1994; **93**: 1072–4

22 Colloff MJ, Taylor C, Merrett TG. The use of domestic steam treatment for the control of house dust mites. *Clin Exp Allergy* 1995; **25**: 1061–6

23 Colloff MJ. House dust mites – part II. Chemical control. *Pestic Outlook* 1990; **1**: 3–8

24 Hayden ML, Rose G, Diduch KB *et al.* Benzyl-benzoate moist powder: investigation of acarical activity in cultures and reduction of dust mite allergens in carpets. *J Allergy Clin Immunol* 1992; **89**: 536–45

25 Colloff MJ. Use of liquid nitrogen in the control of house dust mite populations. *Clin Allergy* 1986; **16**: 411–7

26 Woodfolk JA, Hayden ML, Miller JD. Rose G, Chapman MD, Platts-Mills TAE. Chemical treatment of carpets to reduce allergen: a detailed study of the effects of tannic acid on indoor allergens. *J Allergy Clin Immunol* 1994; **94**: 19–26

27 Kalra S, Owen SJ, Hepworth J, Woodcock A. Airborne house dust mite antigen after vacuum cleaning. *Lancet* 1990; **336**: 449

28 Fletcher A, Pickering CAC, Custovic A, Simpson J, Kennaugh J, Woodcock A. Reduction in humidity as a method of controlling mites and mite allergens: the use of mechanical ventilation in British domestic dwellings. *Clin Exp Allergy* 1996; **26**: 1051–6

29 Custovic A, Taggart SCO, Kennaugh JH, Woodcock A. Portable dehumidifiers in the control of house dust mites and mite allergens. *Clin Exp Allergy* 1995; **25**: 312–6

30 Niven RMcL, Fletcher A, Pickering CAC *et al.* Attempting to control mite allergens with mechanical ventilation and dehumidification in British homes. *J Allergy Clin Immunol* 1999; **103**: 756–62

31 Colloff MJ. Dust mite control and mechanical ventilation: when the climate is right. *Clin Exp Allergy* 1994; **24**: 94–6

32 Custovic A, Simpson BM, Simpson A *et al.* Manchester asthma and allergy study: low allergen environment can be achieved and maintained during pregnancy and in early life. *J Allergy Clin Immunol* 2000; **105**:252–9

33 Custovic A, Taggart SCO, Woodcock A. House dust mite and cat allergen in different indoor environments. *Clin Exp Allergy* 1994; **24**: 1164–8

34 Custovic A, Green R, Taggart SCO *et al.* Domestic allergens in public places II: dog (Can f 1) and cockroach (Bla g 2) allergens in dust and mite, cat, dog and cockroach allergens in air in public buildings. *Clin Exp Allergy* 1996; **26**: 1246–52

35 Custovic A, Fletcher A, Pickering CAC *et al.* Domestic allergens in public places III. House dust mite, cat, dog and cockroach allergen in British hospitals. *Clin Exp Allergy* 1998; **28**: 53–9

36 Zielonka TM, Charpin D, Berbis P, Luciani P, Casanova D, Vervloet D. Effects of castration and testosterone on Fel d 1 production by sebaceous glands of male cats: I. Immunological assessment. *Clin Exp Allergy* 1994; **24**: 1169–73

37 Jalil-Colome J, Dornelas de Andrade A, Birnbaum J *et al.* Sex difference in Fel d 1 allergen production. *J Allergy Clin Immunol* 1996; **98**: 165–8

38 Wood RA, Chapman MD, Adkinson Jr NF, Eggleston PA. The effect of cat removal on allergen content in the household dust samples. *J Allergy Clin Immunol* 1989; **83**: 730–4

39 Tunnicliffe W, Fletcher T, Hammond K *et al.* Sensitivity and exposure to indoor allergens in subjects with differing asthma severity. *Eur Respir J* 1999; **13**: 654–9

40 Klucka CV, Ownby DR, Green J, Zoratti E. Cat shedding is not reduced by washings, Allerpet-C spray, or acepromasine. *J Allergy Clin Immunol* 1995; **95**: 1164–71

41 De Blay F, Chapman MD, Platts Mills TAE. Airborne cat allergen Fel d I: environmental control with cat in situ. *Am Rev Respir Dis* 1991; **143**: 1334–9

42 Hodson T, Custovic A, Simpson A, Chapman MD, Woodcock A, Green R. Washing the dog reduces dog allergen levels (but the dog needs to be washed twice a week). *J Allergy Clin Immunol* 1999; **103**: 581–5

43 Green R, Simpson A, Custovic A, Faragher B, Chapman MD, Woodcock A. The effect of air filtration on airborne dog allergen. *Allergy* 1999; **54**: 484–8

44 Green R, Simpson A, Custovic A, Woodcock A. Vacuum cleaners and airborne dog allergen. *Allergy* 1999; **54**: 403–5

45 Custovic A, Simpson A, Chapman MD, Woodcock A. Allergen avoidance in the treatment of asthma and atopic disorders. *Thorax* 1998; **53**: 63–72

46 Garrett MH, Rayment PR, Hooper MA, Abramson MJ, Hooper BM. Indoor airborne fungal spores, house dampness and associations with environmental factors and respiratory health in children. *Clin Exp Allergy* 1998; **28**: 459–67

47 Charpin D, Kleisbauer JP, Lanteaume A *et al.* Asthma and allergy to house dust mites in population living in high altitudes. *Chest* 1988; **93**: 758–61

48 Charpin D, Birnbaum J, Haddi E *et al.* Altitude and allergy to house dust mites. *Am Rev Respir Dis* 1991; **143**: 983–6

49 Kerrebijn KF. Endogenous factors in childhood CNSLD: methodological aspects in population studies. In: Orie NGM, Van der Lende R. (eds) *Bronchitis III*. The Netherlands: Royal Van Gorcum Assen, 1970; 38–48

50 Platts Mills TAE, Chapman MD. Dust mites: immunology, allergic disease, and environmental control. *J Allergy Clin Immunol* 1987; **80**: 755–75

51 Boner AL, Niero E, Antolini I, Valletta EA, Gaburro D. Pulmonary function and bronchial hyperreactivity in asthmatic children with house dust mite allergy during prolonged stay in the Italian Alps (Misurina 1756 m). *Ann Allergy* 1985; **54**: 42–5

52 Morrison Smith J. The use of high altitude treatment for childhood asthma. *Practitioner* 1981; **225**: 1663–6

53 Boner AL, Peroni DG, Piacentini GL, Venge P. Influence of allergen avoidance at high altitude on serum markers of eosinophil activation in children with allergic asthma. *Clin Exp Allergy* 1993; **23**: 1021–6

54 Simon HU, Grotzer M, Nikolaizik WH, Blaser K, Schoni MH. High altitude climate therapy reduces peripheral blood T lymphocyte activation, eosinophilia, and bronchial obstruction in children with house-dust mite allergic asthma. *Pediatr Pulmonol* 1994; **17**: 304–11

55 Valletta EA, Comis A, Del Col G, Spezia E, Boner AL. Peak expiratory flow variation and bronchial hyperresponsiveness in asthmatic children during periods of antigen avoidance and reexposure. *Allergy* 1995; **50**: 366–9

56 Piacentini GL, Martinati L, Mingoni S, Boner AL. Influence of allergen avoidance on the eosinophil phase of airway inflammation in children with allergic asthma. *J Allergy Clin Immunol* 1996; **97**: 1079–84

57 Sarsfield JK, Gowland G, Toy R, Norman ALE. Mite sensitive asthma of childhood. Trial of avoidance measures. *Arch Dis Child* 1974; **49**: 716–21

58 Burr ML, Leger ASST, Neale E. Anti-mite measures in mite-sensitive adult asthma. A controlled trial. *Lancet* 1976; **i**: 333–5

59 Burr ML, Dean BV, Merrett TG, Neale E, Leger ASST, Verrier-Jones ER. Effect of anti-mite measures on children with mite-sensitive asthma: a controlled trial. *Thorax* 1980; **35**: 506–12

60 Burr ML, Neale E, Dean BV, Verrier-Jones ER. Effect of a change to mite-free bedding on children with mite-sensitive asthma: a controlled trial. *Thorax* 1980; **35**: 513–4

61 Mitchell EA, Elliott RB. Controlled trial of an electrostatic precipitator in childhood asthma. *Lancet* 1980; ii; 559–61

62 Korsgaard J. Preventive measures in house-dust allergy. *Am Rev Respir Dis* 1982; **125**: 80–4

63 Korsgaard J. Preventive measures in mite asthma. A controlled trial. *Allergy* 1983; **38**: 93–102

64 Murray AB, Ferguson AC. Dust-free bedrooms in the treatment of asthmatic children with house dust or house dust mite allergy: a controlled trial. *Pediatrics* 1983; **71**: 418–22

65 Bowler SD, Mitchell CA, Miles J. House dust mite control and asthma: a placebo control trial of cleaning air filtration. *Ann Allergy* 1985; **55**: 498–500

66 Walshaw MJ, Evans CC. Allergen avoidance in house dust mite sensitive adult asthma. *Q J Med* 1986; **58**:199–215

67 Gillies DRN, Littlewood JM, Sarsfield JK. Controlled trial of house dust mite avoidance in children with mild to moderate asthma. *Clin Allergy* 1987; **17**: 105–11

68 Dorward AJ, Colloff MJ, MacKay NS, McSharry CM, Thomson NC. Effect of house dust mite avoidance on adult atopic asthma. *Thorax* 1988; **43**: 98–102

69 Verrall B, Muir DCF, Wilson WM, Milner R, Johnston M, Dolovitch J. Laminar flow air cleaner bed attachment: a controlled trial. *Ann Allergy* 1988; **61**: 117–22

70 Reiser J, Ingram D, Mitchell EB, Warner JO. House dust mite allergen levels and an anti-mite mattress spray (natamycin) in the treatment of childhood asthma. *Clin Exp Allergy* 1990; **20**: 561–7

71 Reisman RE, Mauriello PM, Davis GB, Georgitis JW, DeMasi JM. A double-blind study of the effectiveness of a high-efficiency particulate air (HEPA) filter in the treatment of patients with perennial allergic rhinitis and asthma. *J Allergy Clin Immunol* 1990; **85**: 1050–7

72 Morrow Brown H, Merrett TG. Effectiveness of an acaricide in management of house dust mite allergy. *Ann Allergy* 1991; **67**: 25–31

73 Antonicelli L, Bilo MB, Pucci S, Schou C, Bonifazi F. Efficacy of an air cleaning device equipped with a high efficiency particulate air filter in house dust mite respiratory allergy. *Allergy* 1991; **46**: 594–600

74 Ehnert B, Lau-Schadendorf S, Weber A, Buettner P, Schou C, Wahn V. Reducing domestic exposure to dust mite allergen reduces bronchial hyperreactivity in sensitive children with asthma. *J Allergy Clin Immunol* 1993; **90**: 135–8

75 Huss K, Squire EN, Carpenter GB *et al*. Effective education of adults with asthma who are allergic to dust mites. *J Allergy Clin Immunol* 1992; **89**: 836–43

76 Dietermann A, Bessot JC, Hoyet C, Ott M, Verot A, Pauli G. A double-blind, placebo controlled trial of solidified benzyl benzoate applied in dwellings of asthmatic patients sensitive to mites: clinical efficacy and effect on mite allergens. *J Allergy Clin Immunol* 1993; **91**: 738–46

77 Warner JA, Marchant JL, Warner JO. Double blind trial of ionisers in children with asthma sensitive to the house dust mite. *Thorax* 1993; **48**: 330–3

78 Huss RW, Huss K, Squire EN *et al*. Mite allergen control with acaricide fails. *J Allergy Clin Immunol* 1994; **94**: 27–31

79 Warburton CJ, Niven RMcL, Pickering CAC, Hepworth J, Francis HC. Domiciliary air filtration units, symptoms and lung function in atopic asthmatics. *Respir Med* 1994; **88**: 771–6

80 Marks GB, Tovey ER, Green W, Shearer M, Salome CM, Woolcock AJ. House dust mite allergen avoidance: a randomised controlled trial of surface chemical treatment and encasement of bedding. *Clin Exp Allergy* 1994; **24**: 1078–83

81 Sette L, Comis A, Marcucci F, Sensi L, Piacentini GL, Boner AL. Benzyl benzoate foam: effect on mite allergens in mattress, serum and nasal secretory IgE to *Dermatophagoides pteronyssinus*, and bronchial hyperreactivity in children with allergic asthma. *Pediatr Pulmonol* 1994; **18**: 218–27

82 Geller-Bernstein C, Pibourdin JM, Dornelas A, Fondarai J. Efficacy of the acaricide: Acardust for the prevention of asthma and rhinitis due to dust mite allergy in children. *Allergie Immunol* 1995; **27**: 147–54

83 Carswell F, Birmingham K, Oliver J, Crewes A, Weeks J. The respiratory effect of reduction of mite allergen in the bedroom of asthmatic children: a double-blind, controlled trial. *Clin Exp Allergy* 1996; **26**: 386–96

84 Frederick JM, Warner JO, Jessop WJ, Enander I, Warner JA. Effect of a bed covering system in children with asthma and house dust mite hypersensitivity. *Eur Respir J* 1997; **10**: 361–6

85 van der Heide S, Kauffman HF, Dubois AEJ, de Monchy JGR. Allergen reduction measures in houses of allergic asthmatic patients: effects of air cleaners and allergen-impermeable mattress covers. *Eur Respir J* 1997; **10**: 1217–23

86 Halken S, Niklassen U, Hansen LG *et al*. Encasing of mattress in children with asthma and house dust mite allergy. *J Allergy Clin Immunol* 1997; **99**: S320

87 van der Heide S, Kauffman HF, Dubois AEJ, de Monchy JGR. Allergen avoidance measures in homes of house dust mite allergic asthmatic patients: effects of acaricides and mattress encasing. *Allergy* 1997; **52**: 921–7

88 Gotzsche PC, Hammarquist C, Burr M. House dust mite control measures in the management of asthma: meta analysis. *BMJ* 1998: **317**: 1105–10

89 Roberts DLL. House dust mite allergen avoidance and atopic dermatitis. *Br J Dermatol* 1984; **110**: 735–6

90 August PJ. House dust mite causes atopic eczema. A preliminary study. *Br J Dermatol* 1984; **111 (Suppl 26)**: 10–1

91 Colloff MJ, Lever RS, McSharry C. A controlled trial of house dust mite eradication using natamycin in homes of patients with atopic dermatitis: effect on clinical status and mite populations. *Br J Dermatol* 1989; **121**: 199–208

92 Kniest FM, Young E, Van Praag MCG *et al*. Clinical evaluation of a double-blind dust-mite avoidance trial with mite-allergic rhinitic patients. *Clin Exp Allergy* 1991; **21**: 39–47

93 Howarth PH, Lunn A, Tomkins S. A double-blind, placebo controlled trial of Intervent bedding system in perennial allergic rhinitis. *J Allergy Clin Immunol* 1992; **89**: 305

94 Sanda T, Yasue T, Ooashi M, Yasue A. Effectiveness of house dust-mite allergen avoidance through clean room therapy in patients with atopic dermatitis. *J Allergy Clin Immunol* 1992; **89**: 653–7

95 Tan BB, Weald D, Strickland I, Friedmann PS. Double blind controlled trial of effects of house dust mite allergen avoidance on atopic dermatitis. *Lancet* 1996; **347**: 15–8

96 Wood RA, Johnson EF, Van Natta ML, Chen PH, Eggleston PA. A placebo controlled trial of a HEPA air cleaner in the treatment of cat allergy. *Am J Respir Crit Care Med* 1998; **158**: 115–20

97 Arshad SH, Matthews S, Gant C, Hide DW. Effect of allergen avoidance on development of allergic disorders in infancy. *Lancet* 1992; **339**: 1493–7

98 Hide DW, Matthews S, Tariq S, Arshad SH. Allergen avoidance in infancy and allergy at 4 years of age. *Allergy* 1996; **51**: 89–93

99 Jones CA, Kilburn SA, Warner JA, Warner JO. Intrauterine environment and fetal allergic sensitization. *Clin Exp Allergy* 1998; **28**: 655–9

100 Holt PJ, Sly PD. Allergic respiratory disease: strategic targets for primary prevention during childhood. *Thorax* 1997; **52**: 1–4

101 Brown MA, Halonen MJ, Martinez FD. Cutting the cord: is birth already too late for primary prevention of allergy. *Clin Exp Allergy* 1997: **27**: 4–6

Provision of allergy care for optimal outcome in the UK

Pamela W Ewan

Allergy and Clinical Immunology Clinic, Addenbrooke's Hospital, Cambridge, UK

Allergy is common and the prevalence has increased substantially in the last 2–3 decades. There has been a particular increase in severe allergic disease, including anaphylaxis, food, drug and latex rubber allergy. Provision of allergy services in the NHS is extremely poor and there is a huge unmet need. Allergy is a full speciality, but there are few consultants and few trainees. Whilst other specialists have a role in the management of allergy, it is no longer adequate to devolve most of allergy care to them. Provision of allergy care must be lead by allergy specialists so that adequate standards of care can be achieved. The lack of care leads to morbidity, mortality and substantial cost to the NHS, much of which is avoidable. There is an urgent need for the creation of more consultant posts in allergy and this requires recognition by Trust Managers, Regional Commissioners and the Department of Health.

Disorders dealt with by an allergist

An allergist deals with a wide range of disorders crossing the organ-based disciplines within medicine (Table 1). It is important to emphasise that the expertise of an allergist is unique and distinct from that of organ-based specialists and immunologists. However, in addition, allergists require detailed knowledge of certain areas within some of the organ-based specialities, but not the full breadth of knowledge that these other specialists have, *e.g.* in respiratory medicine, dermatology and ENT.

One of the difficulties in the establishment of this speciality has been to define the need, particularly where there appears to be overlap with an organ-based specialist. Of the disorders an allergist will deal with (Table 1), some of these are clearly specific to allergy, such as drug allergy, food allergy, venom allergy, latex rubber allergy, (disorders categorised by aetiology) as well as some of the disorders defined by symptomatology – anaphylaxis and severe allergic reactions. There are others where there is overlap with the organ-based specialists in terms of appropriate referral. These are asthma, rhinitis, conjunctivitis, eczema, urticaria and angioedema. An allergy opinion may be of great value in these disorders. This is particularly true when they are severe, not readily controlled, part of multi-system allergic disease or where an allergic aetiology is (or should be) suspected.

Correspondence to:
Dr Pamela W Ewan,
Allergy and Clinical
Immunology Clinic, Box
40, Addenbrooke's
Hospital, Hills Road,
Cambridge CB2 2QQ, UK

Table 1 Disorders dealt with by allergists

Disorders	Indication for referral to allergist
Rhinitis Conjunctivitis Asthma Urticaria Angioedema Atopic eczema	(i) Where an allergic aetiology (should be) is suspected (ii) Severe (iii) Not easily controlled (iv) Part of multisystem allergic disorder
Multisystem allergic disease (any combination of the above)	
Anaphylaxis/anaphylactoid reactions Severe allergic reactions	
Venom allergy Food allergy Drug allergy and adverse drug reactions Latex rubber allergy Reactions to vaccines	
C1 inhibitor deficiency* Food intolerance Exclusion of allergy as a cause of disease	

*Hereditary angioedema or acquired C1 esterase inhibitor deficiency.

Appropriate referral

Angioedema is an example of a disorder where the appropriate referral pathway is not clearly defined. Angioedema is often associated with urticaria, and the latter (particularly idiopathic urticaria) was traditionally the province of the dermatologist. However, allergy is increasingly a cause of angioedema/urticaria, particularly the more severe forms and general dermatologists do not have the training to determine allergic aetiology or advise on management (note: this is distinct from contact dermatitis, a T-cell-mediated reaction, where patch testing is the diagnostic test and which is the province of dermatologists). Angioedema is often severe, *e.g.* glottal oedema which may lead to asphyxia and respiratory arrest or facial and laryngeal oedema: problems commonly due to allergy. Referral to ENT or respiratory medicine is also not appropriate. Aspirin, NSAID or ACE-induced angioedema are examples of non-IgE mediated reactions which should be referred to an allergist and where determination of aetiology is essential.

Most asthmatics can be dealt with in primary care or by respiratory physicians. However, the allergic aetiology is often not addressed (although some asthma nurses in general practice are beginning to receive allergy training through the National Asthma and Respiratory Training Centre). Referral to an allergist is appropriate for a proportion of patients with asthma, particularly those with asthma as part of multisystem allergic disease, poorly controlled asthma or severe asthma where an allergic aetiology might be suspected, and in patients with acute life-threatening attacks. The identification of allergic triggers may be important and their avoidance a key part of management. There are examples of fatal anaphylaxis which have been mislabelled as asthma deaths. Asthma was a key part of the syndrome but there had been failure to recognise the allergic aetiology both in life and in the terminal event. Involvement of an allergist in such patients should lead to accurate diagnosis, better management and reduce morbidity and mortality. However, even in more ordinary asthma, allergen avoidance (*e.g.* house dust mite) is often an important part of management and can improve control and/or reduce the need for medication.

The majority of patients with hayfever can be controlled with straight forward medication (oral antihistamines and/or nasal steroids and/or chromoglycate eye drops) and can be dealt with in general practice. However patients with severe hayfever not readily controlled by standard medical treatment should be referred for an allergy opinion. An allergist can usually control the disease either by providing medical treatment under expert direction or by offering desensitisation (immunotherapy). A patient referred to us recently illustrates the consequences of failure to refer appropriately. This man had devastating hayfever symptoms with profuse and uncontrolled nasal discharge. His general practitioner resorted to annual injections of a deposteroid over 14 years. This led to bilateral avascular necrosis of the hip, with the result that a 39-year-old is crippled and faces (in the long term, multiple) bilateral hip replacements[1].

Epidemiology

This will not be described in detail as it is dealt with elsewhere in this issue. It is important to emphasise two key factors: the increase in common allergic disease and the increase in severe allergic disease. It is well known that the prevalence of asthma, rhinitis and eczema have doubled or trebled in the last 2–3 decades[2,3]. Much of this is due to the increase in the allergic component of these diseases. The ISAAC study shows the world-wide increase in allergic disease in children[4]. Following this upsurge in atopy and common allergic disorders, there has been an increase in severe allergic disorders. This is less well documented but clear to those in clinical practice. Peanut and tree nut allergy has become common in the UK since the early 1990s. One study showed the incidence of confirmed peanut allergy was 1 in 200 4-year-olds[5]. A telephone questionnaire study in the US found an incidence of peanut allergy of about 1% (most of the respondents were adults): even allowing for the errors intrinsic in self-diagnosis, peanut allergy is evidently common. Anaphylaxis has become more common and is now a major part of referrals to an allergist (see below). There is lack of previous prevalence data. A study carried out in 1993/94 looking at anaphylaxis occurring in the community (*i.e.* excluding hospital-induced anaphylaxis) found this occurred in 1 in 300,000 of the population each year[6]. Because of the design of this study the authors felt it underestimated the true incidence. Hospital admissions due to anaphylaxis have also risen[7]. Since most patients with anaphylaxis are not admitted from accident and emergency departments, again the extent of the problem is underestimated.

Adverse reactions to drugs seem to be more common, *e.g.* due to aspirin, non-steroidal anti-inflammatory drugs, other analgesics and ACE inhibitors, often presenting with severe reactions such as glottal oedema, laryngeal oedema, severe asthma or severe generalised urticaria and angioedema.

Adverse reactions during anaesthesia, presenting with anaphylaxis, are usually due to allergy to the induction agents used in general anaesthesia. The incidence is reported as 1 in 3500 to 1 in 6000 in France[8], and 1 in 10,000 to 1 in 20,000 in Australia[9]. Extrapolating from these figures, one would expect 175–1000 reactions in the UK each year.

Latex rubber allergy is a relatively new disease, particularly of the last decade. The first case was reported in 1919 and the second case in 1979, but since then large numbers have occurred particularly amongst those exposed to latex rubber, mainly from surgical or other rubber gloves. The main groups affected are health care workers – including doctors, nurses, paramedics and dentists – laboratory staff and patients having multiple surgical procedures[10,11]. The larger studies of hospital staff focus on sensitisation (the presence of latex rubber IgE) rather than clinical allergy and the incidence varies from ~3–17%.[12,13] About half of those sensitised have clinical allergy.

Oral allergy syndrome is a relatively new problem on which there is little prevalence data but which appears to be coming much more common. In this disorder, patients are allergic to fresh fruits and vegetables which cause oedema and pruritus of the oral mucosa, some-times also involving the pharynx and larynx. This disorder is associated with tree pollen allergy and certain types of nut allergy and usually occurs in atopics. The incidence is not known.

The European White Paper on allergy highlights the problem of the impact of allergy across Europe.

Expertise required by an allergist

The knowledge required by an allergist falls into two main areas: (i) that which is unique to allergy; and (ii) expertise in organ-based specialties, covering only part of these specialties but relevant to the problems encountered in allergy.

Specialist knowledge

This includes (Table 2) understanding of:(i) the immunological principles and pathogenesis of allergic disease; (ii) knowledge of allergens; and (iii) the aetiology of disorders (whether they are allergic or non-allergic). They also have expertise in the clinical presentation and patterns of allergic

Table 2 Expertise required by an allergist

Specific to allergy

Immunological mechanisms
Pathogenesis of allergic disease
Allergens
Aetiology of different disorders
Clinical presentations
Patterns of allergic disease
Natural history
Diagnostic tests: use and interpretation of skin prick tests and serum specific IgE assays
Performing skin prick tests
Performing challenge tests (nasal; bronchial)
Food challenges
Drug challenges
Use of diagnostic exclusion diets
Management
      Medical treatment of all disorders
      Allergen avoidance (*e.g.* HDM, animal, latex rubber, food, drug)
      Training in use of medication
      Written treatment plans (*e.g.* for anaphylaxis, glottal oedema)
      Exclusion diet
Immunotherapy

Overlap with other specialities

Respiratory medicine	Asthma – diagnosis, management (acute and chronic)
	BTS management guidelines
	Monitoring peak flow
	Differentiation from other disorders
	COPD, emphysema, bronchitis
	Lung function tests: use and interpretation
	Imaging
Dermatology	Diagnosis and management of eczema
	Urticaria and angioedema
	Differential diagnosis
	Principles of and indications for referral for patch testing
ENT	Rhinitis
	Sinusitis
	Nasal polyps
	Anterior rhinoscopy
	Nasal airway resistance
	Use of investigations: radiology and CT
	Knowledge of surgical options

disease, the use and interpretation of diagnostic tests (an area poorly understood by the medical profession leading to confusion and bad management), and the management of allergic disease.

Knowledge overlapping with organ-based specialists

The allergist must have detailed knowledge of aspects of respiratory medicine, dermatology and ENT (Table 2). However, good knowledge of other areas of medicine is also necessary, particularly gastroenterology (including knowing when to refer) and general (internal) medicine. Paediatrics is another important area of overlap. Whilst the ideal would be for a child to be seen by a paediatric allergist or a paediatrician with an interest in allergy, this is unrealistic at present. There are few paediatric allergists nationally and no formal training programme in paediatric allergy, so there is lack of expertise amongst paediatricians. Allergy is common in children and it is better for a child to be seen by a specialist allergist rather than a paediatrician without appropriate knowledge. It is, therefore, essential for allergists to incorporate paediatric practice into their clinics: (i) awareness of the differences between paediatric and adult practice; (ii) understanding the natural history of disease in children; (iii) knowledge of therapy and doses for children; (iv) providing an appropriate environment including play areas, activities, and having nurses and doctors appropriately dressed in clinics; and (v) handling families sensitively. Adult allergists must liaise with paediatric colleagues so there is ready access to consultation and joint care when required. Close liaison with the community paediatric team is also important for the management of children at risk of anaphylaxis in schools[14].

Demand for allergy services

The need in the community

There is a large unmet need, evident from a number of sources.

Help lines
Two charities, the Anaphylaxis Campaign and the British Allergy Foundation, have set up help lines for the public. They are inundated with calls, the commonest problem being the difficulty patients have in obtaining allergy advice. The British Society for Allergy and Clinic Immunology have published a handbook of allergy clinics in the UK and this has been sent to all general practices.

Allergy Care - An Investment for Life?

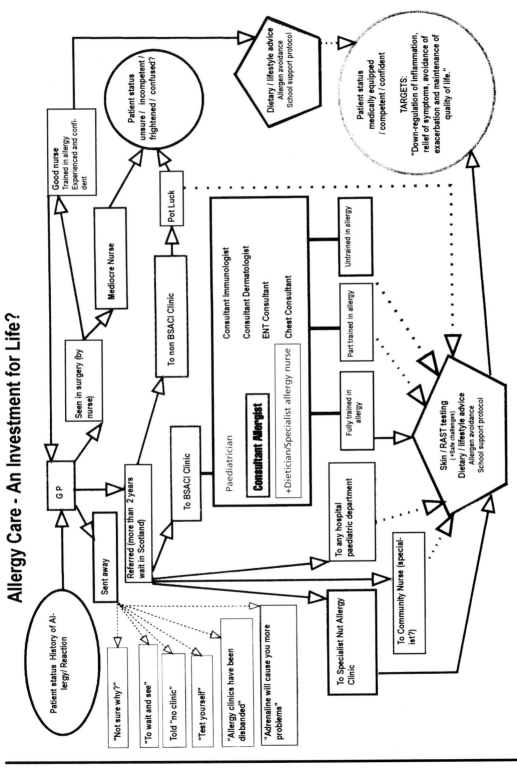

Fig. 1 Difficulty in obtaining quality allergy advice: the patient's perspective. This diagram shows the difficulties a patient (top left) has in obtaining high quality allergy advice (bottom right). In the majority of patients this goal is not achieved. There are few consultant allergists. (Produced by Hazel Gowland for the Anaphylaxis Campaign, and reproduced with permission.)

Table 3 Impact of failure to obtain a specialist allergist opinion or delay in allergy diagnosis

Disorders	Consequence
Anaphylaxis of any cause	Risk of severe or fatal reaction
Adverse reaction during anaesthesia	Risk of general anaesthetic (GA)
Suspected drug allergy, *e.g.*	
Allergy to LA drugs	Unable to have local anaesthetic (LA)
Reactions to opiates	Which potent analgesic can be given?
Reactions to aspirin/NSAID	Risk of severe reaction
Allergy to antibiotics	Which antibiotic can be prescribed?
Latex allergy	Risk of severe reaction (especially if medical intervention required)
Glottal oedema	Risk of asphyxia
Severe urticaria/angioedema	Disabling
Multisystem allergic disease	Attendances at three or more specialist clinics. Allergic aetiology still unlikely to be addressed
Food allergy in infant	Unable to wean
Egg allergy	Inappropriate avoidance of vaccination
Venom allergy	Risk of anaphylaxis
Exercise/cold/heat induced-urticaria, angioedema, anaphylaxis	Other specialists fail to deal with this (inappropriate management, *e.g.* exclusion diets)

Lack of allergy expertise

The difficulty in obtaining allergy advice is illustrated in Figure 1 (prepared by Hazel Gowland for the Anaphylaxis Campaign).

Deaths

Deaths from anaphylaxis occur, mainly in otherwise healthy teenagers or young adults, which should be preventable. Most of these patients knew of their allergy, e.g. a food allergy, but had not been referred to an allergist or received expert advice.

Morbidity

Failure to diagnose and treat allergy leads to enormous morbidity (Tables 3 & 4).

Demand: the experience of an allergy clinic

There is a steady and substantial rise in referrals to specialist allergy centres. The Allergy Clinic in Cambridge serves the Eastern Region (population 5.4 million), yet has a single consultant allergist. Activity for the past 5 years (Figure 2) shows an increase of 440%. This figure underestimates the true increase in work-load, since over the same period there has been a change in case-mix to the more complex. This is reflected in part by the increase in day case activity which includes patients attending for challenge tests (most commonly to drugs or foods,

Table 4 Morbidity, mortality and cost from lack of allergy advice

Unnecessary:	A&E attendances
	Hospital admissions
	GP attendances
	Referrals to other specialties (*e.g.* respiratory, dermatology and ENT)
	ENT surgery (*e.g.* SMR, nasal polypectomy)
Loss of time from work and school (poorly controlled allergic disease; recurrent acute reactions)	
Increased drug costs	
Respiratory arrest	
Death	

where challenge may be the only way to confirm or refute the cause of a severe reaction).

Despite this increase in activity, the waiting list continued to rise and was 16 months in 1998. Referrals to this clinic are triaged on the basis of the referral letter into 'urgent', 'soon' or 'routine'. Urgent and soon patients are given priority and receive appointments but routine patients wait for over 12 months before they are allocated an appointment date. The number of referrals continues to exceed the capacity for new patients, activity exceeds contract levels by about 50% and activity was 20% more in 2000 compared to 1999, and 26% more in 1999 compared to 1998.

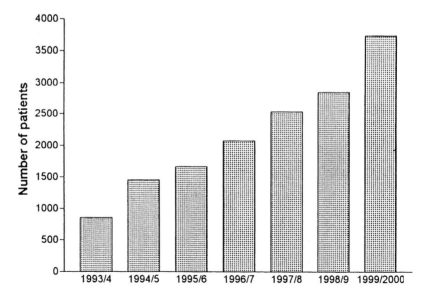

Fig. 2 The number of patients seen in Addenbrooke's Hospital Allergy Clinic between 1993 and 2000. There was a substantial annual increase and activity increased by 440% over this period, reflecting demand. There was a change in case-mix to the more severe. The waiting list also rose.

Value of a specialist allergy service

Control of disease: cost savings to the NHS

A specialist allergy service will be able to deal with the disorders and problems in Table 3. Identification of aetiology prevents or reduces the risk of repeated severe reactions, *e.g.* anaphylaxis or angioedema. In addition, management, including written treatment plans which the patient carries, are invaluable for dealing with future reactions, should these occur. In many areas of allergy, prevention with a system for immediate treatment, means reduced morbidity and substantial cost savings to the National Health Service.

A recent study reported such cost-benefit. A management strategy for nut allergy was developed and then evaluated in 567 patients over 13,610 patient-months[15]. It showed not only a substantial reduction in the incidence of follow-up reactions, but where reactions did occur they were mostly mild. This demonstrated the value of repeated advice on avoidance. Patients also carried medication for self-administration (*e.g.* an adrenaline auto-injector) and this was effective or appropriate in all but one patient. Hospital admission and A&E attendance was avoided.

Identification of aetiology can also lead to better control of chronic diseases, such as asthma, rhinitis and eczema, through allergen avoidance, e.g. house dust mite, cat or a food[16,17]. Knowledge of the allergic trigger also identifies the time when symptoms will begin, *e.g.* in seasonal allergies such as spring hayfever (tree pollen allergy) or severe late summer asthma (allergy to alternaria) or intermittent exposure to an animal, through a planned visit to a relative. Prophylactic treatment can be instituted when symptoms are expected.

Identification of what is safe

If a food or drug is suspected of causing anaphylaxis or an allergic reaction, there is great concern amongst patients and doctors as to what can be safely given. This applies to reactions occurring during general anaesthesia, after local anaesthetic, analgesics or antibiotics and in putative food allergy. An allergist can not only identify the cause, but importantly, also identify which drugs can be safely given. Until the cause of anaphylaxis during general anaesthesia is established, it is likely that all drugs given at induction will be avoided and this may increase the risk of future anaesthesia. Similarly, in putative local anaesthetic allergy, dentists refuse to administer local anaesthetic. The role of the allergist is to confirm, or more often refute, this sensitivity. This usually involves a challenge test in a centre with expertise and the appropriate facilities.

A patient referred with anaphylaxis was known to have morphine allergy, but after a series of day-case challenge tests we found she was also sensitive to all of the potent analgesics tested. During the period of investigation she had an emergency appendicectomy and spinal anaesthesia had to be used for pain relief. This type of patient required urgent referral to a specialist allergy clinic – this type of service is not available in large parts of England.

Cost benefit

Allergy services are largely outpatient based and involve few investigations (skin prick tests are the main investigation). They are, therefore, relatively cheap. There are substantial cost savings to the Health Service as a result of employing specialist allergists (Tables 3 & 4).

Training

Allergy has suffered a period of difficulty because of the Calman changes. Previously, the training scheme for allergy was within the Clinical Immunology and Allergy training programme. The curriculum was provided by the Royal College of Physicians speciality committee in Clinical Immunology and Allergy and training regulated by the Joint Committee on Higher Medical Training (JCHMT). All entrants to this scheme were senior registrars.

When the Calman changes in training were introduced, a new programme was written, with entry at specialist registrar level. Up to this time, immunology (immunopathology) training had been regulated by the Royal College of Pathologists and not the JCHMT, the key requirement being the MRCPath examination. A Working Party, then Joint Committee, was set up between the Royal College of Physicians and the Royal College of Pathologists to look at areas of overlap between physicians and pathologists dealing with immunological problems. A joint training scheme was considered but abandoned, a fundamental difference being the requirement of the Royal College of Pathologists training scheme, for the MRCPath examination and training to run a diagnostic laboratory service. Two separate Calman training programmes therefore emerged, Allergy and Immunology. Allergy was not on the initial specialist list so this programme was not formally recognised until the second specialist list was accepted by the Specialist Training Authority in 1999.

Throughout this period of uncertainty the number of trainees in post fell (from 13 whole time equivalents on the Clinical Immunology and

Allergy programme to 4 on the new Allergy programme). Manpower training positions in allergy were lost, and numbers are now at an all time low. This is despite the fact that allergic disease is common, there is a great need for more specialists and there is geographical inequality of provision of care, most specialist allergists being in London or the south-east of England.

It is important to recognise that Immunology and Allergy are not the same. Allergy services in hospitals should be provided primarily by trained allergists.

A real problem is how do small specialties expand. Training numbers are dictated by a formula, which depends on expected opportunities, calculated from the number of consultants and expected retirements, *etc.* This is controlled by the Specialist Advisory Working Group (SWAG) in the Department of Health. It is, therefore, difficult to increase the number of trainees, unless we can demonstrate consultant growth. The latter of course requires trainees. Trainees will also be reluctant to enter a speciality where prospects are poor. Pump-priming of a relatively small number of consultant allergist posts is needed.

Existing provision of allergy services in the UK

There are only six centres providing full-time allergy services run by a specialist allergist in the UK. All of these are in England mainly in the south and east: in Cambridge, Leicester, Southampton, and London (Guy's Hospital, Royal Brompton Hospital and St Mary's Hospital). There are also 15 clinics staffed by part-time specialist allergists.

There are no allergy posts in Scotland and Wales. A review of the service provision for Immunology and Allergy in Scotland for the Scottish Executive, identified 4 consultant immunologists and no allergists, and recommended an immediate increase in immunologists and a later increase in allergists[18]. The expertise of immunologists is different from that of allergists, and it is inappropriate for them to be asked to cover for allergy. A better solution would be to plan to appoint four allergists, to work alongside the immunologists.

In addition there are 81 'allergy clinics', where the service is provided by an organ-based specialist with an interest in allergy (data from *BSACI Allergy Clinic Handbook 1998*[19]). These vary, but the majority are not dedicated allergy clinics (allergy patients are seen within another speciality clinic, *e.g.* respiratory medicine or immunology). They operate from weekly to monthly, specialist services are lacking and commonly they were set up to deal with a restricted area of allergy (usually related to the consultant's own area, *e.g.* asthma for respiratory physicians or rhinitis for an ENT specialist). The reality, and a problem in terms of clinical governance, is that the nature of referrals is not restricted so that these clinics receive referrals they are ill-equipped to deal with, for example food allergy, drug allergy and anaphylaxis, much of which will be outwith the competence of the specialists running these clinics.

There are 27 consultant allergists in the UK (Manpower data 2000), so that there is only 1 consultant per 2.1 million population of UK.

Provision of allergy services in the future

Previous recommendations

The Royal College of Physicians Committee on Clinical Immunology and Allergy produced a report, *The Physician Immunologist: Future Role and Manpower Needs* in 1989 (20). This was commissioned before the substantial rise in allergic disease, particularly severe allergic disease and anaphylaxis in the last decade. The model suggested was that most (about 80%) of allergic disease will be dealt with in primary care and that about 20% of patients should be referred to a specialist (allergist). It was proposed that the manpower provision should be one specialist allergist for three health districts, *i.e.* about 750,000 population.

Good Allergy Practice, a joint document of the Royal College of Physicians and Royal College of Pathologists in 1994, defined standards of care[21]. Requirements for a good allergy clinic were described, so that purchasers would better informed when contracting for allergy services.

Current model

An Allergy Task Force was set up in 1998, between the British Society of Allergy and Clinical Immunology and the Department of Health to discuss provision of allergy services in the NHS. The proposal is for 4 levels of provision of allergy care (Table 5).

There would be regional allergy centres, with a minimum of one per region, each with a minimum of two consultant allergists and appropriate support staff. These would provide specialist services for the Region, as

Table 5 Provision of allergy care

1.	Regional allergy centres
2.	Allergists (in teaching hospitals and DGHs)
3.	Organ-based specialists with an interest
4.	Primary care

At present most care is provided by 3 and 4.
The balance should shift from 3 to 2 as new allergists are appointed.

well as services in all areas of allergy for their local population (a definition of specialist services is available to Regional Specialist Services Commissioning Groups). The regional centre would provide special diagnostic facilities (challenge tests, *etc*) and immunotherapy and act as an education and liaison resource for other doctors in the region.

Throughout each region, general allergy services will also be provided in other teaching hospitals and district general hospitals, by allergists and by organ-based physicians with an interest in allergy. These allergists might have joint appointments in two hospitals, to provide geographical spread of expertise. In time, the balance should shift from organ-based specialists with an interest to trained allergists (with the Allergy CCST). The majority of allergic disease would be dealt with in primary care.

It should be noted that this model: (i) provides the minimum in specialist care; and (ii) assumes adequate expertise/knowledge of allergy at primary and secondary care levels. Unfortunately this does not exist at present.

References

1 Nasser SMS, Ewan PW. Depot corticosteroid causing avascular necrosis of both hips in hayfever – is this treatment still appropriate? *BMJ* 2001; In press
2 Robertson CF, Heycock E, Bishop J *et al*, Prevalence of asthma in Melbourne school children: changes over 26 years. *BMJ* 1991; **303**: 1116–8
3 Aberg N. Asthma and allergic rhinitis in Swedish conscripts. *Clin Exp Allergy* 1989; **19**: 59–63
4 ISAAC. Worldwide variation in prevalence of symptoms of asthma, allergic rhinoconjunctivitis, and atopic eczema: *Lancet* 1998: **351**: 1225–32
5 Tariq SM, Stevens M, Matthews S *et al*, Cohort study of peanut and tree nut sensitisation by the age of 4 years. *BMJ* 1996; **313**: 514-7
6 Stewart AG, Ewan PW. The incidence, aetiology and management of anaphylaxis presenting to an accident and emergency department. *Q J Med* 1996; **89**: 859–64.
7 Sheikh A, Alves B. Hospital admissions for acute anaphylaxis: time trend study. *BMJ* 2000; **320**: 1441
8 Fisher MMcD, Baldo BA. The incidence and clinical features of anaphylactic reactions during anaesthesia in Australia. *Ann Fr Anesth Reanim* 1993; **12**: 97–104
9 Laxenaire MC, Mouton C, Moneret-Vautrin DA *et al*. Drugs and other agents involved in anaphylactic shock occurring during anaesthesia. A French multicentre epidemiological inquiry. *Ann Fr Anesth Reanim* 1993; **12**: 91–6
10 Turjanmaa K, Alenius H, Makinen-Kiljunen S *et al*, Natural rubber latex allergy. *Allergy* 1996; **51**: 593–602
11 Wagner A, Ewan PW. Latex allergy: clinical associations and evaluation of diagnostic tests. In preparation.
12 Leung R, Chan HJ, Choy D, Lai CKW. Prevalence of latex allergy in hospital staff in Hong Kong. *Clin Exp Allergy* 1997; **27**: 167–74.
13 Liss GM, Sussman GL, Deal K *et al*. Latex allergy: epidemiological study of 1351 hospital workers. *Occup Environ Med* 1997; **54**: 335–42
14 Vickers DW, Maynard L, Ewan PW. Management of children with potential anaphylactic reactions in the community: a training package and proposal for good practice. *Clin Exp Allergy* 1997; **27**: 898–903
15 Ewan PW, Clark AT. Long-term prospective observational study of patients with peanut and nut allergy after participation in a management plan. *Lancet* 2001; **357**: 111–15

16 Platts-Mills TAE, Tovey ER, Mitchell EB *et al*. Reduction of bronchial hyperreactivity during prolonged allergen avoidance. *Lancet* 1982; ii: 675–8

17 Tan BB, Weald D, Strickland I, Friedmann PS. Double-blind controlled trial of effect of housedust-mite allergen avoidance on atopic dermatitis. *Lancet* 1996; 347:15–8

18 Anon. *Immunology and Allergy Services in Scotland*. Edinburgh: Scottish Medical and Scientific Advisory Committee, Scottish Executive, 2000

19 Anon. *National Health Service Allergy Clinics (1998–1999)*. London: British Society for Allergy and Clinical Immunology, 2000

20 Anon. Physician immunologist: future role and manpower needs. Report by Royal College of Physicians Committee on Clinical Immunology. *Clin Exp Immunol* 1987; 70: 664–75

21 Anon. *Good allergy practice – Standards of care for providers and purchasers of allergy services within the National Health Service*. Royal College of Physicians and Royal College of Pathologists. *Clin Exp Allergy* 1995; 25: 586–95

Index

Type 2 diabetes: the thrifty phenotype

Scientific Editor: David J P Barker